Forensic Mental Health Nursing: Forensic Aspects of Acute Care

Note

Health care practice and knowledge are constantly changing and developing as new research and treatments, changes in procedures, drugs and equipment become available.

The author and publishers have, as far as is possible, taken care to confirm that the information complies with the latest standards of practice and legislation.

Forensic Mental Health Nursing: Forensic Aspects of Acute Care

Edited by the

National Forensic Nurses' Research and Development Group

Alyson Kettles (Chair), Phil Woods, Richard Byrt, Mary Addo, Michael Coffey and Mike Doyle

Chapter reviews by Mary Addo, Richard Byrt, Michael Coffey, Mike Doyle, Alyson Kettles and Phil Woods

QUAY BOOKS

A division of MA Healthcare Ltd

Quay Books Division, MA Healthcare Ltd, St Jude's Church, Dulwich Road, London SE24 0PB

British Library Cataloguing-in-Publication Data
A catalogue record is available for this book

ISBN-10: 1 85642 320 4
ISBN-13: 978 1 85642 320 5

Printed by Ashford Colour Press Ltd, Gosport, Hampshire

Contents

Erratum notice

Forensic Mental Health Nursing: Forensic Aspects of Acute Care

Chapter 5, Page 75 first bullet point; and page 77, last line 7,

In both the above pages, hyperglycaemia (raised blood sugar) should read hypoglycaemia (lowered blood sugar). We would like to apologise for any confusion caused.

Acknowledgements

Thanks to:

Mave Holmes
Catherine Sanders
Minal Sikotra
Library Staff, School of Nursing and Midwifery, De Montfort University

Contributors

Mary Addo

Mary Addo, MEd, MA Soc Sci (Aberdeen), DMS, PgCertTLT (Aberdeen), RMN, EN (G) (Aberdeen) is a Lecturer/Practice Education Lecturer in Mental Health Nursing for The Robert Gordon University based at Aberdeen, Scotland. She has completed her PhD by research at the Centre for Advanced Studies in Nursing, University of Aberdeen, on the experience of trained nurses working with sex offenders in secure care settings. Mary has published on forensic nursing and related issues in books and journals, and is a member of the National Forensic Nurses' Research and Development Group.

Anne Aiyegbusi

Anne Aiyegbusi, RMN, MSc, PGCE, PGCert Social Science Research Methods, Diploma in Forensic Psychotherapeutic Studies, trained in the use of the Adult Attachment Interview, is Consultant Nurse for Women's Secure Services at West London Mental Health NHS Trust. Anne has a special interest in personality disorder and complex mental health needs and has extensive clinical experience in these areas. She has published articles and presented at conferences for many years, focusing most recently on the emotional impact on nurses of working on the frontline of forensic mental health services with service users who have experienced early psychological trauma. Anne is completing a PhD and the subject is managing the nurse–patient relationship with people who have personality disorders.

Richard Byrt

Richard Byrt, RMN, RNLD, RGN, PhD, BSc (Hons), is Lecturer-Practitioner, Nursing, at Arnold Lodge medium secure unit, Nottinghamshire Healthcare NHS Trust and the School of Nursing and Midwifery, De Montfort University, Leicester. Richard's publications include work on forensic mental health nursing and empowerment and participation in health care.

Michael Coffey

Michael Coffey is Lecturer in Community Mental Health Nursing at Swansea University. He previously worked as a community mental health nurse in both generic and forensic mental health services. His research focuses upon aspects of community mental health nursing and particularly people's experiences of receipt of these services. He has co-edited (with Chris Chaloner) the textbook *Forensic Mental Health Nursing: Current Approaches* and (with Ben Hannigan) *The Handbook of Community Mental Health Nursing*.

Mike Doyle

Michael is a Forensic Nurse Consultant in Manchester, England. He is also undertaking a Post-Doctoral Research Fellowship investigating risk assessment in mental health services. A qualified RMN, he also has a BSc (Hons) in Community Health and an MSc in Individual and Family Cognitive Therapy from the University of Manchester, and he completed his PhD in 2003. He has provided extensive training in risk and related subjects since 1996 and has a particular interest in systematic approaches to risk assessment and management.

Stephen Fyffe

Steve Fyffe has over 20 years' experience as a mental health nurse and nurse manager, mainly in secure settings. Steve is currently a Senior Nurse at Arnold Lodge medium secure unit, Leicester.

Tina Gronow

Tina Gronow, RMN, BSc (Hons), is a Forensic Community Mental Health Nurse at the Caswell Clinic medium secure unit, Bro Morgannwg NHS Trust. Tina has an interest in working with women with complex needs.

Stuart Guy

Stuart Guy, RN, MSc, PG Dip Soc L, Dip HE Hs, Nurse Consultant Psychiatric Intensive Care, BABCP Accredited Cognitive Behavioural Psychotherapist, Leicestershire Partnerships NHS Trust. Stuart is currently in his first post as Nurse Consultant in Acute Psychiatry, having held a previous position in forensic psychiatry in London. He has extensive experience of working in forensic mental health settings, spanning high, medium, low and community forensic settings. His clinical expertise is working with complex patient presentations utilising cognitive behavioural therapy as the vehicle for change.

Paula Hall

Paula Hall, RMN, Dip Professional studies, PG Dip Counselling, is a Community Psychiatric Nurse working in the Out of Hours Crisis Intervention Team in NHS Grampian. She has been with the team since its inception in 1997 and has a keen interest in crisis prevention and counselling using the person-centred approach. Paula is very keen to see the use of psychological therapies in mental health services increase and has completed a study (currently being written up) as part of a research fellowship, to ascertain staff qualifications and what facilitates or inhibits their use of these skills in the workplace within mental health services in Grampian.

Tim Hardie

Dr Tim Hardie is a consultant forensic psychiatrist at Arnold Lodge medium secure unit, Leicester. Amongst other interests, he has a commitment to issues concerning culture, equality and diversity, including services for individuals who are deaf.

Linda Hart

Linda Hart is a mother, writer, artist and campaigner. Linda is the author, amongst other works, of the 1996 MIND Book of the Year: *Phone at Nine, Just to Say You're Alive*, based on her experience as a service user.

Wendy Ifill
Wendy Ifill is an author who has written about various aspects of mental health and other topics, based, in part, on her experience as a service user.

Linnette James
Linnette James, RN, BSc (Hons), is a staff nurse who is working in an acute mental health setting. Linnette is also a poet and songwriter during her spare time.

Alyson McGregor Kettles
Dr Alyson M. Kettles, PhD, MSc (London), BSc (Dundee), RMN, RGN, RNT, PGCEA (Surrey), AMIBiol, ILTM, is Research and Development Officer (Mental Health) for NHS Grampian and is based at the Royal Cornhill Hospital in Aberdeen, Scotland. She is also Honorary Lecturer for the Centre for Advanced Studies in Nursing at the University of Aberdeen, where she coordinates and teaches on modules for the postgraduate taught Masters degrees. Her personal portfolio of research has had a forensic focus for the last decade. She is a well-known author of mental health and forensic nursing articles and books. Her specific research interests include the relationship between education and practice, specific assessment and interventions, such as observation, and related management issues such as operational competency development.

Michele McGunnigle
Michele McGunnigle, RMN, qualified as a registered psychiatric nurse in 2004. Since qualifying she has worked for NHS Grampian. Previous to this, she worked with people with learning difficulties for five years. This is her first book chapter contribution.

Julie Morgan
Julie Morgan, RMN, BSc (Hons), is a Forensic Community Mental Health Nurse working in South Wales Forensic Psychiatric Service, Caswell Clinic, Bridgend. She has interests in drug and alcohol issues and relapse prevention through early intervention.

Helen Walker
Helen Walker, BEd, RMN, BSc, MSc in CBT, is currently acting senior nurse for practice development at the State Hospital, Carstairs, Scotland. She qualified as a mental health nurse in 1991 and has experience of working in a variety of mental health settings, predominantly community, acute admissions and a high secure forensic unit. Throughout most of her career, she has been actively involved in research and the many posts she has held have been evenly divided between clinical and research activities.

Carol Watson
Carol Watson, RMN, RGN, RNT, MPhil, is the Associate Director of Nursing and Midwifery NHS Education for Scotland. Carol has worked in research, education and practice in high-secure settings. Her main focus has been in facilitating the development of post-registration clinical competencies in mental health, generally, and forensic mental health nursing, particularly.

Jean Woodally

Jean Woodally, RMN, is a Senior Staff Nurse for NHS Grampian at the Blair Unit, Royal Cornhill Hospital, Aberdeen. She has over 20 years in psychiatry, 10 of them in the forensic area. Jean has participated in research activities within the BEST-Index.

Phil Woods

Dr Phil Woods, RMN, RPN, PhD, is an Associate Professor at the College of Nursing, University of Saskatchewan. He has an extensive personal portfolio of forensic-related research. He is a well-known author of mental health and forensic nursing articles and books. His specific research interests are risk assessment and management, and violence prediction.

CHAPTER 1

Introduction

Alyson McGregor Kettles, Richard Byrt and Phil Woods

Introduction

Welcome to this book on issues related to individuals who are forensic mental health patients being nursed on acute mental health units. We hope that you will find it enjoyable and practically relevant. This book is one of a series that emerged from a discussion, in a National Forensic Nurses' Research and Development Group meeting, about how the Group could contribute to the development of forensic nursing, and more widely, mental health nursing. As with the first book, a seed was planted and this book was born! This text is aimed at helping nurses working in acute areas to care for and to manage those forensic patients who, for whatever reason, find themselves in an acute inpatient area.

Forensic means 'of the law', and is based on the Latin word *forum*, meaning 'what is out of doors' (Soanes, 2002). The Ancient Romans met outside in fora (the plural of forum) for public meetings, political debates and public legal hearings to try offenders (Parker, 1985). In the United Kingdom, forensic mental health nurses work with the relatively small proportion of individuals whose mental health problems are associated with offending behaviours. Forensic mental health nurses work in a variety of settings. These include: high secure hospitals and medium and low secure units; court diversion schemes (e.g., in magistrates' courts); prisons and young offender institutions and police stations (Kettles *et al.*, 2002; McClelland *et al.*, 2001; Wix and Humphreys, 2005). Some nurses registered in learning disability nursing work in these services (Rowe and Lopes, 2003).

Forensic mental health patients in acute admission wards

However, the majority of mental health nurses work with individuals with histories of offending in (non-forensic) settings (including acute admission wards; services for children and young people and older people; therapeutic communities; and facilities for treatment and recovery), as well as with individuals with problematic substance use (Kettles *et al.*, 2002; Woods, 2004).

There is an increasing need for forensic knowledge in acute mental health care. Acute inpatient psychiatric care services provide safety and security for patients and others. Amongst other reasons, patients are admitted to acute inpatient areas because of the risk to self and others; self-neglect; and serious mental health problems (Bowers, 2005, p. 1).

As more forensic units are commissioned, and more patients who have been discharged from forensic areas are being cared for in the community, there is an increasing likelihood that these individuals may re-enter services through the acute inpatient areas. There is also the transition for some forensic patients, either up or down through differing security levels, as they enter forensic services or are rehabilitated from high, medium and low security services (Collins, 2000; Collins and Davies, 2005). Some patients are brought in to a place of safety by the police and this place of safety is the local acute mental health ward. Other patients are diverted from custody or admission is arranged by social workers and their colleagues. Not only this, but substantial demands are being made on acute inpatient services caused by the more challenging symptoms of those who are admitted. Howard (2004, p. 1) points out that community staff are supporting less severely ill patients. Consequently, individuals with high levels of risk to self and/or others are admitted. Furthermore, there is an increase in the number of admissions complicated by problematic substance use (Higgins *et al.*, 1999; Watson, 2001), which is a known compounding and co-morbidity factor in criminal behaviour (Hawkins *et al.*, 1992; Champney-Smith, 2002; McMurran, 2002).

The links between ensuring safety, respect for the individual and relief of distress

Nursing and other staff aim to prevent and reduce disturbed behaviour and manage an environment where patients can comfortably stay. The aims of nursing acute mental health patients (including those whose mental health problems are associated with offending behaviours) include the following (Dale *et al.*, 2001; Kettles *et al.*, 2002; National Forensic Nurses' Research and Development Group, 2006; Wix and Humphreys, 2005):

- Holistic assessment and care, based on respect for the individual and his or her unique needs, including those related to culture, spirituality and diversity.
- Relieving individuals' distress, particularly through therapeutic nurse–patient relationships and communication.
- The assessment of risk of harm to self and others and of self-neglect, with observation with engagement and specific nursing/multidisciplinary interventions to reduce this risk.

> ...In a forensic mental health setting... the maintenance of a safe and secure environment is the essential basis for all other psychotherapeutic work, rather than being in opposition to it (Dale and Gardner, 2001, p. 256).

Whilst there can be tensions and ethical dilemmas concerning the balance between enabling individuals' autonomy and ensuring the safety of the individual patient and other people (Byrt, 1993; Clarke, 1996; Mason and Mercer, 1998), it is suggested that these three aspects of assess-

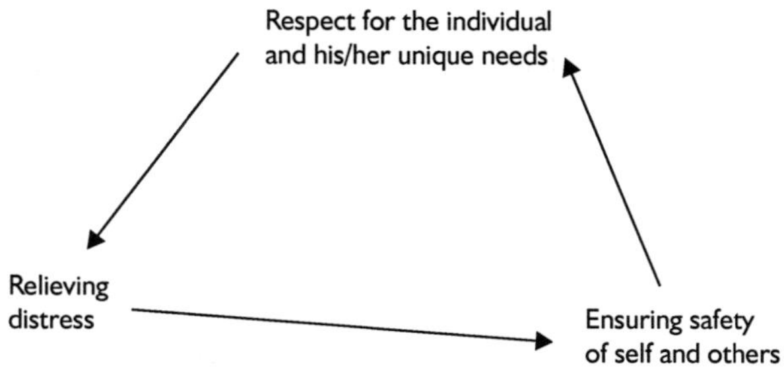

Figure 1.1 The links between ensuring safety, respect for the individual and relieving distress.

ment and care are interlinked in the care of forensic and other mental health patients and clients (Dale *et al.*, 2001; Kettles *et al.*, 2002; McClelland *et al.*, 2001, National Forensic Nurses' Research and Development Group, 2006). Often, as examples in this book indicate, interventions that respect the individual and relieve distress also have implications for reducing risk to others and improving public safety (Kettles *et al.* 2002, 2006). This is illustrated in the following example, based on the nursing practice experience of one of the authors, but with details changed to ensure anonymity.

'Ms Pam Purple': reduced distress and reduced risk

'Ms Pam Purple' was very distressed by voices commanding her to attack other people (auditory command hallucinations). After she had assaulted a neighbour, Pam was admitted to an acute mental health unit, where a thorough risk assessment and other assessments were carried out. These informed a multidisciplinary care plan, which was devised with Pam's participation, and took into account her individual needs, including those related to her vegetarian diet, and needs for space to be with women only and to pray daily.

In addition, the care plan contained strategies to reduce both Pam's distress related to the voices and the risk to others, based on psychosocial interventions. Interventions included: opportunities to talk to a nurse and ventilate feelings; relaxation techniques; antipsychotic medication (when required), as well as Olanzapine, 10 mg daily; and the use of activities that were diversionary and channelled aggression. Pam enjoyed these activities, which included drawing and aerobic exercises.

The effects of these interventions were carefully assessed, in relation to both Pam's well-being and the risk of harm to others. Eventually, Pam was able to monitor her own levels of distress in response to the voices and the likely effectiveness of particular interventions at any one time. For example, she would say to a member of her nursing team: 'I don't think it would be helpful to talk at the moment, but could you go through some relaxation techniques with me?'. Over time, both the frequency of Pam's voices and her associated distress diminished. Risk assessment revealed that the likelihood of Pam's assaulting others also diminished, mainly because she rarely had voices commanding her to do so. When these hallucinations did occur, she had a range of strategies to deal with them, instead of harming others.

'Acute' and 'forensic' – a matter of degree

Like other service users in acute settings, forensic patients are suffering from a variety of mental state disorders, resulting in considerable distress and risk to self and/or others (Bowers, 2005). However, in addition, forensic patients have either committed an offence or are charged with doing so.

Bowers (2005) identifies that the reasons for admission to acute inpatient care include dangerousness, assessment, medical treatment, self-care deficits, respite for carers and respite for the patient. From his review of the literature, Bowers (2005, p. 234) states that:

> Seven reasons for admission have been identified... of which dangerousness was the most prominent, carrying the implication that the premier task of acute psychiatric inpatient wards is to keep patients safe.

So if the two most prominent acute nursing issues are dangerousness and assessment, then this does relate to forensic nursing care, where major issues are also about the index offence (i.e. the offence leading to admission; McClelland, 2001), risk assessment and dangerousness. However, *risk* is seen as a more useful term in forensic care, as its features can form the basis of risk assessment. It is those features or risk items which the nurse then concentrates on for assessment purposes (Woods, 2001). In addition, 'dangerousness' is considered by some authors to be a more stigmatising term than risk (Morgan and Wetherell, 2004; see Box 1.1).

Box 1.1 Valid and reliable, but non-stigmatising risk assessments

In implementing clinical risk assessment and clinical risk management, nurses and other professionals need to take into account:

- The importance of not stigmatising or labelling people with avoidance of a tendency to see them only as someone with a mental health problem or an offending history (Morgan and Wetherell, 2004). Whilst risk assessment and risk management are fundamental to all forensic mental health nursing (Jones and Plowman, 2005; Woods, 2001), there is also a need to assess, and provide care that meets, or is sensitive to, a variety of patients' needs, including those related to diversity.

However, there is also a need to make thorough assessments of individuals' mental health problems and associated offending as accurately as possible – and provide effective interventions to reduce the individual's risk. Clinical risk assessment cannot be 100% accurate, but efforts are made to make assessments using measures that are valid and reliable (Jones and Plowman, 2005; Woods, 2001). (Validity refers to the extent that a risk assessment scale or other instrument actually measures risk. Reliability refers to the extent that it measures risk accurately: Carter and Porter, 2000).

The varying definitions of forensic nursing all have some common features with Bowers' (2005) statement (quoted on p. 4), as can be seen from the following definitions of forensic nursing:

- 'Forensic nursing is becoming more recognised as a speciality of mental health nursing, and has a specific group of skills and interventions developing around patient offending and anti-social behaviour in a range of settings from high security to community care' (Kettles *et al.*, 2002, p. 13).

In North America, in particular, 'forensic nursing' also concerns victims or survivors of crime (International Association of Forensic Nurses, 1999; Lynch and Standing Bear, 2000), as the following definitions indicate:

- Lynch and Standing Bear (2000, p. 258) define the forensic nurse as 'a nurse specialising in the application of clinical or community-based nursing practice, involving victims or those accused or convicted of intentional or non-intentional injury or other criminal acts.... The nurse who is qualified by education and experience in the specialised treatment of victims of violent crime, suspects or perpetrators of criminal acts, or patients with liability-related injuries, and whose primary focus, during assessment, is on the evaluation of mental status or competency, the investigation of trauma, whether physical or psychological, at the crime scene or in the clinical environs, or through review of medical records, involving evidence or assessment data for use in a court of law, is practising forensic nursing – whether the patient is living or dead.'
- '... the application of the forensic aspects of health care combined with the bio-psychosocial education of the registered nurse in the scientific investigation and treatment of trauma, and/or death of victims and perpetrators of violence, criminal activity, and traumatic accidents. The forensic nurse provides direct services to individual clients, consultation services to nursing, medical, and law-related agencies, as well as providing expert testimony in areas dealing with questioned death investigative processes, adequacy of service delivery, and specialised diagnoses of specific conditions as related to nursing.' (International Association of Forensic Nurses, 1999, p. 2).

These differing definitions all indicate the need for risk and other assessment; they all indicate some level of violence or other index offence; and they all indicate that the patient is in serious need of care in a safe environment. The definition from Kettles *et al.* (2002) enables the reader to see that forensic nursing is carried on in a range of settings and this includes acute inpatient mental health areas.

However, risk assessment is somewhat different from standard mental state assessment, and in acute care areas, it is generally standard mental state and general mental health nursing assessments that are conducted. These can be inadequate for forensic patients in acute areas. An appropriate risk assessment should be made, depending upon the circumstances of the admission and the potential risk that the patient may pose. Forensic risk is substantially different from a standard mental state assessment. In some ways, it can represent one end of the spectrum of assessment.

Kettles (2004, p. 491) gives a modified version of Woods' (2001) definition of forensic risk as:

> the clinical probability of a negative consequence, related specifically to the behaviour of those patients who are committed by law, or who are diverted from custody, to forensic settings and who have the potential to cause serious physical and psychological harm to others. This includes those fear-inducing, impulsive, intimidating, manipulative and destructive behaviours that are displayed or have been known to be displayed. This risk can either be pure or speculative in nature and is directly attributable, as the unwanted outcome occurs when the risk factor is present.

Assessment is a part of all nursing care and is now carried out in all areas. Where forensic risk differs lies in the issues of probability, outcome and the likelihood that an adverse event will occur. The chronology of adverse events is important, and Woods (2001, p. 86) gives an outline of this in terms of the risk posed in the past, the risk now and the likely risk in the future.

Holistic assessments and interventions

As has been indicated, all aspects of forensic mental health nursing are concerned with risk assessment and risk management, which aim both to relieve the individual's distress associated with specific problems and symptoms and to ensure the safety of self and others (Jones and Plowman, 2005; Woods, 2001; Woods, 2004). Related to risk assessment and risk management are holistic assessments and interventions concerned with the individual's physical, psychological, spiritual, cultural, social, psychosexual, economic and legal needs; and those related to diversity, including ethnicity, gender, sexual orientation, gender identity, and varying physical, sensory and intellectual abilities (Addo, 2006; Aiyegbusi and Byrt, 2006).

Specific aspects of nursing forensic mental health patients in acute settings

Much of this book is concerned with specific aspects of nursing and multidisciplinary risk assessment and risk management. In summary, risk management with forensic (and, to a large extent, with other) mental health patients is concerned with the areas listed below, which are covered in this book. The nurse's skills, in working with forensic mental health patients, include those that are used in all areas of mental health nursing, as well as skills specific to forensic mental health nursing. The latter include specialist areas of risk assessment, interventions concerned with reducing the risk of offending behaviours, and maintaining both physical and relational security (Woods, 2001).

Nursing forensic mental health patients in acute settings involves the following, in collaboration with the patient, as far as possible; his or her carers at home, with the patient's agreement; and in close liaison with various members of the multidisciplinary team (McClelland *et al.*, 2001; Wix and Humphreys, 2005). (Most of the following areas are covered in later chapters in this book.)

- Risk assessment: evaluation of the extent and nature of harm to others and to self (Jones and Plowman, 2005; Woods, 2001).
- Using risk assessment, and other assessments to inform the nursing/multidisciplinary interventions outlined below:
  - Ensuring a safe, and, in some instances, physically secure environment (Dale and Gardner, 2001).
  - Skills in admitting patients and in developing empathetic appreciation of the many crises and problems with which they are faced (Walsh *et al.*, 2001).
  - Skilled observation with engagement, which maintains both safety and the individual's dignity as much as possible (Jones and Jackson, 2004; Kettles and Woodally, 2006).
- Relational security, involving:
  - Developing in-depth knowledge of the individual, especially in relation to risk (Dale and Gardner, 2001).
  - Establishing trust, a therapeutic alliance and negotiation (including establishing 'common ground') with individuals who may be 'reluctant patients' and find it difficult to trust staff (see Box 1.2). Developing in-depth knowledge of the individual, especially in relation to risk (Dale and Gardner, 2001).
  - Approachability, and establishing good non – verbal and verbal communication, including active listening and empathy (Arnold and Boggs, 2003; Dale and Gardner, 2001; West and Abolins, 2001).
  - In the present authors' experience, the keeping of promises and the translation of the nurse's concern and empathy into practical help (Kunyk and Olson, 2001) are also important.
- Facilitating a ward environment which is:
  - Safe. (If patients and staff feel unsafe, this is likely to increase their anxiety, and nursing and other interventions are less likely to be therapeutic: Bowers *et al.*, 2002; Dale and Gardner, 2001.)
  - Therapeutic in other ways, with the provision of opportunities for individuals to discover positive qualities, skills and abilities (Campling *et al.*, 2004).
- The administration and monitoring of antipsychotic and other medication (Robson *et al.*, 2005).
- Specific nursing/multidisciplinary interventions to reduce distress, develop positive coping skills and reduce risk of future offending. The latter is achieved partly through individuals learning about themselves, their relationships and problems, particularly in relation to their offending behaviours (Kettles *et al.*, 2002). Specific interventions include:
  - Psychosocial interventions for individuals with mental illness, including cognitive behavioural therapy, psychoeducation and provision of 'low expressed emotion' ward environments which minimise stress (McKeown and McCann, 2000; Gamble and Brennan, 2006).
  - Specific cognitive behavioural therapies and other psychotherapies concerned with particular skills and problems, including those related to offending behaviours. Examples of areas addressed include anger management, social problem solving and issues concerning problematic substance use (Byrt *et al.*, 2005; Doyle *et al.*, 2006).
  - The application of therapeutic community principles (Byrt, 2006).
  - The use of particular activities, so that individuals can gain skills, positive coping strategies and fulfilment (Byrt, 2006). (For example, research has found that exercise can increase individuals' self-esteem and decrease and channel aggressive behaviours (Adams, 2002).

- Enabling the patient to access independent advocates from legal, voluntary and other organisations (Garman *et al.*, 2003; Kenny, 2005).
- Providing assessments and interventions that are culturally sensitive and culturally competent, in relation to the individual's ethnicity, gender, disability, sexual orientation and gender identity (Addo, 2006; Aiyegbusi and Byrt, 2006).
- In relation to the spiritual needs of patients, enabling the latter to find hope and 'explanation' (Swinton, 2002, p. 209) is particularly important, given the crisis, uncertainty and considerable problems that they face.
- Self-awareness is essential for nurses to work effectively with forensic mental health patients (Kirby and Hart, 2004). For example, in order to be non-judgemental and establish therapeutic communication, nurses need to be aware of their feelings in relation to particular patients and their past offending. An awareness of professional boundary issues and of counter-transference is particularly important, especially with patients with 'personality disorders' (Bowers, 2002; Peternelj-Taylor, 2003; Tennant *et al.*, 2000).
- Ethical and legal awareness is also essential, given the many moral dilemmas related to the care and treatment of forensic mental health patients; for example, balancing the needs and rights of patients with those of the general public (Kettles *et al.*, 2006; Nolan, 2005).
- Sociological and political awareness enables nurses to be aware of the impact of social factors, media influence and government policies on decisions about the care, treatment and rehabilitation of forensic mental health patients. Arguably, one role of nurses working in this area is to influence government policy that impacts on forensic patients' lives (Kettles *et al.*, 2006).
- Of crucial importance are high-quality support, clinical supervision, education and training related to practice issues (Watson and Kettles, 2006).

Box 1.2 An example of negotiation: 'Mr Barry Blue'

This example is based on the experience of one of the authors of this chapter. However, pseudonyms have been used, and details changed, to ensure confidentiality and anonymity.

Forensic mental health nurses can establish therapeutic alliances with patients who do not see themselves as ill or as putting others at risk through negotiation. For example, in one acute admission ward that admitted forensic patients, one man ('Mr Barry Blue'), who experienced very frightening paranoid delusions, was happy to play card games with his Named Nurse ('Rani'), although he did not wish to speak to her. These games led to Barry trusting Rani sufficiently to state his concerns at what he saw as inappropriate detention. Rani checked, without arguing with Barry, that he was aware of staff views about his need for treatment, and gave him further information about how to contact an independent advocate and organisations concerned with patients' rights. Eventually, Barry felt able to trust Rani sufficiently to tell her about his frightening persecutory voices and delusions. Rani was ready to listen when Barry wished to talk, but recognised his need for space and did not press him to speak.

Between them, and with other members of the clinical team, Barry and Rani were gradually able to agree a multidisciplinary care plan to relieve the distress caused by his symptoms, reduce associated stress, and continue to assess and reduce risk and prevent harm to others. This included continued risk assessment (e.g. assessing the extent of persecutory voices and delusions, which potentiated Barry's risk of harming others). Psychosocial interventions and the administration and monitoring of Clozapine were also included in Barry's care plan, as was his spiritual need for quiet time for reflection in the unit's inter-faith room. Barry said that this helped him to relax and to gain hope. At his suggestion, Barry's need to exercise regularly was also included in his care plan. In line with research findings reported by Adams (2002), this helped him to feel better physically and increased his self-esteem. This and other interventions relieved the intensity and frequency of voices and other distressing symptoms, and associated stress, and also reduced the risk of harm to others.

From Barry's initial wish not to be involved at all in plans for nursing and multidisciplinary interventions, it became possible to gradually negotiate interventions and involve him in care planning with his agreement. This started with Rani's attempt to respond to Barry's requests for games, help with issues concerning his rights and readiness to listen as soon as he wished to talk.

Geographical variations in acute and forensic services

Whilst forensic nursing shares common features in different parts of the UK, geographical area is important in terms of both acute care and forensic care. Some acute wards take patients from rural populations, while others are very urban in nature and take inner city populations. In contrast, the four high-security hospitals (Broadmoor, Rampton and Ashworth in England; the State Hospital, Carstairs, in Scotland) either take patients from large national regions or from whole countries. Carstairs admits patients from the whole of Scotland and has taken patients from Northern Ireland. Therefore, in some acute units, the patient population can be relatively homogeneous, as they are from similar circumstances; while in other units, the population can vary considerably. In forensic units, the patients may have similar social problems, such as being unemployed, on benefits and lonely, but their backgrounds can be very different.

There are also differences in acute wards and the care they provide, as opposed to forensic areas. In some ways it is a matter of degree, and in other ways it can be quite different. For example, both acute and forensic areas now provide psychosocial interventions (PSI) as a form of care that is important and beneficial for patient recovery and well-being. However, the extent to which Thorn or PSI trained staff carry out this form of intervention varies. In acute wards, one or two staff may be PSI trained, whereas in forensic areas there are generally more staff who have a PSI qualification. Also, specialised interventions are now practised in forensic areas, such as dialectical behaviour therapy, domestic violence therapies and sex offender therapies that are rarely, if ever, seen in acute wards.

Transition through different levels of security

Skelly (2001, p. 234) states that there are two routes of discharge from a high-security hospital: discharge to the community or transfer to a lower level of hospital security. He goes on to say that some patients will be transferred to low secure units, which may or may not offer the security of a locked door, or to 'open' wards which may offer little physical security at all.

Patients can go in either direction. They can enter an acute ward and then continue on through increasing levels of security, or they can enter high-security areas and go through the transition to low secure areas. Whichever direction the patient is going in, it is the role of the nurse to care for the patient who is enduring distress, disorientation, difficulty and often stigma or dislike by others.

Policy and legal contexts in forensic aspects of acute care

The work presented in this book is set against the ever-changing backdrop of major legal and policy contexts. (H. M. Government, Scotland, 2003; Office of the Leader of the House of Commons, 2006). This includes a change in legal status for those suffering from personality disorder (H. M. Government, Scotland, 2003); and readers are directed to the first book in this series (National Forensic Nurses' Research and Development Group, 2006). The National Reviews of Mental Health Nursing in both Scotland (2006) and England (2006) have been conducted, and there is no doubt that key messages coming from the two National Reviews of Mental Health Nursing (2006) include the following:

- The complexity of users' and carers' needs must determine the role and focus of mental health nursing.
- Intensive, acute and crisis care are areas where extended and advanced roles need to be developed to meet patient need.
- There is a need to develop whole systems ways of working.
- Mental health nurses will continue to have a key role in supporting people with long term and complex mental health problems.

These particular messages relate very strongly to forensic aspects of acute care, given that the complex nature of forensic clients' problems often presents through acute and crisis areas and teams. Acute care services need to change to rise to the challenge of admitting individuals with personality disorder, problematic substance use and histories of offending if they want to give appropriate therapeutic care rather than just holding patients until the worst of the crisis is past and then discharging them. Whole systems and recovery models are likely to help people with these types of problem and acute care needs to embrace such ideas as quickly as possible, so as to enable appropriate care to take place.

Evidence-based practice and best practice

Bowers (2005) is clear that acute inpatient services have suffered from a lack of nursing research in recent years, whereas forensic areas have been well funded, in this respect, in the last ten years. Woods *et al.* (2002) suggest that forensic nursing research findings may be low down in the hierarchy of research evidence, but that what has been done gives a strong foundation for development. Perhaps this indicates that what is now required is some joint working between the two areas of acute and forensic nursing to consider what is relevant from one to the other and to develop material (such as appropriate assessments) and interventions that complement each other for patients in transition from one area to another. Evidence-based practice is a developing issue that will take time to mature and best practice can only be improved upon with professional, caring nurses in both areas communicating to the benefit of the patient and the safety of the community.

Topics covered in this book

Carol Watson and Alyson McGregor Kettles deal with the educational and policy aspects of forensic and acute care in Chapter 2.

In Chapter 3, Richard Byrt, with a contribution by Linnette James, discusses the problems and challenges related to social and physical environments of acute and forensic mental health settings. Chapter 4 considers ways to facilitate beneficial and therapeutic environments, for example through measurements of ward atmosphere and the application of therapeutic community principles and psychosocial interventions. In Chapter 5, Richard Byrt and Mike Doyle discuss the assessment, prevention and reduction of violence and aggression. This chapter includes a consideration, by Mike Doyle, of risk assessment measures that are used in forensic services, and their applicability to acute mental health care.

In Chapter 6, Mike Doyle and Michael Coffey further consider aspects of risk assessment and other areas of assessment.

Phil Woods and Alyson McGregor Kettles, in Chapter 7, outline the measurement of health and social functioning using standardised instruments such as the Health of the Nation Scale (HoNOS) – Secure Version 2 and the Behavioural Status (BEST) Index.

In Chapter 8, Stuart Guy, Steve Fyffe and Wendy Ifill discuss the forensic issues that relate to patients in Psychiatric Intensive Care Units (PICU in England or IPCU in Scotland). This chapter includes a review of the beneficial results of changes made in one Psychiatric Intensive Care Unit, including the introduction of low-conflict high-therapy nursing (Bowers *et al.*, 2006).

Alyson McGregor Kettles and Paula Hall, in Chapter 9, deal with crisis interventions teams and other forms of acute care that the forensic patient may encounter.

In Chapter 10, Michael Coffey and his colleagues, Tina Gronow and Julie Morgan, give an excellent view of the transition of the forensic patient from acute to community services.

Linda Hart gives us a thought-provoking discussion, in Chapter 11, of her experiences as a service user and her transition through acute care: an account of considerable relevance to nursing and multidisciplinary interventions with forensic patients in acute settings.

Chapter 12 is written by Jean Woodally and Michelle McGunnigle, with their considerable experience of individuals with personality disorder. Jean and Michelle outline the application, to acute settings, of forensic aspects of care for this group of patients.

Richard Byrt, Tim Hardie, Anne Aiyegbusi and Mary Addo write in Chapter 13 about cultural and diversity issues. Following on in Chapter 14, Richard Byrt and Tim Hardie discuss cultural sensitivity and cultural competence relevant to the care of forensic patients in acute mental health areas.

Alyson McGregor Kettles and Richard Byrt write about the nature of observation and engagement and apply the forensic issues to acute care in Chapter 15.

Helen Walker, from the State Hospital, Carstairs, in Scotland, delineates multi-professional working in Chapter 16. She goes on to write, with Mike Doyle in Chapter 17, about the application of psychosocial interventions to forensic patients in acute areas.

Finally, the conclusions, with 15 identified themes from the text, are presented by Richard Byrt, Alyson McGregor Kettles and Phil Woods in Chapter 18.

References

Adams, L. (2002) Nursing interventions and future directions for exercise therapy. In: *Therapeutic Interventions for Forensic Mental Health Nurses* (eds. A. M. Kettles, P. Woods and M. Collins), Chapter 8. Jessica Kingsley, London.

Addo, M. (2006) Culture, spirituality and ethical issues in caring for clients with personality disorder. In: *Forensic Mental Health Nursing: Interventions with People with 'Personality Disorders'* (ed. National Forensic Nurses' Research and Development Group), Chapter 5. Quay, London.

Aiyegbusi, A. and Byrt, R. (2006) Gender and sexuality. In: *Forensic Mental Health Nursing: Interventions with People with 'Personality Disorders'* (ed. National Forensic Nurses' Research and Development Group), Chapter 8. Quay, London.

Arnold, E. and Boggs, K. U. (eds.) (2003) *Interpersonal Relationships*, 4th edn. Saunders, St Louis.

Bowers, L. (2002) *Dangerous and Severe Personality Disorder. Response and Role of the Psychiatric Team.* Routledge, London.

Bowers, L. (2005) Reasons for admission and their implications for the nature of acute inpatient psychiatric nursing. *Journal of Psychiatric and Mental Health Nursing*, **12**(2), 231–6.

Bowers, L., Crowhurst, N., Alexander, J., Callaghan, P., Eales, S., Guy, S., McCann, E. and Ryan, C. (2002) Safety and security policies on psychiatry acute admission wards: results from a London-wide survey. *Journal of Psychiatric and Mental Health Nursing*, **9**, 427–33.

Bowers, L., Brennan, G., Flood, C., Lipang, M. and Oladapo, P. (2006) Preliminary outcomes of a trial to reduce conflict and containment on acute psychiatric wards: city nurses. *Journal of Psychiatric and Mental Health Nursing*, **13**, 165–72.

Byrt, R. (2006) Nursing interventions in therapeutic communities. In: *Forensic Mental Health Nursing: Interventions with People with 'Personality Disorders'* (ed. National Forensic Nurses' Research and Development Group), Chapter 14. Quay, London.

Byrt, R., Wray, C. and 'Tom' (2005) Towards hope and inclusion: nursing interventions in a medium secure service for men with 'personality disorders'. *Mental Health Practice*, **8**(8), 38–43.

Campling, P., Davies, S. and Farquharson, G. (eds.) (2004) *From Toxic Institutions to Therapeutic Environments: Residential Settings in Mental Health Services*. Gaskell, London.

Champney-Smith, J. (2002) Dual diagnosis. In: *Working with Substance Misusers: a Guide to Theory and Practice* (eds. T. Petersen and A. McBride), pp. 267–75. Routledge, London.

Clarke, L. (1996) Covert participant observation in a secure forensic unit: care, conflict and control. *NT Research*, **1**(6), 431–40.

Collins, M. (2000) The practitioner new to the role of forensic psychiatric nurse in the UK. In: *Forensic Nursing and Multidisciplinary Care of the Mentally Disordered Offender* (eds. D. Robinson and A. Kettles), pp. 39–50. Jessica Kingsley, London.

Collins, M. and Davies, S. (2005) The security needs assessment profile: a multidimensional approach to measuring security needs. *International Journal of Forensic Mental Health*, **4**(1), 39–52.

Dale, C. and Gardner, J. (2001) Security in forensic environments: strategic and operational issues. In: *Forensic Mental Health: Issues in Practice* (eds. C. Dale, T. Thompson and P. Woods), Chapter 23. Baillière Tindall/Royal College of Nursing, Edinburgh.

Dale, C., Thompson, T. and Woods, P. (eds.) (2001) *Forensic Mental Health: Issues in Practice*. Baillière Tindall/Royal College of Nursing, London.

Doyle, M., Aiyegbusi, A. and Burbery, P. (2006) Personality disorder: specialist psychological approaches. In: *Forensic Mental Health Nursing: Interventions with People with 'Personality Disorders'* (ed. National Forensic Nurses' Research and Development Group), Chapter 15. Quay, London.

Gamble, C. and Brennan, W. (eds.) (2006) *Working with Serious Mental Illness*, 2nd edn. Baillière Tindall, Edinburgh.

Garman, G., Kelly, R. and Waldron, S. (2003) Setting up a successful patients' council. *Mental Health Practice*, **6**(7), 20–2.

Hawkins, J. D., Catalano, R. F. and Miller, J. Y. (1992) Risk and protective factors for alcohol and other drug problems in adolescence and early adulthood: implications for substance abuse prevention. *Psychological Bulletin*, **112**, 64–105.

Higgins, R., Hurst, K. and Wistow, G. (1999) Nursing acute psychiatric inpatients: a quantitative and qualitative study. *Journal of Advanced Nursing*, **29**(1), 52–63.

H. M. Government, Scotland (2003). *Mental Health (Care and Treatment) (Scotland) Act*, 2003.

Howard, D. (2004) An introduction to acute mental health care: from acute concerns to capable practitioner. In: *Acute Mental Health Nursing: From Acute Concerns to Capable Practitioner* (eds. M. Harrison, D. Howard and D. Mitchell), pp. 1–28. Sage, London.

International Association of Forensic Nurses (1999) [[Please complete]]

Jones, J. and Jackson, A. (2004) Observation. In: *Acute Mental Health Nursing: From Acute Concerns to the Capable Practitioner* (eds. M. Harrison, D. Howard and D. Mitchell), Chapter 8. Sage, London.

Jones, J. and Plowman, C. (2005) Risk assessment: a multidisciplinary approach to estimating harmful behaviour in mentally disordered offenders. In: *Multidisciplinary Working in Forensic Mental Health Care* (eds. S. Wix and M. Humphreys). Elsevier, China.

Kenny, P. J. (2005) The place of a legal representative or advocate working for the client. In: *Multidisciplinary Working in Forensic Mental Health Care* (eds. S. Wix and M. Humphreys), Chapter 4B. Elsevier Churchill Livingstone, Edinburgh.

Kettles, A. M. (2004) A concept analysis of forensic risk. *Journal of Psychiatric and Mental Health Nursing*, **11**, 484–93.

Kettles, A. M. and Woodally, J. (2006) Observation and engagement with people with personality disorder. In: *Forensic Mental Health Nursing: Interventions with People with 'Personality Disorders'* (ed. National Forensic Nurses' Research and Development Group), Chapter 12. Quay, London.

Kettles, A. M., Woods, P. and Collins, M. (2002) Introduction. In: *Therapeutic Interventions for Forensic Mental Health Nurses* (eds. A. M. Kettles, P. Woods and M. Collins), pp. 13–20. Jessica Kingsley, London.

Kettles, A. M., Woods, P. and Byrt, R. (2006) Conclusions: themes, action and research for the future. In: *Forensic Mental Health Nursing: Interventions with People with 'Personality Disorders'* (ed. National Forensic Nurses' Research and Development Group), Chapter 16. Quay, London.

Kunyk, D. and Olson, J. K. (2001) Clarification of conceptualisations of empathy. *Journal of Advanced Nursing*, **35**(3), 317–25.

Lynch, V. and Standing Bear, Z. (2000) A global perspective in forensic nursing: challenges for the 21st century. In: *Forensic Nursing and Multidisciplinary Care of the Mentally Disordered Offender* (eds. D. Robinson and A. M. Kettles), pp. 249–66. Jessica Kingsley, London.

Mason, T. and Mercer, D. (eds.) (1998) *Critical Perspectives in Forensic Care: Inside Out*. Macmillan, Basingstoke.

McClelland, N. (2001) Aessesment and clinical risk. In: Forensic Nursing and Mental Disorder in Clinical Practice (eds. N. McClelland, M. Humphreys, L. Conlon and T. Hillis), Chapter 2. Butterworth-Heinemann, Oxford.

McClelland, N., Humphreys, M., Conlon, L. and Hillis, T. (eds.) (2001) *Forensic Nursing and Mental Disorder in Clinical Practice*. Butterworth-Heinemann, Oxford.

McKeown, M. and McCann, G. (2000) Psychosocial interventions. In: *Forensic Mental Health Nursing: Current Approaches* (eds. C. Chaloner and M. Coffey), Chapter 12. Blackwell Science, Oxford.

McMurran, M. (2002) Expert Paper: *Dual Diagnosis of Mental Disorder and Substance Misuse*. NHS National Programme on Forensic Mental Health Research and Development, Liverpool.

Morgan, S. and Wetherell, A. (2004) Assessing and managing risk. In: *The Art and Science of Mental Health Nursing: a Textbook of Principles and Practice* (eds. I. Norman and I. Ryrie), Chapter 8. Open University Press, Maidenhead.

National Forensic Nurses' Research and Development Group (2006) *Forensic Mental Health Nursing: Interventions with People with 'Personality Disorder'*. Quay, London.

Nolan, P. (2005) The historical context. In: *Multidisciplinary Working in Forensic Mental Health Care* (eds. S. Wix and M. Humphreys), Chapter 1. Elsevier Churchill Livingstone, Edinburgh.

Office of the Leader of the House of Commons (2006). `http://www.commonsleader.gov.uk/`.

Parker, E. (ed.) (1985) The development of secure provision. In: *Secure Provision* (ed. L. Gostin), Chapter 1. Tavistock Publications, London.

Skelly, C. (2001) Transition from higher to lower levels of security. In *Forensic Mental Health: Issues in Practice* (eds. C. Dale, T. Thompson and P. Woods), pp. 233–41. Baillière Tindall/Royal College of Nursing, London.

Swinton, J. (2002) Spiritual care in forensic nursing: spiritual interventions and future directions for care. In: *Therapeutic Interventions for Forensic Mental Health Nurses* (eds. A. M. Kettles, P. Woods and M. Collins), Chapter 13. Jessica Kingsley, London.

Tennant, A., Davies, C. and Tennant, I. (2000) Working with the personality disordered offender. In: *Forensic Mental Health Nursing: Current Approaches* (eds. C. Chaloner and M. Coffey). Blackwell Science, Oxford.

Watson, A. (2001) *Detained: Inspection of Compulsory Mental Health Admissions*. Stationery Office, London.

Watson, C. and Kettles, A. M. (2006) Education, training and support for staff working with clients with a diagnosis of personality disorder: some thoughts. In: *Forensic Mental Health Nursing: Interventions with People with 'Personality Disorders'* (ed. National Forensic Nurses' Research and Development Group), Chapter 7. Quay Books, London.

West, M. and Abolins, D. (2001) Dealing with hostility. In: *Forensic Nursing and Mental Disorder in Clinical Practice* (eds. N. McClelland, M. Humphreys, L. Conlon and T. Hillis), Chapter 4. Butterworth-Heinemann, Oxford.

Wix, S. and Humphreys, M. (eds.) (2005) *Multidisciplinary Working in Forensic Mental Health Care*. Elsevier Churchill Livingstone, Edinburgh.

Woods, P. (2001) Risk assessment and management. In *Forensic Mental Health: Issues in Practice* (eds. C. Dale, T. Thompson and P. Woods), pp. 85–97. Baillière Tindall/Royal College of Nursing, London.

Woods, P. (2004) The person who uses forensic mental health services. In: *The Art and Science of Mental Health Nursing: a Textbook of Principles and Practice* (eds. I. Norman and I. Ryrie), Chapter 20. Open University Press, Maidenhead.

Woods, P., Collins, M. and Kettles, A. M. (2002) Forensic nursing interventions and future directions for forensic mental health practice. In: *Therapeutic Interventions for Forensic Mental Health Nurses* (eds. A. M. Kettles, P. Woods and M. Collins), pp. 240–5. Jessica Kingsley, London.

CHAPTER 2

Forensic educational aspects of acute mental health care: policy, characteristics, skills and knowledge

Carol Watson and Alyson McGregor Kettles

Introduction

The education of mental health nurses has to change to meet the significant paradigm shift (Forrest *et al.*, 2005) that is signposted for the future mental health nursing policy agenda. This is driven both by the need to redesign services in line with service user demands and government policies, and by the significant recruitment and retention issues arising from the changing demographic. The latter affects all public services and the range of employment and other lifestyle choices available to people of all ages, who may previously have been attracted to them. This chapter aims to discuss some of the issues affecting the recruitment, education, training and ongoing professional development of mental health nurses. It will focus, in particular, on the needs of the workforce in acute mental health settings, who increasingly have responsibility for individuals who have a forensic history or background, as well as complex mental health needs.

Despite Whyte's (2000) view that forensic nursing does not exist as a specialist entity and the converse views held by others (NHS Education for Scotland, 2000; Robinson and Kettles, 2000) the contemporary view is that all mental health practitioners, in particular nurses, should have, and be able to use, a range of sound evidence-based therapeutic skills, and operate from a recovery-focused values-based approach. Should service design take the challenge of enabling nurses and other practitioners to follow patients/clients throughout their (often long) journey to recovery, then education must equip the workforce to deliver a greater range of interventions in both acute and primary care settings, ensuring that only individuals with the most complex needs are referred to specialist services which deliver complex care and psychological interventions. The Mental Health (Care and Treatment) (Scotland) Act 2003 provides the option of compulsory treatment orders in the community as well as in inpatient units, and nursing education must respond with undergraduate, postgraduate and continuing professional development opportunities which deliver a workforce that is fit for purpose. This is an enormous opportunity for nurses to enhance their knowledge and skills around an array of interventions, and to reclaim the core of mental health practice: i.e. in the daily use of psychosocial skills, family and individual therapeutic skills and psychological interventions.

The relationship between nursing education and mental health nursing policy

The Nursing and Midwifery Council (NMC) sets the standards for the content and outcomes of all undergraduate and statutory postgraduate nursing and midwifery programmes. Concerns have been increasing around nursing, in particular – about fitness for practice at the point of registration. Employers, practitioners and service users have all questioned whether the current structure and content of mental health nursing education does, in fact, prepare nurses to meet the needs of service users and their carers/families as they really are, at all stages of the patient journey, and within an increasingly diverse range and configuration of service delivery. More than ever, there is an imperative for educationalists to work up their curricula, not just in partnership with service providers, but with service users and carers (experts by experience), and with representatives of all client groups, especially those with the most complex needs, including children and young people, those with dual diagnosis and those with forensic histories and needs related to these. All of these issues are reflected in the acute population, and at any one time, practitioners in acute care will be dealing with individuals who have potential, as well as current, actual needs, and who are at risk of developing more complex, and certainly forensic, histories if basic elements of risk, vulnerability, resilience factors and response to interventions are not looked at through a prism of:

- Meeting current mental ill health needs/response to interventions
- Preventing further deterioration or the development of additional/more complex needs
- Promoting mental health well-being and optimum social functioning for the individual and those of significance around him/her

Key messages from mental health service policy (Scottish Executive Health Department, 2006a; Department of Health, 2006), mental health legislation (Scottish Executive, 2003; Mental Welfare Commission for Scotland, 2005) and individual practitioner groups across the UK (e.g. Scottish Executive Health Department, 2006b; Department of Health, 2006; Scottish Executive, 2006; National Institute for Mental Health in England and Royal College of Psychiatrists, 2005) all reinforce the same themes:

1. The individual and his/her needs as the centre of service/treatment/care planning
2. Rights-based approaches to practice and service delivery
3. The imperative of positive relationships as the starting point to all interventions with service users and their carers and families
4. Recovery as the underpinning principle of therapeutic interventions
5. Ensuring a focus on promotion of mental health and well-being and prevention of mental ill health, as well as the delivery of high-quality care and evidence-based interventions

6. In addition, the Mental Health (Care and Treatment) (Scotland) Act 2003 is underpinned by a set of principles which reflect this rights-based approach and the treatment of individuals in the least restrictive environment that ensures safe and effective care (see Table 2.1). This applies in respect of all individuals receiving treatment under the Act.

Table 2.1 Adapted from Millan principles.

Non-discrimination	People with mental disorder should, whenever possible, retain the same rights and entitlements as those with other health needs
Equality	All powers under the Act should be exercised without any direct or indirect discrimination
Respect for diversity	Service users should receive care, treatment and support in a manner that accords respect for their individual qualities, abilities and diverse backgrounds, and which properly takes account of their age, gender, sexual orientation, ethnic group and social, cultural and religious background
Reciprocity	Where society imposes an obligation on an individual to comply with a programme of treatment or care, it should impose a parallel obligation on health and social care authorities to provide safe and appropriate services
Informal care	Wherever possible, care, treatment and support should be provided to people with mental disorder without recourse to compulsion
Participation	Service users should be fully involved to the extent permitted by their individual capacity, in all aspects of their assessment, care, treatment and support. Account should be taken of their past and present wishes, so far as they can be ascertained. They should be provided with all of the information and support necessary to enable them to participate fully
Respect for carers	Those who provide care to service users on an informal basis should receive respect for their role and experience, receive appropriate information and advice and have their views and needs taken into account
Least restrictive alternative	Service users should be provided with any necessary care, treatment and support, both in the least invasive manner and in the least restrictive manner and environment compatible with the delivery of safe and effective care, taking account, where appropriate, of the safety of others
Benefit	Any intervention under the Act should be likely to produce, for the service user, a benefit that cannot reasonably be achieved other than by the intervention
Child welfare	The welfare of a child with mental disorder should be paramount in any interventions imposed on the child under the Act

National reviews of mental health nursing

The recent reviews in England and Scotland of Mental Health Nursing (Scottish Executive Health Department, 2006b; Department of Health, 2006) also make significant criticisms of current undergraduate preparation of mental health nurses. The reviews reflect the view that students are insufficiently prepared or skilled for the real challenges of practice at the point of registration. The Nursing and Midwifery Council (NMC) has the statutory (UK) responsibility to set the standards for education, including the Standards of Proficiency (previously competencies) (Nursing and Midwifery Council, 2004). The latter need to be achieved at the point of registration to demonstrate a nurse's fitness to practice, set generic nursing standards for all four branches of nursing (adult, mental health, child health and learning disability), and it is left to curriculum developers and their partner service organisations to interpret these within the context of each specific branch. The mental health nursing reviews have argued that these proficiencies do not describe the skills, knowledge, attitudes, values and approaches necessary to deliver contemporary mental health care and treatment, as it needs to be delivered in the increasing range of service delivery models. In response to this, and to address general concerns within Council, the NMC is currently working up six Essential Skills Clusters (ESCs) to better describe the core clinical skills which nurses will require to demonstrate at the point of registration. These are:

1. Care and compassion
2. Communication
3. Hygiene and infection control
4. Nutrition and fluid management
5. Medication management
6. Management of care

However, this may not address the concerns around mental health nursing. The Scottish Review particularly makes a strong case for using the Ten Essential Shared Capabilities (Sainsbury Centre for Mental Health, 2004) and has a range of recommendations targeted at influencing higher education institutions (through monitoring and encouraging greater clinical involvement for academic staff) and undergraduate programmes (a national framework for pre-registration programmes to reflect the priorities in the report). Both will involve influencing the direction of travel of the NMC itself. In addition, NHS Education for Scotland and the Scottish Recovery Network are to develop a national framework for training in recovery-based practice, and health boards are charged to implement whole-systems ways of working with planned rotation of nursing staff across boundaries and service settings. The education, training and workforce development agenda for such radical change in ways of working and delivering care and treatment is enormous. The culture of nursing will have to continue to change, and practitioners will face both opportunities and challenges to their existing professional self-concepts and knowledge and skills sets.

Using the stepped approach to care described in Delivering for Health (Scottish Executive Health Department, 2006a), patients should expect more care delivered within primary care, with only complex problems being referred to secondary or tertiary services. There is also an expectation that patients will have a continuity of care, and examples of best practice cite models where nurses follow patients through primary care, hospital, and back to community care (see for example Perinatal Mental Health Service, p. 29 in Scottish Executive Health Department, 2006b).

This kind of individualised approach is promoted as one which is not only more satisfying and effective for clients and practitioners, but also provides continuity around risk assessment and risk management. Given the complex long-term patient journeys for those with severe and enduring mental health problems, taking them through inpatient acute settings, day care, or low/medium secure settings as well as community care, it is ever less tenable for nurses to expect to develop a knowledge and skills set which differentiates between these settings, with an identity as a specialist acute care, community or forensic nurse. Teams of practitioners must be prepared to look at their individual client as a whole person, addressing promotion of mental (and general) health and well-being, prevention of further ill health and the care and treatment of a broad range of issues, defined and prioritised in partnership with the patient/client themselves. This model requires a much more collaborative and flexible range of approaches and skills, along with the autonomy to utilise them. Specialist tertiary services will always be required, but for fewer individuals, and with nurses and other practitioners in acute and community settings retaining and developing what may have been previously regarded as specialist skills. Many nurses working in acute inpatient settings report feeling deskilled, and there is evidence that investment in further training and development around 'specialist skills', such as cognitive behaviour therapy, family therapy and anger management, is lower in these settings than in specialist settings. This can leave some acute care nurses and their clients in an effectively therapy-free environment, including those with some of the most severe and complex problems (Mental Welfare Commission for Scotland, 2005). For many patients, coming in to forensic services is their first exposure to specific psychological interventions, often delivered by nurses, as well as psychologists and occupational therapists. This is clearly not what rights-based, needs-led care and treatment means.

Forensic domains of competency and integrated service delivery

The basis of all care and treatment is a core set of attitudes and values, whether we are caring for children with leukaemia, adults with severe depressive episodes or those individuals suffering from mental illness who also have offending histories and requisite needs. In any NHS setting, we provide treatment at the point of need, and NHS practitioners are both contractually and (where professionally regulated via their codes of conduct) committed to a set of ethical principles and values which is dominated by 'Respect for the Person'. Not just respect for the person we like or approve of, the free person who comes in of his/her own volition seeking care and treatment with which he/she will cooperate fully, but with the difficult, the confused, the prisoner, and those from the socially excluded of our society who often have the most complex and pressing bio-psychosocial needs. Services must be equipped to deal with all of these, and practitioners need constantly to remember their professional commitments to them. Values are not just about statements, philosophies or charters. Values are demonstrated in the day-to-day working practices of staff, in the policies and guidelines used by staff, and in the structures and processes available to staff to support their practice and ensure its quality and effectiveness (Watson, 2002). Having a forensic history does not make an individual a 'forensic patient', only to be cared for in specialist forensic settings or by specialist forensic practitioners for all time. That is rather like saying that if you have diabetes, no matter what other health problem you encounter you must be treated by a diabetologist and specialist diabetes nurse. This approach of stereotyping individuals and seeing them in a box that says 'mentally disordered offender' (or 'over 65 year old', or 'alcoholic' or 'personality disorder') minimises, as well as stigmatises, the individual and his/her health needs. It has also contributed to the deskilling of nurses working in generic services. By all means ask for a specialist opinion, but there is no excuse for failing to carry out a full assessment of needs, rather than just a risk assessment with a view to a quick referral to someone else.

The attitudes and values espoused in the Forensic Competency Framework (NHS Education for Scotland, 2000) apply equally to all mental health professionals. The domains of competencies described also have relevance to acute and community care. These are currently being updated, but the core remains the same:

- Interpersonal/relationship competencies
- Risk assessment/risk management
- Professional, legal and ethical aspects of care

In the process of updating this framework to take account of new legislation and contemporary service re-design, colleagues in Glasgow have added a set of non-clinical competencies, linked to the Knowledge and Skills Framework, for all staff who are new to working with forensic clients. In addition, competencies described for practitioners working with individuals who have severe and/or enduring mental health needs (NHS Education for Scotland, 2002) considerably overlap with these and equally apply to many with a forensic history (see Box 2.1).

These two competency frameworks differed in relation to their target audiences only in quite minor ways:

- The first described competencies to be primarily utilised by those working with Mentally Disordered Offenders (MDOs) in a range of settings, and were in addition to fundamental core competencies for all mental health practitioners. Furthermore, the values are applicable in all settings and reflect the view that all mental health nurses should have experience in forensic mental health care.
- The second described a development pathway, with the first stage of competence for newly qualified practitioners consolidating their knowledge and skills during their first post-registration year. The second stage is for practitioners who are focusing specifically on this severe/enduring client group in any setting and the third is for specialist practice.

Box 2.1 Competency domains for working with people suffering from severe/enduring mental health problems

- Professional ethical practice
- Care delivery
- Treatment-specific competencies
- Care management
- Personal/professional development

What the frameworks have in common is that they focus on the client and the nature of the client's needs, irrespective of the setting. The content of the competencies in each of the frameworks is complementary, and together they provide a more comprehensive competency set for practitioners in any setting, but particularly in acute care, as this is where the key assessments, the therapeutic interventions and the management and evaluation of holistic care must begin. In addition, if we move towards nurses following the service user throughout his/her journey of care, then a broader range of competencies will enable all practitioners to function autonomously and meet the needs of their clients in a much more pro-active and satisfying way.

Interpersonal/relationship competencies

This domain deals with the nature of the therapeutic relationship with the service user, who may find it difficult to comply with care, treatment and support. The emphasis is on the need to establish clear communication strategies with both clients and their carers and families to ensure they have as complete an understanding as possible of the nature of, and rationale for, their detention, compulsory treatment and stage/environment of care delivery. In addition, it highlights the need to define roles and boundaries with clients and to undertake supervision. Whilst written with a secure environment in mind, it is wholly applicable to acute care or community care, especially since contemporary care emphasises more active treatment and interventions accessible from primary care through to specialist services (Scottish Executive Health Department, 2006a).

Risk assessment/risk management

The profile of risk assessment and risk management has been raised significantly over recent years, in part due to a number of high profile cases within the public domain. From the murder of Jonathon Zito, to the latest investigation by the Mental Welfare Commission for Scotland (2006) the failure of professionals, services and agencies to work together, share information and consistently assess and mange risk, has been a consistent theme. The theoretical concepts as well as the skills and methodologies around risk assessment, the safety of the public as well as the safety of the service user and his/her immediate family, are now a core competency in all mental health work, with all client groups. Nor is it solely the discharge or ongoing community support for individuals that are the focus of risk assessment and management. Acute inpatient settings are increasingly perceived by both staff and patients as dangerous environments, where both the interpersonal skills of staff and the environmental/organisational culture, systems and processes are not sufficiently robust to ensure individual safety. Many women still report sexual assaults in acute settings (Byrt *et al.*, 2001; Mental Welfare Commission for Scotland, 2005) and the intimidation of patients and staff from visitors and patients who would seek to prey on the vulnerable around issues such as illegal substances, bullying, theft and assault, is reportedly increasing. Some of the core risk management strategies from forensic services are relevant, ethical and useful, in terms of maintaining a safe environment, prevention and management of violence, searching of individuals and areas, and observation for interpersonal/therapeutic purposes, as well as environmental safety and security. In forensic environments, these elements are controlled by policy and protocols and supported by professional education and training so that procedures are transparent and appropriate to the context of a health care environment and are carried out in ways that are legal and ethical and minimise the damage to therapeutic relationships with client and their families/carers. Acute settings need to formulate similar policies which maintain and enhance the safety of the environment so that staff and patients can feel confident and secure. Competencies in risk assessment and risk management ensure that staff understand and can demonstrate a systematic approach to the various risk factors, assessment tools/methodologies and risk management strategies at both individual and environmental levels. This would enable a smoother transition for many patients on their journey back from secure settings towards community-based care treatment and support.

Professional, legal and ethical aspects of care

The percentage of detained patients in acute settings has continued to grow in recent years, and it has always been recognised that mental health nurses utilise a significant knowledge of the application of mental health legislation on a daily basis. However, the amount of relevant legislation and policy is ever growing; in Scotland, practitioners need to understand the Human Rights (Scotland) Act, the Mental Health Act, the Criminal Procedures Act, the Adults with Incapacity Act and the Children's Act, as well as benefits and housing legislation and local authority social work policies and procedures. Practitioners need to develop considerable networks within both health and a range of other agencies in the statutory and voluntary sectors, in order to provide information and support to their patients/clients and their families and carers. Multiprofessional and multiagency working, as well as understanding of the patient and carer experience, would be enhanced if practitioners were to follow their patients/clients throughout the many transitions and pathways through care.

Treatment-specific competencies

The previous discussion may seem all well and good when the focus is on generic skills and evidence-based interventions, e.g. psychosocial interventions such as psycho-education and cognitive behaviour therapy for psychosis, brief interventions (solution-focused therapy), relapse prevention, family therapy, anger management or dialectical behaviour therapy for self-harming behaviour. It most certainly should be the case that these therapies are available, and delivered by appropriately trained, skilled and supervised clinicians. However, should staff in acute settings be expected to deliver forensic and specialist interventions, such as sex offender treatment programmes? The evidence base for these treatments will tend to have been obtained from the treatment milieu of a secure environment, so consideration would have to be given as to whether they would be effective in different settings. Since there will still be a need for specialist settings, and also for experienced specialist or advanced practitioners, then perhaps the availability of that treatment by an experienced and accredited practitioner will be more important than the setting in which the therapy takes place. If staff are crossing boundaries and service settings, there would be increased opportunities to develop specific advanced skills, based on the needs of their clients, rather than a narrowly defined service setting. If we are to recruit and retain mental health nurses, then these opportunities for professional development and meeting individual clients' needs will be of crucial importance, and will strengthen career pathways for those who want professional progression without leaving frontline clinical practice.

Governance

A widely used definition of clinical governance is (Scally and Donaldson, 1998):

> A framework through which NHS organisations are accountable for continually improving the quality of their services and safeguarding high standards of care by creating an environment in which excellence in clinical care will flourish.

Clinical governance, staff governance and research governance are currently seen as separate though connected functions. However, given that future service re-design will focus on 'continuous whole systems care' (Forrest *et al.*, 2005, p. 6), a disjointed approach to governance will also have to change. If, as suggested above, there are opportunities for staff to have planned rotational experiences across services, an integrated approach to forensic and acute care, including risk assessment and management, might be one of the early benefits. From an education/workforce development perspective, rotational placements offer excellent opportunities for the development of enhanced and new competencies and ways of working. In addition, given that service users, carers and practitioners/service providers are to be partners in the planning and delivery of care and treatment, a new approach to governance, where risk is shared across all of the partners, needs to be developed. It is no longer sustainable that only the services and practitioners carry all of the risk. The over-emphasis of governance, evidence-based, protocol-driven practice and risk avoidance in relation to care and treatment has led to much defensive (but perhaps less defensible) practice amongst clinicians. All mental health practice involves risk, and that must be acknowledged with service users and their families. Then, in partnership with them, it can be assessed, managed and shared amongst the team.

Integrated governance can be instituted at the earliest opportunity to begin the process of whole systems care:

- Organisational strategy and corporate philosophy as underpinnings to practice
- Risk assessment and management strategies integral to acute inpatient (and community) assessment
- Forensic clinical effectiveness methodologies applied to acute clinical practice
- Integrated and cost-effective education, training and workforce development activities focused on client needs, and improving standards of care, accessibility, waiting times for psychological interventions, early discharge, physical health and well-being, crisis interventions etc.

Conclusion

There are a number of critical factors which both service and education providers need to address in relation to mental health nursing. Firstly, undergraduate nurses need to be given opportunities and guidance to develop and demonstrate the values, as well as knowledge and skills to equip them to work in partnership with service users and their families to meet their mental health (not just illness) needs. If this isn't addressed, we may continue to see dissatisfied practitioners and service users, and significant attrition from undergraduate programmes, as students recognise the dissonance between what should be and what is, in relation to their own experience and the experiences of those in their care. Secondly, if mental health nurses are not given opportunities to develop new ways of working which reflect rights-based, recovery-focused approaches, and are not equipped to deal ethically, honestly and effectively with their clients, the NHS may continue to have difficulty in retaining staff, putting further pressure on existing stretched services.

Thirdly, if we do not change and adapt our working practices as individuals, teams and service providers, service users may continue to prefer to access their care from non-statutory sector organisations, and the future of statutory mental health services will be threatened. More nurses in acute services need to develop their understanding and skills at a generic level without seeing themselves as specialists. Some specialist nurses and services will always be needed, but care, compassion and the right to access psychological interventions are fundamental to a therapeutic environment, as is anti-discriminatory practice. Acute care mental health nurses must access opportunities to improve their range of skills to understand and manage the care of all of their client groups.

References

Byrt, R., Lomas, C., Gardiner, G. and Lewis, D. (2001) Working with women in secure environments. *Journal of Psychosocial Nursing*, **39**(9), 42–50.

Department of Health (2006) *From Values to Action: The Chief Nursing Officer's Review of Mental Health Nursing*. Department of Health, London.

Forrest, S., Martin, P. and Samuels, S. (2005) *National Review of Mental Health Nursing in Scotland: Interim Report (1)*: July. http://www.show.scot.nhs.uk/sehd/nrmhns/

Mental Welfare Commission for Scotland (2005) *Unannounced Visit Report*. Mental Welfare Commission for Scotland, Edinburgh.

Mental Welfare Commission for Scotland (2006)*Report of Inquiry into the Care and Treatment of Mr L and Mr M*. Mental Welfare Commission for Scotland, Edinburgh.

National Institute for Mental Health in England and Royal College of Psychiatrists (2005) *New Ways of Working for Psychiatrists: Enhancing Effective Person Centred Services Through New Ways of Working in Multidisciplinary and Multi-agency Contexts*. CSP/NIMHE/RCP/CWP, London.

NHS Education for Scotland (2000) *Continuing Professional Development Portfolio – A Route to Enhanced Competence in Forensic Mental Health Nursing*. NHS Education for Scotland, Edinburgh.

NHS Education for Scotland (2002) *Continuing Professional Development Portfolio – A Route to Enhanced Competence for Nurses Working with People Suffering From Severe/Enduring Mental Illness*. NHS Education for Scotland, Edinburgh.

Nursing and Midwifery Council (2004) *Standards of Proficiency for Pre-Registration Nursing*. Nursing and Midwifery Council, London.

Robinson, D. and Kettles, A. M. (eds.) (2000) *Forensic Nursing and Multidisciplinary Care of the Mentally Disordered Offender*. Jessica Kingsley, London.

Sainsbury Centre for Mental Health (2004) *Ten Essential Shared Capabilities. A Framework for the Whole Mental Health Workforce*. Sainsbury Centre for Mental Health, London.

Scally, G. and Donaldson, L. J. (1998) Clinical governance and the drive for quality improvement in the new NHS in England. *British Medical Journal*, **317**(7150), 61–5.

Scottish Executive (2003) *The Mental Health (Care and Treatment) (Scotland) Act 2003*. HMSO, Edinburgh.

Scottish Executive (2006) *Changing Lives: The Report of the 21st Century Social Work Review Group*. Scottish Executive, Edinburgh.

Scottish Executive Health Department (2006a) *Delivering for Health*. Scottish Executive Health Department, Edinburgh.

Scottish Executive Health Department (2006b) *Rights, Relationships and Recovery: The Report of the National Review of Mental Health Nursing in Scotland*. Scottish Executive Health Department, Edinburgh.

Watson, C. (2002) Exploring the interface of competence and clinical effectiveness. In *Therapeutic Interventions for Forensic Mental Health Nurses* (eds. A. Kettles, P. Woods and M. Collins), Chapter 3. Jessica Kingsley, London.

Whyte, L. A. (2000) Educational aspects of forensic nursing. In: *Forensic Nursing and Multidisciplinary Care of the Mentally Disordered Offender* (eds. D. Robinson and A. Kettles), Chapter 1. Jessica Kingsley, London.

CHAPTER 3

Towards therapeutic environments: challenges and problems

Richard Byrt with Linnette James

Introduction

This chapter and the next are concerned with nursing interventions related to physical and social environments of acute admission wards, other acute services, and forensic secure hospitals and units. In a busy service, with a requirement to respond to emergencies, it may be difficult to provide therapeutic environments, yet research findings suggest that these are essential to clients' safety, health and well-being, and the relief of both stress and distress (Barker, 2005; Campling *et al.*, 2004; Faulkner, 2004). In addition, there is evidence that therapeutic social environments (for example, those based on psychosocial interventions and therapeutic community principles) can enable some individuals to address factors associated with violent and other offending behaviours (Byrt, 2006; McKeown and McCann, 2000).

The present chapter will consider challenges and problems, highlighted in the literature, with the physical and social environments of acute admission and secure forensic services. Ways to overcome these problems are considered in Chapter 4.

Similarities between acute admission and secure mental health services

The literature suggests that wards in acute admission units and in secure units and hospitals share similar features, including the following:

- A multitude of functions, which, in relation to forensic and other patients, include the need to ensure safety and undertake risk assessment and risk management, with the provision of therapeutic interventions (Bowers, 2005; Harrison *et al.*, 2004; Kettles and Robinson, 2000; Woods *et al.*, 2002).

- Related to these diverse functions are the (sometimes conflicting) expectations of different stakeholders (e.g. service users, the public, politicians) about the extent that, for example, both acute admission and secure units should meet needs for public safety and patients' needs and rights (Byrt, 2001; Kettles *et al.*, 2006).
- These conflicting expectations, and the diverse needs of patients, may make it difficult to ensure an environment which both ensures patient and public safety and is therapeutic (Byrt, 2001; Kettles *et al.*, 2006).
- Much of the research-based and other literature is critical of both acute admission and secure services. Criticisms include observations that nurses in both types of service have largely social control, rather than therapeutic functions. Wards in acute and high secure settings, in particular, have often been described as anti-therapeutic, with criticisms concerning negative staff attitudes; nurses spending limited amounts of time with patients; boredom and a lack of fulfilling activities for patients; and drab, under-stimulating ward environments (Campling *et al.*, 2004; Kilshaw, 1999; Mason and Mercer, 1998). Research findings concerning types of ward environment that are beneficial to patients are applicable to acute, secure forensic and other wards (Timko and Moos, 2004). This includes research related to therapeutic communities (Byrt, 2006) and psychosocial interventions (McKeown *et al.*, 2002).

Components of mental health nursing in acute admission and secure forensic wards

Acute admission wards have been identified as serving many essential functions with benefits to patients (Bowers, 2005; Firth, 2004; Harrison *et al.*, 2004; Higgins *et al.*, 1999; Quirk and Lelliott, 2004). Bowers (2005) considered several components of mental health nursing in these environments, including those related to: ensuring safety; assessing and reducing risk to self and others; other aspects of assessment and treatment, especially of individuals with 'severe mental disorder' (p. 233); and respite for both service users and informal carers. In addition, Bowers (2005) emphasised various communication and therapeutic skills and the nurse's role in relation to psychotherapies and application of therapeutic community principles to acute admission areas.

A wide variety of nursing skills in specialist forensic services have also been identified, with some research on the nature of these skills. Many of the latter are similar to those identified as important for nursing in acute admission wards: for example, communication and establishment of therapeutic relationships with (often reluctant) patients; and ensuring safety. Forensic nurses have also been identified as having very specific roles in relation to higher levels of security; specialised aspects of risk assessment and risk management; rehabilitation in the community; and specific interventions to prevent future offending behaviours. In addition, forensic nurses often work with patients who are in a hospital environment for comparatively long periods of time (Kettles and Robinson, 2000; Niskala, 1986; Woods *et al.*, 2002; Woods, 2004).

Several authors stress the importance of nurses in both acute and secure forensic services working collaboratively with patients/clients, where possible, and with colleagues as part of a multidisciplinary team (Dale *et al.*, 2001; Harrison, *et al.*, 2004; McClelland *et al.*, 2001; Wix and Humphreys, 2005).

Patients' experiences at the time of admission: sources of stress

The need for beneficial and social environments is related, in part, to the (often considerable) crises and related distress experienced by patients admitted to both acute (Bowers, 1999; Repper and Perkins, 2004) and secure (Lees and Withington, 2001) forensic settings. Individuals who are compulsorily admitted lose freedom over important aspects of their lives; and this is sometimes compounded by their experiences of adverse ward environments (Repper and Perkins, 2004):

> ...Is it possible that if you did not have PTSD [post-traumatic stress disorder] before you went into hospital, you certainly might have it now? A... study by Morrison *et al.* (1999) found that *44% of the patient sample developed PTSD symptoms as a result of psychiatric admission.* One of the contributory factors in the report is that hospitalization and treatment involve a *global loss of control for the individual...* (Lees and Withington, 2001, p. 115; emphasis added)

Patients' concerns are related to a variety of problems, including those listed below. These problems can considerably impact on the individual and contribute to his/her feelings of despair, anxiety, uncertainty, disempowerment and loss of control (Repper and Perkins, 2004). Stress can be related to any of the following factors:

- Admission to both acute and secure forensic services, with their restrictions to ensure safety, can be a shock for some patients (George, 1998; Hart, 1999). However, some patients may experience a sense of relief on their admission, and feel that, at last, something will be done to help with their problems (Higgins *et al.*, 1999).
- Patients in secure forensic services, and some in acute admission wards, experience understandable anxiety and uncertainty about the eventual outcome of court proceedings. This includes patients remanded by courts for assessment under Section 38 of the Mental Health Act 1983 (Woods, 2004).
- Some patients face rejection from partner/spouse and/or other family members. In some cases, people who were close to a patient find it difficult to maintain contact with him/her: e.g. because their offences, related to mental illness or 'personality disorder', involved a partner or family member (McKeown and McCann, 2000).
- Some separation from partner, family and children occurs even if they maintain contact, particularly for patients who are admitted to secure forensic services a long way from home. In addition, although it is necessary for nursing staff to supervise visits for safety reasons, this may make it hard for patients and their loved ones to express how they feel (Aiyegbusi and Byrt, 2006).
- Visits by patients' children may not be possible, either because of lack of legal access or as a result of a decision by the clinical team, with reference to child protection procedures, that the visit of a child or young person is not in his/her best interests (Aiyegbusi and Byrt, 2006).

- Some patients lose their homes, sometimes because they cannot afford mortgage repayments, or more usually, as a result of loss of council or housing association tenancy. In addition, individuals may (understandably) be anxious about their homes being burgled, especially in inner city areas with high crime rates (Bowers *et al.*, 1999).
- Patients may also lose a job or place on a course and the opportunity to engage in activities that are of importance to them, including their roles in their families (Bowers *et al.*, 1999).
- Loss of income or benefits, with little or no finances, is a common problem. Patients transferred from prisons and young offender institutions to secure hospitals/units find it particularly hard to obtain benefits. This may make it hard for patients to purchase items (such as trainers and other clothes) that are important to their feelings of positive identity and self-esteem (Aiyegbusi and Byrt, 2006).
- Losses of accommodation, work, education, income and other material goods may increase the likelihood of forensic patients' further involvement in offending following discharge (Gilligan, 2001).
- Symptoms of mental illness are likely to result in considerable stress and distress (Harris *et al.*, 2002).

The tale of Mr King and Ms Kaur

Social and physical environments of wards and other services can either increase or reduce patients' stress, as is illustrated in the tale of Mr King and Ms Kaur, and their admission, as patients with forensic mental health needs, to two acute wards serving inner city areas. Both Mr King and Ms Kaur are admitted soon after making threats towards individuals, about whom they have paranoid delusions. (Although the following accounts are based on the author's experience, the individuals described are fictitious.)

Mr Gladstone King is admitted to 'Ward X'. When he arrives, accompanied by his partner, they are shown to a dingy room with faded wallpaper and flaking paint. They can see, at a distance, staff in a ward office, completing paperwork. Mr King and his partner are not offered a drink, although Gladstone's mouth is particularly dry because of his understandable anxiety and the medication prescribed by his GP. It is 45 minutes before Mr King and his partner are seen by the admitting nurse, who, without apologising or explaining the reasons for the delay, asks various questions, but does little to explain why Gladstone has been admitted, or the care and treatment he will receive.

During Mr King's stay on Ward X, he receives antipsychotic medication and is occasionally assessed by a psychiatrist and by his primary nurse. He is invited into a ward round, but feels overwhelmed by the large number of professionals present. Issues related to Gladstone's threats and the associated delusions are assessed and addressed only cursorily. His main experiences on Ward X are of feeling isolated and having no one to talk to, as nurses are busy dealing with crises, observing other patients and involved in paperwork. Gladstone experiences boredom: long periods of sitting around with nothing to do, often with patients whose behaviours he finds threatening and stressful. His surroundings are drab, with threadbare carpets and dingy walls.

A television set is left on most of the day, whether or not anyone is watching it, and there is no private space for the quiet and reflection that Gladstone craves. He feels oppressed by the cacophony of noises from the television, patients' loud CD players and the constantly ringing phone, which compete with persistent intrusive thoughts and derogatory voices. Gladstone likes to be out in the fresh air, especially on his allotment, but there are no opportunities for him to go out, and he feels confined and oppressed by the narrow space available to him. When Gladstone is discharged, there is minimal liaison with the community forensic mental health team who will be working with him.

Ms Rani Kaur is admitted to Ward Y, also accompanied by her partner. The ward is attractively and recently decorated, with pot plants and pictures, including a mural produced by patients with a local community artist. Ms Kaur and her partner are welcomed by the admitting nurse and offered a drink. She also receives an explanation and apology when the nurse is temporarily called away.

On Ward Y, staff share the aim that the whole of each patient's stay should be beneficial and therapeutic. A ward secretary is available for much of the paperwork, with periods of the day when telephone calls are diverted, so that nursing staff have dedicated time to spend with patients (Kent, 2005). The Tidal Model, with its emphasis on patients' experiences and perspectives (Barker, 2002) is implemented. The ward also has an interdisciplinary commitment to risk assessment, using valid and reliable tools, and to psychosocial interventions. The latter are used mainly to reduce Rani's distress related to her paranoid delusions, and to reduce risk to others, by helping her to develop coping strategies other than threatening behaviour. In addition, there are attempts on Ward Y to provide a low expressed emotion environment, including a social milieu that is relaxed, does not place excessive pressure on patients (Baker, 2000) and endeavours to reduce noise. Thus, Rani has a choice to eat a meal in a quiet environment on the ward, rather than having to go to a noisy and stressful communal dining area. Her ward is on the ground floor, and she has access to a garden, within safe parameter walls, and space for prayer.

Meaningful and potentially enjoyable activities are provided, and there are opportunities for patients to suggest ideas related to the ward in low-key community meetings. When Rani is discharged, after careful risk assessment and risk management, there is clear communication with her local Community Forensic Mental Health Team.

The physical environment

Given that you needed admission to an acute mental health unit, would you prefer to be Rani Kaur or Gladstone King? Part of their differing experiences relates to the physical environments of their wards. The importance of first impressions of the physical environment on admission is emphasised by Jones (1988). The term *physical environment* is used here to refer to all aspects of the individual's physical surroundings, in both acute and secure forensic services, including:

- The extent that it is safe
- The appearance of a ward or other facility, including its décor and furnishings

- The extent that the service provided, including the physical environment, reflects individuals' culture
- The amount of physical space and the presence or absence of crowding (Whittington, 2000)
- Rooms available to both patients and staff, including those for single-sex use, activity and recreation; and space for privacy (within the parameters of safety): e.g. for personal telephone calls or for prayer, meditation and reflection (NHS Executive, 1999)
- Lighting, heating, ventilation and odour (Von Sommaruga, 2004; Whittington, 2000)
- Opportunities for fresh air and exercise and access to gardens and other outdoor spaces (Von Sommaruga, 2004)

The social environment

The term *social environment* refers to the following, in both acute and secure mental health services. (*Social environment* is sometimes referred to as *organisational environment* or *milieu* in the literature.)

- The extent that all aspects of the patient's stay are seen by patients and staff as potentially therapeutic (one feature of a therapeutic community; Byrt, 2006)
- Professionals' attitudes and availability to, and communication with, patients (Byrt, 2006)
- Staff and patients' relationships and roles (e.g. whether individuals are seen only as 'patients' and treated as passive recipients of care; or as people with strengths, talents and significant relationships, as well as problems; Campling *et al.*, 2004; Byrt, 2006)
- The organisational structures of the ward, and the absence or presence of 'dehumanizing and unnecessary regimes, routines, rules and restrictions' in the service (Byrt, 2006, p. 193, citing Kilshaw, 1999)
- Other aspects of the 'atmosphere' of the acute service, that is, what it feels like to the individual, including the extent that it:
  - Is noisy or relaxed
  - Provides space for quiet and privacy (within the parameters of safety)
  - Is structured, with purposeful and meaningful activities, or with time hanging heavily with nothing to do (Goffman, 1968)
  - Enables and values patients' opinions, experiences and perspectives
  - Provides opportunities for patients to safely express feelings and problems
  - Is sensitive to each individual's specific needs, including those related to her/his spirituality, culture, age, gender, sexual orientation, gender identity and specific disabilities and problems (Byrt, 2006; Timko and Moos, 2004)

Earlier studies of the physical and social environments of mental health services

In large psychiatric hospitals, therapeutic communities and other improvements in social environments developed from the 1950s onwards (Firth, 2004; Gale and Sanchez, 2005). These changes occurred partly in response to research on adverse effects of life in institutions (Barton, 1966; Caudill, 1958; Cumming and Cumming, 1962; Goffman, 1968; Stanton and Schwartz, 1954). The problems described included many of those identified in more recent studies of acute admission and secure forensic services and outlined later in this chapter. Several earlier studies considered the all-pervasive nature of institutions, where the needs of individuals were sometimes subordinated to those of the hospital. Regimes were often custodial and authoritarian, sometimes with rules which were unnecessarily restrictive (Goffman, 1968; Rowden, 2002; Pilgrim and Rogers, 2005). People were often treated as passive 'patients', without opportunities to assert choices or preferences, or recognition of their abilities or positive coping strategies. In some hospitals, there was a lack of respect for individuals, ill treatment and a denial of basic rights and needs and of healthy expression of feelings and views (Rowden, 2002; Sang, 2003). Anger was sometimes pathologised, or discouraged, rather than being seen as a natural, creative and healthy response (Goffman, 1968).

Erving Goffman's concept of 'total institutions' was influential. In *Asylums*, he described ways in which certain psychiatric hospitals and other organisations were all-pervasive: i.e. they controlled all aspects of the lives of patients, who were offered little choice or autonomy. Goffman (1968) stated that total institutions had several features, including those listed below. Sadly, some of Goffman's account appears to be relevant to more recent criticisms of both acute and forensic secure environments (Kilshaw, 1999):

- **Mortification of self**: The individual is stripped of his/her identity. This refers not only to storage of possessions and wearing of hospital clothing, but to an expectation that the person will conform and behave in accordance with staff's expectations. In mortification of self there is a denial of individuality and a subjection of the person to the (often unnecessary) routines, rules and regimes of institutional life (Goffman, 1968).
- **Pathologising all patient behaviours and actions**: Everything the individual says or does is perceived as evidence of mental illness. In relation to institutional processes, individuals either withdraw and conform to the institution, or express anger, which is then pathologised and perceived to be the result of his/her illness. Thus, an individual's assertive questioning of his/her nursing care, or failure to conform with task-orientated regimes and rituals, could be seen as evidence of being 'difficult' (Duxbury, 2000; Goffman, 1968).
- **Lack of purpose and activities**: Goffman (1968) described long periods of inactivity, boredom and exclusion from life outside the institution and from everyday concerns (Jones, 1993).
- **'Working the system'**: Whilst some patients conformed and became institutionalised (e.g. apathetic and finding it difficult to take the initiative), others found ways of getting round the unreasonable rules without staff's knowledge (Goffman, 1968).

Goffman's (1968) account of total institutions enables nurses and other professionals to consider the extent that inpatient settings are therapeutic. However, his observations are based on

Box 3.1 Rules, regimes and routines, roles, responsibilities and relationships: beneficial or harmful (Byrt, 1999)?

In any mental health service known to you:

1. To what extent do the rules, regimes and routines exist:
- For good clinical and safety reasons?
- For the convenience of the organisation/staff?
- Or does no one know why they exist?

2. To what extent are patients' roles, responsibilities and relationships beneficial? Are patients:
- Expected to be passive and comply, with nothing to do – or do they have opportunities to express views, develop aptitudes and talents and engage in meaningful activities?
- Ignored and seen only as a 'patient' – or listened to and taken seriously?

a study of one secure psychiatric hospital, and it is unclear how far his findings are based on patients' views or generalisable to other mental health services. Goffman (1968) made it clear that no ward had all the features of a total institution.

Rules, regimes and routines

The questions in Box 3.1 can guide us (in relation to the findings of Goffman (1968)) in considering whether or not particular services have therapeutic social environments. Some of the questions are considered by Kilshaw (1999) in relation to medium secure units.

Recent research on acute admission and secure forensic mental health wards

Some patients have reported benefits from their admission: e.g. in relation to respite and the provision of a safe environment. However, several more recent studies have found that some wards, in both acute and secure forensic mental health settings, have social and/or physical environments that are anti-therapeutic. Relevant research and other writing includes Beardsmore *et al.* (1998), Garcia *et al.* (2005), Hart (1999), Higgins, *et al.* (1999), Royal College of Psychiatrists Audit Team (2005) and Walton (2000) in relation to acute admission wards. Ryan and Bowers (2005) outline environmental problems in a psychiatric intensive care unit. Relevant studies of secure forensic settings include Clarke (1996), Mason and Mercer (1998) and Mercer *et al.* (1999). The following problems have been identified.

Some acute services are described as being over-stretched, admitting people with a wide range of disparate and desperate needs, including an increasing number of people with problems related to the use of alcohol and/or other drugs, and/or violent behaviours (Quirk and Lelliott, 2001). In some parts of the country, a lack of acute mental health services has been identified, in relation to both the numbers of beds in acute admission wards and a shortage of alternatives (Clarke and Flanagan, 2003). The latter include specific community mental health services (Hannigan and Coffey, 2003) and various alternative crisis services (Barker, 2005; Mental Health Foundation and Sainsbury Centre for Mental Health, 2002). In addition, there is a shortage of services to which patients can be transferred from high secure hospitals, and medium and low secure units, with some patients being detained in conditions of security greater than is warranted by their assessed levels of risk (Collins and Davies, 2005).

The lack of acute beds and other viable alternatives has resulted in pressures to discharge patients rapidly, and sometimes prematurely, from acute mental health services, possibly leading to a need for readmission which, in some instances, might have been avoided if there had been more time to plan discharge and community interventions and services. In addition, a shortage of suitable treatment and recovery and other services to which patients can be discharged or transferred has been reported (Clarke and Flanagan, 2003).

Social and political groups impinging on the role of nurses in acute admission and secure forensic units

The services provided by both forensic and acute mental health units have been said to be adversely affected by political and social factors and a variety of stakeholders with conflicting interests and expectations. These stakeholders include (often unwilling) patients, their carers at home, politicians, a variety of mental health professionals, members of the public and the media (Byrt, 2001; Byrt with Dooher, 2006; Faulkner, 2004) (see Figure 3.1), with a political and media tendency to emphasise public safety at the expense of the rights of individual service users (Faulkner, 2004; Kettles *et al.*, 2006). Goffman (1968) stated that mental health inpatients experienced environments that were untherapeutic, and served the needs of individuals with power in wider society (Jones, 1993); a point that has been made by several more recent authors (Mason and Mercer, 1998).

Forensic mental health nurses, and, to some extent, nurses working in acute admission units, are subject to (often conflicting) expectations in wider society (Byrt, 2001), including:

- Members of the public, media and politicians who think that some patients should be ‘locked up for life’
- Voluntary organisations and other pressure groups who argue that patients’ rights are infringed
- Contradictory government policies: e.g. that patients should be ‘empowered’, but, in some cases, be subject to considerable (and arguably, sometimes excessive) restrictions (Byrt, 2001; Byrt with Dooher, 2006)

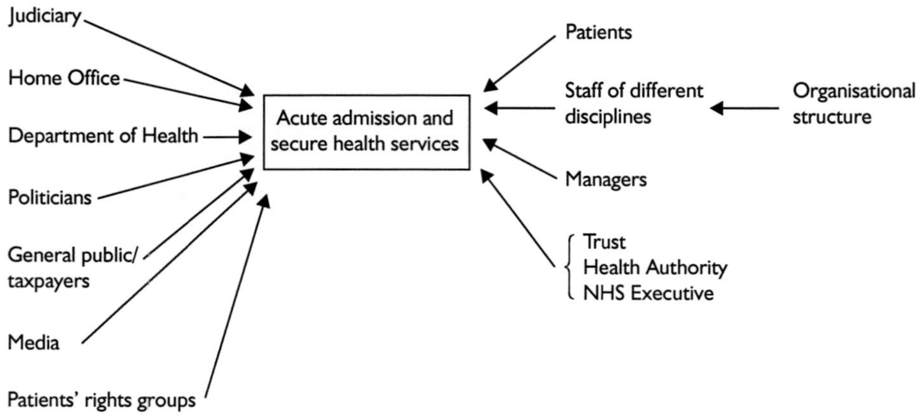

Figure 3.1 Service users/stakeholders in acute admission and secure units. Adapted, with kind permission of Quay Books, MA Healthcare Ltd, from: Byrt, R. (2001) Power, influence and control in practice development. In: *The Handbook of Practice Development* (eds. A. Clark, J. Dooher and J. Fowler), p. 86. Quay, Salisbury.

It can be argued that mental health nurses have a responsibility to endeavour to influence central government policy that impacts on the life and care of patients, and to draw to the attention of government instances of policy that are to the detriment of patients and do not contribute to public safety (Byrt, 2001; Kettles *et al.*, 2006).

Limited nursing time with patients

Several studies of acute admission wards have found that nursing staff in some units spend comparatively little time interacting and communicating with patients and considerable time in ward offices, partly to deal with paperwork (Faulkner, 2004; Higgins *et al.*, 1999). Studies from the 1970s onwards have found that this is especially the case with more senior nurses, with health care assistants being more involved in direct patient care (Altschul, 1972; Cormack, 1976; Robinson, 1996; Higgins *et al.*, 1999). Several reasons for this have been identified, including the following:

- The pressure on beds and the emergency admission of many individuals with complex needs and problems have meant less time for nurses to spend with each patient (Clarke and Flanagan, 2003; Higgins *et al.*, 1999).
- Nurses have been expected to complete an increasing amount of paperwork: e.g. in reporting critical incidents. This has been said to be associated with increasing managerial concern to monitor risk and a shortage of secretarial help (Higgins *et al.*, 1999).
- In addition, one study found that nurses were expected by other professional colleagues to engage in various administrative tasks: e.g. answering telephone calls and liaising with other disciplines and agencies (Clarke and Flanagan, 2003).

Forensic nurses in some secure settings also spend a considerable amount of time away from direct patient contact on security checks (Collins *et al.*, 2006), which, arguably, could be performed by non-nursing staff.

In both acute and secure forensic services, service user accounts, including those given in research studies, describe both nurses with helpful interactions and communication skills, but, in addition, staff dismissal of patients' problems and concerns, with a lack of active listening and engagement with patients or an appreciation of their perspectives and experiences of distress (Coffey, 2006; Duxbury, 2002; Faulkner, 2004; Meehan *et al.*, 2006; Repper and Perkins, 2004). This can occur, despite research findings that service users desire opportunities to talk to and to receive support from staff (Faulkner, 2004, citing various studies). Lack of such opportunities and a poor quality physical environment may result in lowered self-esteem (Faulkner, 2004). In addition, the establishment of a therapeutic relationship and regular communication is seen as an important aspect of 'relational security' with forensic patients, as a means to effectively assess and manage risk, including risk related to offending behaviours (Dale and Gardner, 2001).

Coercive measures

Coercive and punitive treatment has been described by some service users (Faulkner, 2004) and identified in the Blom-Cooper Inquiry into Ashworth High Secure Hospital (Blom-Cooper, 1992). Duxbury (2002) described a 'lack of staff engagement with clients' (p. 172) before, during and after incidents of violence and aggression. Studies have found both positive and negative attitudes of nurses towards patients, including individuals with antisocial personality disorder, in high secure hospitals (Bowers, 2002; Byrt *et al.*, 2006; Mason *et al.*, 1999; Meehan *et al.*, 2006).

Related to lack of staff engagement during observation (Buchanan-Barker and Barker, 2005), some researchers, in both acute and secure forensic settings, have reported tendencies to deal with violent incidents with what patients sometimes see as coercive measures, such as control and restraint and seclusion, instead of using communication skills to prevent or reduce violence and aggression. This was particularly emphasised in the Blom-Cooper (1992) Inquiry into Ashworth Hospital and by Duxbury (2002), Meehan *et al.* (2006) and Secker *et al.* (2004, p. 174). The latter authors reported:

> ...There was *little evidence of the staff... simply spending time with, and thus being available to clients* before the reported incidents [of violence and aggression] took place, and no evidence at all of anyone spending time with the clients who later became involved in the incidents...
>
> In those cases where some discussion with the client was described, the overriding aim appeared to have been to correct the client's behaviour, rather than exploring what happened from the client's perspective or considering together how it might have been avoided... (*emphasis added*)

Secker *et al.* (2004) emphasise findings, from their own and other studies, of the importance of 'staff–client relationships', 'powerlessness', environmental factors and 'the organisation of care' (p. 173) as contributory factors to violence and aggression in acute admission wards. A concentration on coercive measures, with a lack of opportunity for discussion, contrasts with interventions to enable patients to understand the reasons for offending behaviours, and to find practical means to prevent their recurrence (Byrt *et al.*, 2005; Davies *et al.*, 2005; Doyle *et al.*, 2006; Hartman and Smith, 2002).

Some studies have reported that nursing staff spend time dealing with crises and emergencies, including those related to violence and self-harm, rather than on interventions to prevent such occurrences (Norton and Dolan, 1995; Secker *et al.*, 2004). These and other problems are often related to staff shortages and the use, in acute admission units, of 'bank' and agency nurses (Garcia

Box 3.2 'How acute' by Linnette James

There are 15 strangers amongst me here.
They say that this could be my home for the next 6 months, as I am on a section 3.

I'm delusional, I was told, I could be of threat to my self and others.
However, I've made no attempts to hurt any one.
I've told my family that I wanted a change of career; something that will bring in more finances.

I dream of becoming a successful business man and in order to pursue my dreams...
I've booked a flight to America. For this reason I'm classed as delusional.
My dreams are no different to the next individual.

Since my admission, I've been threatened by one of the patients, when I report this to a member of staff they dismissed my concerns.
'It's a part of his delusions,' I overheard one staff member saying.

I have to share my bedroom with 2 other males: a dormitory they call it.

This environment is daunting, frightening and completely new to me.
However, staff are not that empathic about my plight.
They seem to think that I should be able to settle in easily and treat it as if it was my home.
Do they ever wonder why for some of us we appear so frightened
No they see this as being paranoid.

I've been robbed of my autonomy, my dignity and pride
All I'm left with is my self respect and even that...
Even that I'm struggling to keep a hold of.

et al., 2005; McMillan and Allen, 2005). In addition, acute admission work, unlike forensic nursing, has not been seen as a specialised area of care. Some acute wards have had high proportions of relatively inexperienced nurses, with more experienced staff tending to move to community work or to what are seen as 'specialist' services (Sainsbury Centre for Mental Health, 2006).

Boredom and lack of worthwhile activities

Many studies and service user accounts report boredom and insufficient opportunities for worthwhile, meaningful activities: factors found to be associated with increased incidences of violence and aggression (Faulkner, 2004; National Institute for Health and Clinical Excellence, 2005; Royal College of Psychiatrists Audit Team, 2005; Walton, 2000; Whittington, 2000). A lack of fulfilling and meaningful activities has also been identified in relation to women in secure settings (Storey and Murdock, 2001) and individuals transferred from high secure to medium secure settings (Skelly, 1994, 2001).

> [There are] high levels of boredom: many wards/units are unable to offer service users a structured and therapeutic system of care. This is linked to low staffing levels and high volumes of paperwork. As well as the obvious link between 'boredom' and 'violence', this seems to have an impact on recovery rates for service users, and on job satisfaction for staff. Ways have to be found of supporting staff to spend more time on face-to-face contact with service users... (Royal College of Psychiatrists Audit Team, 2005, p. 7)

Other patients' threatening or violent behaviours

In both acute admission and secure forensic settings, whilst some patients have felt supported by their peers, others report being understandably frightened of others' threatening or violent behaviours (Bailey, 2000; Bowers *et al.*, 1999; Byrt and Reece, 1999; Ifill, 2002). Bowers *et al.* (1999) found that patients sometimes absconded from acute admission wards, partly for this reason and also because of realistic concerns about their families or that their empty homes, in inner London, would be burgled (Bowers *et al.*, 1999). Some women patients have experienced sexual harassment or chauvinism from male patients in both acute admission and secure forensic services (Aiyegbusi, 2002; Byrt *et al.*, 2001; Ifill, 2002; Jeffcote and Watson, 2004).

The quality of physical environments

Drab and dingy physical environments have been described, with comments that acute admission wards have been financially under-resourced in relation to both the physical environment and staffing. The physical environment of some secure forensic services has also been criticised (Bailey, 2000; Davies, 2004). The moral management reformers of the late 18th and early 19th centuries stressed the importance of beneficial hospital grounds with gardens, as well as pleasant ward environments. Ideas about therapeutic milieux influenced the design of the asylums built in England and Wales under the County Asylums Acts of 1808 and 1845 (Jones, 1993; Nolan, 1993). Whilst former patients at the high secure hospitals have described their physical and social environments as grim and unpleasant (Bailey, 2000; Laing with McQuarrie, 1989; Thompson, 1972), they have offered a range of activities and eventual access to extensive grounds far greater than has been the case with many medium and low secure units (Collins *et al.*, 2006; Skelly, 2001).

Whilst the closure of the Victorian psychiatric hospitals led to the welcome disappearance of some ugly buildings, they also resulted in the loss of many beautiful hospital grounds, as well as a variety of facilities such as concert halls, social clubs and accessible hospital shops. The new district general hospital mental health units have often been built with more limited facilities, less space and less access to gardens and other outdoor facilities (Von Sommaruga, 2004). Similarly, many low and medium secure units have afforded less space and outdoor and indoor facilities than the older high secure hospitals (Collins and Davies, 2005; Skelly, 2001). Barefoot (1992), an architect, has emphasised the importance of the physical environment in acute admission units, in relation to homely colours, décor, furnishings, ward design and gardens.

Safety in the ward environment

Many authors have commented that safety, including prevention of behaviours associated with offending, is amongst the most important functions of both acute admission units (Bowers, 2005; Firth, 2004; Harrison *et al.*, 2004) and secure forensic services (Collins *et al.*, 2006; Dale and Gardner, 2001; Kettles and Robinson, 2000). Arguably, some of the literature on safety in secure settings (Collins *et al.*, 2006) may be applicable to acute areas. Many acute wards have design features that increase the risk of harm to self and others (Bowers *et al.*, 2002; National Institute for Health and Clinical Excellence, 2005). The Guideline on Violence of the latter organisation recommends ward designs, CCTV cameras and mirrors to facilitate safe observation, although the possibly adverse effects on clients and staff and the acceptability of such methods of surveillance would need to be considered. Bowers *et al.* (2002), citing the Standing Nursing and Midwifery Advisory Committee (1999), suggest the following to reduce risks of suicide, self-harm, aggression and violent behaviours in acute admission wards:

- Windows made of materials that are difficult to break
- Avoidance of 'ligature points': i.e. places on which patients can tie items (e.g. belts, ties) to try to hang themselves
- Design of wards to avoid hidden corners, so that patients can be observed to ensure the safety of themselves and/or others easily and unobtrusively.
- Offices with large windows centrally placed to enable observation of patients – but situated so that this can be as unobtrusive as possible.

- Use of attractive and culturally appropriate colours, décor, furnishings and pictures – but with furniture and pictures made of relatively safe materials (Bowers *et al.*, 2002, citing the Standing Nursing and Midwifery Advisory Committee, 1999).

'Therapy' and 'security': complementary or conflicting?

Authors vary in their views of whether or not it is possible to combine safety and security and therapeutic interventions in secure forensic services, and, to some extent, in acute admission units. This has been referred to as the 'therapy versus security' debate (Burrow, 1998). Some authors have argued that 'therapy' and 'security' are opposed and cannot coexist (Clarke, 1996; Mercer and Mason, 1998). For example, Szasz (1963) has expressed concern about the rise of forensic psychiatry, and has argued that diagnosing mental disorder in people who offend, or admitting people compulsorily, is damaging. He argued that (Jones, 1993, p. 177, quoting and citing Szasz, 1963):

> ... liberty was 'an inalienable right', and that the mental health movement, by providing excuses for abnormal behaviour, was eroding moral standards and extending the power of the state... [Szasz] described... compulsory detention as a crime on the grounds that the Declaration of Rights guaranteed 'life, liberty and the pursuit of happiness' to all American citizens.'

Conversely, several authors, on both forensic and acute mental health nursing, have argued that, despite some conflicts, it is possible to provide services which are both safe (and, in some instances, secure) and beneficial to the patient. In many acute and forensic units and hospitals, there is an 'integration' model, where all or most aspects of care and treatment are considered to be concerned both with reducing risk and ensuring safety (including prevention of reoffending), and with therapeutic benefit to the patient (Dale *et al.*, 2001; Harrison *et al.*, 2004; Kettles and Robinson, 2000).

Is treatment just medication – or the whole social environment?

As Linda Hart indicates in Chapter 11, some studies in both forensic and acute settings have found an adherence to narrow ideas that 'treatment' consists solely or completely of medication, with a predominance of medical models (Faulkner, 2004; Mason and Mercer, 1998) and an absence of approaches based on psychological or social, rather than biological, methods of treatment, or of interventions designed to meet individuals' needs holistically (Barker, 2005) or validate them as individuals (Faulkner, 2004).

In some admission and secure forensic services, 'treatment' has been seen solely in terms of medication and occasional sessions with a nurse or a psychiatrist, rather than the social environment being considered an important component of treatment (Faulkner, 2004). In addition, in acute admission units, there has sometimes been a lack of therapeutic models or frameworks to inform care (Gournay, 2004). These factors may be influenced by limited staffing and other resources that have to be devoted to emergency admissions and dealing with crises (Higgins *et al.*, 1999). There may be rapid patient turnover (often of over 30 patients on a ward), with individuals with very different needs that require a variety of therapeutic frameworks and social environments. For example, there is evidence that individuals with acute mental illness, with personality disorder, and problems related to drug use all require different treatment approaches, therapeutic frameworks and social environments (Campling *et al.*, 2004). Yet, at present, they are likely to all be admitted to the same acute admission ward, rather than to specialist services. It can be very difficult to adequately meet everyone's needs in such a circumstance (Beardsmore *et al.*, 1998; Bowles *et al.*, 2001; Garcia *et al.*, 2005; Hart, 2001; Higgins *et al.*, 1999; Walton, 2000). In contrast, patient turnover is generally much slower in secure forensic services, with a greater preponderance of specialist services catering for individuals with specific problems and informed by a therapeutic framework (Kettles *et al.*, 2002).

Conclusion

This chapter has considered aspects of the physical and social environments of acute admission and secure forensic services. Problems in these environments have been identified since at least the 1950s. Recently identified concerns have included: conflicting social and political expectations concerning the functions of services; pressure on beds, particularly in acute admission units; lack of opportunities for patients to communicate with nursing staff; aspects of work that remove nurses from direct patient care; staffing problems; and drab, under-resourced physical environments.

The next chapter considers the organisation of care and the application of therapeutic frameworks to ensure beneficial social environments in acute and secure forensic mental health services

References

Aiyegbusi, A. (2002) Nursing interventions and future directions with women in secure services. In: *Therapeutic Interventions for Forensic Mental Health Nurses* (eds. A. M. Kettles, P. Woods and M. Collins), Chapter 9. Jessica Kingsley, London.

Aiyegbusi, A. and Byrt, R. (2006) Gender and sexuality. In: *Forensic Mental Health Nursing: Interventions with People with 'Personality Disorders'* (ed. National Forensic Nurses' Research and Development Group), Chapter 8. Quay, London.

Altschul, A. (1972) *Patient–Nurse Interactions: a Study of Interaction Patterns in Acute Psychiatric Wards.* Churchill Livingstone, Edinburgh.

Bailey, T. (2000) A personal experience. In: *Forensic Mental Health Care: a Case Study Approach* (eds. D. Mercer, T. Mason, M. McKeown and G. McCann). Churchill Livingstone, Edinburgh.

Baker, J. A. (2000) Developing psychosocial care for acute psychiatric wards. *Journal of Psychiatric and Mental Health Nursing*, **7**, 95–100.

Barefoot, P. (1992) Psychiatric wards in DGHs? An architect's comments. *Psychiatric Bulletin*, **16**, 99–100.

Barker, P. (2002) The Tidal Model: the healing potential of metaphor within the patient's narrative. *Journal of Psychosocial Nursing and Mental Health Services*, **40**(7), 42–50.

Barker, P. (2005) Putting acute care in its place. *Mental Health Nursing*, **23**(1), 12–15.

Barton, R. (1966*) Institutional Neurosis*, 2nd edn. John Wright, Bristol.

Beardsmore, A. *et al.* (1998) *Acute Problems: A Study of the Quality of Care in Acute Psychiatric Wards*. The Sainsbury Centre for Mental Health, London.

Blom-Cooper, L. (1992) *Report of the Committee of Inquiry into Complaints about Ashworth Hospital. Volumes 1 and 2. Cmnd 2028-1*. HMSO, London.

Bowers, L. (2002) *Dangerous and Severe Personality Disorder. Response and Role of the Psychiatric Team*. Routledge, London.

Bowers, L. (2005) Reasons for admission and their implications for the nature of acute inpatient psychiatric nursing. *Journal of Psychiatric and Mental Health Nursing*, **12**, 231–6.

Bowers, L., Jarrett, M. and Clark, N. (1999) Absconding. Part 1. Why patients leave. *Journal of Psychiatric and Mental Health Nursing*, **6**(3), 199–205.

Bowers, L., Crowhurst, N., Alexander, J., Callaghan, P., Eales, S., Guy, S., McCann, E. and Ryan, C. (2002) Safety and security policies on psychiatric acute admission wards: results from a London-wide survey. *Journal of Psychiatric and Mental Health Nursing*, **9**, 427–33.

Buchanan-Barker, P. and Barker, P. (2005) Observation: the original sin of mental health nursing? *Journal of Psychiatric and Mental Health Nursing*, **12**, 541–9.

Burrow, S. (1998) Therapy versus security: reconciling healing and damnation. In: *Critical Perspectives in Forensic Care: Inside Out* (eds. T. Mason and D. Mercer), Chapter 11. Macmillan, Basingstoke.

Byrt, R. (1999) Nursing: the psychosocial environment. In: *Therapeutic Communities: Past, Present and Future* (eds. P. Campling and R. Haigh), Chapter 5. Jessica Kingsley, London.

Byrt, R. (2001) Power, influence and control in practice development. In: *The Handbook of Practice Development* (eds. A. Clark, J. Dooher and J. Fowler), Chapter 10, Quay, Salisbury.

Byrt, R. (2006) Nursing interventions in therapeutic communities. In: *Forensic Mental Health Nursing: Interventions with People with 'Personality Disorders'* (ed. National Forensic Nurses' Research and Development Group), Chapter 14. Quay, London.

Byrt, R. with Dooher, J. (2006) The social consequences of a 'personality disorder' diagnosis. In: *Forensic Mental Health Nursing: Interventions with People with 'Personality Disorders'* (eds. National Forensic Nurses' Research and Development Group), Chapter 3. Quay, London.

Byrt, R. and Reece, J. (1999) Patients' perspectives of self-harm in a medium secure unit. *Mental Health Practice*, **3**(3), 30–4.

Byrt, R., Wray, C. and 'Tom' (2005) Towards hope and inclusion: nursing interventions in a medium secure service for men with 'personality disorders'. *Mental Health Practice*, **8**(8), 38–43.

Campling, P., Davies, S. and Farquharson, G. (eds.) (2004) *From Toxic Institutions to Therapeutic Environments: Residential Settings in Mental Health Services*. Gaskell, London.

Caudill, W. A. (1958) *The Psychiatric Hospital as a Small Society*. Harvard University Press, Cambridge, MA.

Clarke, L. (1996) Covert participant observation in a secure forensic unit: care, conflict and control. *NT Research*, **1**(6), 431–40.

Clarke, L. and Flanagan, T. (2003) *Institutional Breakdown: Exploring Mental Health Nursing Practice in Acute Inpatient Settings.* APS Publishing, Salisbury.

Coffey, M. (2006) Researching service user views in forensic mental health: a critical review. *The Journal of Forensic Psychiatry and Psychology*, **17**(1), 73–107.

Collins, M. and Davies, S. (2005) The security needs assessment profile: a multidimensional approach to measuring security needs. *International Journal of Forensic Mental Health*, **4**(1), 39–52.

Collins, M., Davies, S. and Ashwell, C. (2006) The assessment of security need. In: *Forensic Mental Health Nursing: Interventions with People with 'Personality Disorders'* (ed. National Forensic Nurses' Research and Development Group), Chapter 11. Quay, London.

Cormack, D. (1976) *Psychiatric Nursing Observed.* Royal College of Nursing, London.

Cumming, J. and Cumming, E. (1962) *Ego and Milieu.* Atherton Press, New York.

Dale, C. and Gardner, J. (2001) Security in forensic environments: strategic and operational issues. In: *Forensic Mental Health: Issues in Practice* (eds. C. Dale, T. Thompson and Woods, P.), Chapter 23. Baillière Tindall/Royal College of Nursing, Edinburgh.

Dale, C., Thompson, T. and Woods, P. (eds.) (2001) *Forensic Mental Health: Issues in Practice.* Baillière Tindall/Royal College of Nursing, Edinburgh.

Davies, S. (2004) Secure psychiatric services. In: *From Toxic Institutions to Therapeutic Environments. Residential Settings in Mental Health Services* (P. Campling, S. Davies and G. Farquharson), Chapter 23. Gaskell, London.

Davies, S., Bennion, L., McPhee, D., Osgerby, C. and Wylie, B. (2005) Cedars Community: using a therapeutic community approach in a high security hospital. *Therapeutic Communities*, **26**(2), 139–49.

Doyle, M., Aiyegbusi, A. and Burbery, P. (2006) Personality disorder: specialist psychological approaches. In: *Forensic Mental Health Nursing: Interventions with People with 'Personality Disorders'* (ed. National Forensic Nurses' Research and Development Group), Chapter 15. Quay, London.

Duxbury, J. (2000) *Difficult Patients.* Butterworth-Heinemann, Oxford.

Duxbury, J. A. (2002) An evaluation of staff and patients' views of, and strategies employed to manage patient aggression and violence on one mental health unit. *Journal of Psychiatric and Mental Health Nursing*, **9**, 325–37.

Faulkner, A. (2004) Strategies for surviving acute care. In: *Acute Mental Health Nursing: From Acute Concerns to the Capable Practitioner* (eds. M. Harrison, D. Howard and D. Mitchell), Chapter 4. Sage, London.

Firth, W. (2004) Acute psychiatric wards: an overview. In: *From Toxic Institutions to Therapeutic Environments: Residential Settings in Mental Health Services* Campling, P., Davies, S., Farquharson, G. (eds.), Chapter 17. Gaskell, London.

Gale, J. and Sanchez, B. (2005) Reflections on the treatment of psychosis in therapeutic communities. *Therapeutic Communities*, **26**(4), 485–94.

Garcia, I., Qugaishi, M., Kennett, C. and Duncan, C. (2005) *Acute Care, 2004: a National Survey of Adult Psychiatric Wards in England.* Sainsbury Centre for Mental Health, London.

George, S. (1998) More than a pound of flesh: a patient's perspective. In: *Critical Perspectives in Forensic Care: Inside Out* (eds. T. Mason and D. Mercer), Chapter 7. Macmillan, Basingstoke.

Gilligan, J. (2001) *Preventing Violence.* Thames and Hudson, London.

Goffman, E. (1968) *Asylums: Essays on the Social Situation of Mental Patients and Others.* Penguin, Harmondsworth.

Gournay, K. (2004) Cognitive behaviour therapy in in-patient care. In: *Acute Mental Health Nursing: From Acute Concerns to the Capable Practitioner* (eds. M. Harrison, D. Howard and D. Mitchell), Chapter 9. Sage, London.

Hannigan, B. and Coffey, M. (eds.) (2003) *The Handbook of Community Mental Health Nursing.* Routledge, London.

Harris, N., Williams, S. and Bradshaw, T. (eds.) (2002) *Psychosocial Interventions for People with Schizophrenia: A Practical Guide for Mental Health Workers*. Palgrave Macmillan, Basingstoke.

Harrison, M., Howard, D. and Mitchell, D. (eds.) (2004) *Acute Mental Health Nursing: From Acute Concerns to the Capable Practitioner*. Sage, London.

Hart, L. (1999) The reliable kettle. *OpenMind*, **96**, 20–1.

Hartman, D. and Smith, L. (2002) Developing community groupwork on a locked psychiatric intensive care unit. *Therapeutic Communities*, **23**(1), 5–16.

Higgins, R., Hurst, K., Wistow, G. (1999) *Psychiatric Nursing Revisited: The Care Provided for Acute Psychiatric Patients*. Whurr, London.

Ifill, W. (2002) Therapeutic communities. *The Joint Newsletter of the Association of Therapeutic Communities and the Planned Environment Trust*, **6**, 4.

Jeffcote, N. and Watson, T. (eds.) (2004) *Working Therapeutically with Women in Secure Mental Health Settings*. Jessica Kingsley, London.

Jones, K. (1988) *Experience in Mental Health: Community Care and Social Policy*. Sage, London.

Jones, K. (1993) *Asylums and After*. Athlone Press, London.

Kent, M. (2005) My mental health. *Mental Health Practice*, **8**(8), 22.

Kettles, A. M. and Robinson, D. K. (2000) Overview and contemporary issues in the role of the forensic nurse in the UK. In: *Forensic Nursing and Multidisciplinary Care of the Mentally Disorder Offender* (eds. D. K. Robinson and A. M. Kettles). Jessica Kingsley, London.

Kettles, A. M., Woods, P. and Collins, M. (eds.) (2002) *Therapeutic Interventions for Forensic Mental Health Nurses*. Jessica Kingsley, London.

Kettles, A. M., Woods, P. and Byrt, R. (2006) Conclusions: themes, action and research for the future. In: *Forensic Mental Health Nursing: Interventions with People with 'Personality Disorders'* (ed. National Forensic Nurses' Research and Development Group), Chapter 16. Quay, London.

Kilshaw, J. (1999) Can medium secure units avoid becoming total institutions? In: *Forensic Mental Health Nursing: Strategy and Implementation* (eds. P. Tarbuck, B. Topping-Morris and P. Burnard). Whurr, London.

Laing, J. with McQuarrie, D. (1989) *Fifty Years in the System*. Mainstream, Edinburgh.

Lees, N. and Withington, J. (2001) Involving service users. In: *Forensic Mental Health: Issues in Practice* (eds. C. Dale, T. Thompson and P. Woods), Chapter 11. Baillière Tindall/Royal College of Nursing, Edinburgh.

McClelland, N., Humphreys, M., Conlon, L. and Hillis, T. (eds.) (2001) *Forensic Nursing and Mental Disorder in Clinical Practice*. Butterworth- Heinemann, Oxford.

McKeown, M. and McCann, G. (2000) Psychosocial interventions. In: *Forensic Mental Health Nursing: Current Approaches* (eds. C. Chaloner and M. Coffey), Chapter 12. Blackwell Science, Oxford.

McKeown, M. *et al.* (2002) PSIs in institutional settings. In: *Psychosocial Interventions for People with Schizophrenia: A Practical Guide for Mental Health Workers* (eds. N. Harris, S. Williams and T. Bradshaw), Chapter 16. Palgrave Macmillan, Basingstoke.

McMillan, I. and Allen, D. (2005) National guidelines needed for ward staffing levels. *Mental Health Practice*, **8**(9), 4.

Mason, T. and Mercer, D. (eds.) (1998) *Critical Perspectives in Forensic Care: Inside Out*. Macmillan, Basingstoke.

Meehan, T., McIntosh, W. and Bergen, H. (2006) Aggressive behavior in high-secure settings: the perceptions of patients. *Journal of Psychiatric and Mental Health Nursing*, **13**(1), 19–25.

Mental Health Foundation and Sainsbury Centre for Mental Health (2002) *Being There in a Crisis: A Report of the Learning from Eight Mental Health Crisis Services*. Mental Health Foundation and Sainsbury Centre for Mental Health, London.

Mercer, D., Mason, T. and Richman, J. (1999) Good and evil in the crusade of care. *Journal of Psychosocial Nursing and Mental Health Services*, **37**(9), 13–17.

National Health Service Executive (1999) *Safety, Privacy and Dignity in Mental Health Units: Guidance on Mixed Sex Accommodation for Mental Health Services*. Department of Health, London.

National Institute for Clinical Excellence (NICE) (2005) *Violence Guideline*. NICE, London. Available on: http://www.nice.org.uk/.

Niskala, H. (1986) Competencies and skills required by nurses working in forensic area. *Western Journal of Nursing Research*, **8**(4), 400–13.

Nolan, P. (1993) *A History of Mental Health Nursing*. Chapman & Hall, London.

Norton, K. and Dolan, B. (1995) Acting out and the institutional response. *Journal of Forensic Psychiatry*, **6**(2), 317–32.

Pilgrim, D. and Rogers, A. (2005) *A Sociology of Mental Health and Illness*, 3rd edn. Open University Press, Maidenhead.

Quirk, A. and Lelliott, P. (2001) What do we know about life on acute psychiatric wards in the UK? A review of the research evidence. *Social Science and Medicine*, **53**, 1565–74.

Quirk, A. and Lelliott, P. (2004) Users' experiences of inpatient experiences. In: *From Toxic Institutions to Therapeutic Environments: Residential Settings in Mental Health Services* (eds. P. Campling, S. Davies and G. Farquharson), Chapter 5. Gaskell, London.

Repper, J. and Perkins, R. (2004) Social inclusion and acute care. In: *Acute Mental Health Nursing: From Acute Concerns to the Capable Practitioner* (eds. M. Harrison, D. Howard and D. Mitchell), Sage, London.

Robinson, D. K. (1996) Measuring psychiatric interventions: how much care is individualised? *NT Research*, **1**(1), 13–21.

Rowden, R. (2002) Empowerment in forensic mental health. In: *Empowerment and Participation: Power, Influence and Control in Contemporary Health Care* (eds. J. Dooher and R. Byrt), Chapter 11. Quay, Salisbury.

Royal College of Psychiatrists Audit Team (2005) *The Health Care Commission National Audit of Violence, 2003 – 2005*. Royal College of Psychiatrists, London.

Ryan, C. J. and Bowers, L. (2005) Coercive manoeuvres in a psychiatric intensive care unit. *Journal of Psychiatric and Mental Health Nursing*, **12**, 231–6.

Sainsbury Centre for Mental Health (2006) *The Search for Acute Solutions. Improving the Quality of Care in Acute Psychiatric Wards*. Sainsbury Centre for Mental Health, London.

Sang, B. (2003) Patient and public participation in health systems. In: *Empowerment and the Health Service User* (eds. J. Dooher and R. Byrt), Chapter 3. Quay, Salisbury.

Secker, J., Benson, A., Balfe, E., Lipsedge, M., Robinson, S. and Walker, J. (2004) Understanding the social context of violent and aggressive incidents on an inpatient unit. *Journal of Psychiatric and Mental Health Nursing*, **11**(2), 172–8.

Skelly, C. (1994) From special hospital to regional secure unit: a qualitative study of the problems experienced by patients. *Journal of Advanced Nursing*, **20**, 1056–63.

Skelly, C. (2001) Transition from higher to lower levels of security. In: *Forensic Mental Health: Issues in Practice* (eds. C. Dale, T. Thompson and P. Woods), Chapter 21. Baillière Tindall/Royal College of Nursing, Edinburgh.

Standing Nursing and Midwifery Advisory Committee (SNAMC) (1999) *Mental Health Nursing: 'Addressing Acute Concerns'*. Department of Health, London.

Stanton, A. and Schwartz, M. (1954) *The Mental Hospital*. Basic Books, New York.

Storey, L. and Murdock, D. (2001) Women in secure care. In: *Forensic Mental Health: Issues in Practice* (eds. C. Dale, T. Thompson and P. Woods), Chapter 17. Baillière Tindall/Royal College of Nursing, Edinburgh.

Szasz, T. (1963) *Law, Liberty and Psychiatry: An Inquiry into the Social Uses of Mental Health Practice*. Macmillan, New York.

Thompson, P. (1972) *Bound for Broadmoor*. Hodder & Stoughton, London.

Timko, C. and Moos, R. H. (2004) Measuring the therapeutic environment. In: *From Toxic Institutions to Therapeutic Environments: Residential Settings in Mental Health Services* (eds. P. Campling, S. Davies and G. Farquharson), Chapter 14. Gaskell, London.

Von Sommaruga, T. (2004) The physical environment and use of space. In: *From Toxic Institutions to Therapeutic Environments: Residential Settings in Mental Health Services* (eds. P. Campling, S. Davies and G. Farquharson), Chapter 7. Gaskell, London.

Walton, P. (2000) Psychiatric hospital care – a case of the more things change, the more they remain the same. *Journal of Mental Health*, **9**(1), 77–88.

Whittington, R. (2000) Changing the environment in the management of aggression. In: *Forensic Mental Health Care: A Case Study Approach* (eds. D. Mercer, T. Mason, M. McKeown and G. McCann). Churchill Livingstone, Edinburgh.

Wix, S. and Humphreys, M. (eds.) (2005) *Multidisciplinary Working in Forensic Mental Health Care*. Elsevier Churchill Livingstone, Edinburgh.

Woods, P. (2004) The person who uses forensic mental health services. In: *The Art and Science of Mental Health Nursing: a Textbook of Principles and Practice* (eds. I. Norman and I. Ryrie), Chapter 20. Open University Press, Maidenhead.

Woods, P., Collins, M. and Kettles, A.M. (2002) Forensic nursing interventions and future directions for forensic mental health practice. In: *Therapeutic Interventions for Forensic Mental Health Nurses* (eds. A. M. Kettles, P. Woods and M. Collins), Chapter 15. Jessica Kingsley, London.

CHAPTER 4

Towards therapeutic environments: alternatives and solutions

Richard Byrt

Introduction

This chapter considers ways to ensure beneficial social environments in order to overcome the problems outlined in Chapter 3, and reduce patients' stress, distress and risk of reoffending. This will be considered with particular reference to:

- The organisation of care and other developments in practice
- Therapeutic community principles
- Therapeutic environments based on psychosocial interventions

The effects of social environments will be considered in Chapter 5, in relation to preventing and reducing violence and aggression.

Changes in the reorganisation of nurses' work and other practice developments

Several authors have outlined changes in the organisation of care, and in particular the work of nurses, in attempts to enable them to spend more time with patients and to use a variety of interventions to prevent incidents such as self-harm and violence (McMillan, 2006; Sainsbury Centre for Mental Health, 2006), including behaviours associated with previous offending (Byrt *et al.*, 2005; Doyle *et al.*, 2005). The initiatives reported are all in acute mental health services, and have relevance for interventions with patients with forensic mental health needs.

The value of measures to improve social environments has been described for patients in both acute and secure forensic mental health services (Firth, 2004; Holmes, 2004; Kirby, 1997; McKeown and McCann, 2000; McKeown *et al.*, 2002; Sainsbury Centre for Mental Health, 2006). Kent (2005) has outlined the setting aside of 'protected therapeutic engagement time' for staff to work with patients on acute admission wards, with arrangements at set times to divert telephone calls and to ensure freedom from visitors, meetings and administrative work. *The Search for Acute Solutions* (Sainsbury Centre for Mental Health, 2006) described changes in the organisation of wards and innovative projects to improve social environments for patients and their informal carers. Changes in different services included less intimidating ward rounds; a daily meeting to plan ward activities to meet individuals' needs; a centre for families visiting patients; and arrangements to ensure that patients' meals were not interrupted (McMillan, 2006, citing Sainsbury Centre for Mental Health, 2006).

Many of these recent organisational changes appear to be essential, not only to ensure that patients with forensic mental health needs feel valued, but also to allow sufficient time for interventions to reduce both distress and specific symptoms and problems associated with offending behaviours, and the consequent risks of reoffending (Kettles *et al.*, 2002).

The Clinical Governance Support Team and changes in North Essex Mental Health Partnership NHS Trust

The Clinical Governance Support Team has a website which includes examples of improving mental health and other health services, using clinical governance principles. Sue Champion, a Nurse Consultant in North Essex Mental Health Partnership NHS Trust, asked both service users and staff for their views on areas of good practice and what areas they thought needed particular improvement. Various projects were identified, and implemented, to effect improvements (Modernisation Agency Clinical Governance Support Team, 2005). These included:

- Providing staff to deal with administrative work, so that professionals spent less time on this activity – with more time for patient care.
- In response to patients' views that more activities should be provided, budget flexibility was used to create a 'Therapeutic and Recreational Activities Team', with 'a purpose-built Therapy and Recreational Centre', accessible to individuals who were compulsorily detained under the Mental Health Act 1983 (Modernisation Agency Clinical Governance Support Team, 2005).
- A team to respond to individuals in crisis was created, with developments to improve liaison with clients when they were discharged home: an initiative of particular relevance to clients with forensic mental health needs (Riordan, 2005).
- Ways to improve communication between staff were implemented.
- It was found that patients found ward reviews unsatisfactory. Changes were made to increase patient participation.

Changes in an acute admission ward in inner city Bradford

Dodds and Bowles (2001) outline changes they made, as ward managers, in an acute admission ward in inner city Bradford. The nurses' work changed from dealing with crises, 'observing' (without engaging with clients); and large amounts of paperwork. Of particular relevance to nursing interventions with patients with forensic mental health needs is the observation (below) of Dodds and Bowles (2001) concerning the reduction of violence and aggression:

> We gradually reduced formal observation over a six-month period... Nurses stopped using observation levels... and spent more time with patients in one-to-one settings, developing collaborative therapeutic relationships that may not have been previously possible. After six months, formal observations were hardly used. After eighteen months, one-to-one observations were no longer used and haven't been used since...
>
> With the nursing time released, we began to provide a weekly programme of activities for patients. Patients are now more involved in their care, and with decisions that affect the ward as a whole. Nurses are better supported, audit and clinical supervision have been introduced to maintain and promote clinical standards.
>
> After eighteen months, the nature of nurse–patient relationships, the atmosphere on the wards and the patients' experience are markedly improved. Deliberate self harm has reduced by two-thirds, violence and aggression by over a third, staff sickness has reduced by almost two-thirds, and absconding has reduced by almost half. In the same period, there has not been an increase in suicides on the ward.
>
> Audit data show that patients are more engaged with their named nurses, better informed and more involved in their care. All patients now hold their own copies of care plans. Nurses are now able to make a 'gift of time' to patients, this may be social or therapeutic.
>
> ... 95% of patients receive daily, structured one-to-one time with a nurse...
>
> Financial savings have also been significant... largely through reduced sickness and reduced need for agency nurses...
>
> (Dodds and Bowles, 2001, p. 187)

The application of therapeutic community principles

Therapeutic community principles can also contribute positively to mental health service environments, including those for individuals with offending histories (Byrt, 2006; Rawlings, 2005). The features of social environments, listed in Chapter 3, relate to the characteristics of therapeutic communities. Therapeutic communities in acute and secure forensic services and in psychiatric intensive care units have the following features (Byrt, 2006; Firth, 2004; Hartman and Smith, 2002):

- The whole of the resident's stay in the ward or other service is seen as potentially therapeutic. Treatment is not just seen to be the medication round or occasional sessions with a primary nurse or a psychiatrist. Everything that happens within the service is intended to be therapeutic, including interactions with staff, activities, and opportunities to relax and recover (Byrt, 2006; Kelly *et al.*, 2004).
- In contrast to findings that some patients in acute and secure forensic settings have limited communication with staff (Meehan *et al.*, 2006; Mental Health Foundation and Sainsbury Centre for Mental Health, 2002), in services with therapeutic community principles there are many opportunities for communication in non-threatening ways, including the safe expression of feelings and exploration of problems, both informally and at structured times. People are enabled to gradually find solutions to problems (Bree *et al.*, 2003; Kelly *et al.*, 2004), including those related to offending behaviours (Byrt, 2006; Rawlings, 2005).
- Staff attempt to understand, and take seriously, people's experiences, concerns and perspectives, including those related to hallucinations and delusions and other experiences of mental illness (Gale and Sanchez, 2005).
- Whilst the facilitation of community meetings and types of group psychotherapy may be suitable for some individuals in acute and forensic secure settings, there is recognition of the need for flexibility, and that certain patients may find it easier to talk individually to staff (Byrt, 2006; Holmes, 2004).
- Residents' views, e.g. about everyday life in the ward or other service, are invited and taken seriously by staff (Liderth, 2003).
- Whilst it is recognised that many individuals may be acutely ill, and need a low expressed emotion environment, without excessive and stressful pressure, residents are encouraged to gradually make decisions and take on responsibility for aspects of their lives, and to be involved in decisions related to life on the ward (Byrt, 2006). An example of the latter could be involvement, with staff, in plans for a ward social event or shared recreational activity. This approach contrasts with situations where staff impose activities on residents without their participation; and is intended to enable residents to gradually make decisions about their lives (Liderth, 2003).
- Related to involvement in decision making is the recognition that, besides having problems, residents have positive qualities and coping strategies, talents and abilities, which they are enabled to use and develop (Byrt, 2006). In particular, increased educational opportunities for people with histories of violent offending have been found to be statistically significantly related to reductions in recidivism (Gilligan, 2001).

Acute and secure mental health services with therapeutic community principles

Therapeutic communities have been established in secure forensic settings for people with 'personality disorders' (Byrt, 2006; McMurran *et al.*, 1998; Reiss *et al.*, 1996) and in a ward for individuals with enduring mental illness in a high secure hospital (Davies, 2004; Davies *et al.*, 2005).

A number of prison wings (for example, at Grendon, Gartree and Dovedale Prisons) are run as therapeutic communities, within the parameters of security (Rawlings, 2005). Few present-day acute admission wards apply therapeutic community principles, although several of these services have functioned, with reported benefits to patients, in the 1970s (Firth, 2004; Gale and Sanchez, 2005), and recently, in an acute day hospital (Crockford *et al.*, 2003) and a psychiatric intensive care unit (Hartman and Smith, 2002; see also McKenzie, 2001).

Most NHS and therapeutic communities are run on democratic-analytic lines (Kennard, 1998; Kelly *et al.*, 2004) and specialise in the treatment of people with 'personality disorders' (although not all therapeutic communities apply this diagnostic category to residents) (Byrt, 2006). Individuals are often admitted following periods of acute and intense crisis, and some, particularly at the Henderson Hospital, have histories of offending (Warren *et al.*, 2004). A structured programme of psychodynamic psychotherapy and other groups is offered, with intensive opportunities to use the social environment to learn about, and resolve, relationship difficulties and other problems; take on responsibility; and develop positive attributes, abilities and talents. The individual is enabled to understand and find solutions to problems (including those related to violence and offending behaviours) and, with staff, contribute positively to the treatment of other residents and the day to day life of the community. The nurse's role includes facilitation of a therapeutic social environment and the application of various skills in psychotherapy groups and various shared activities (Bree *et al.*, 2003; Byrt, 2006; Kelly *et al.*, 2004).

Psychiatric medication is never or rarely prescribed in democratic-analytic therapeutic communities. However, in acute and secure settings for people with mental illness, therapeutic community principles are usually combined with other treatments such as medication. This is the case in an acute day hospital (Crockford *et al.*, 2003) and a psychiatric intensive care unit (Hartman and Smith, 2002) run as modified therapeutic communities, as well as in a high secure therapeutic community for individuals with enduring mental illness (Davies, 2004; Davies *et al.*, 2005). It has been suggested that, whilst some features of the democratic-analytic therapeutic community, such as psychodynamic psychotherapy groups, are suited to only a minority of patients, other characteristics of these organisations are applicable to every inpatient, day or residential mental health service (Byrt, 1999; Holmes, 2004).

Research findings suggest that therapeutic communities relieve some individuals' anxiety, self-harm and underlying distress, and lead to increases in self-esteem, confidence and positive coping strategies, including those related to the prevention of offending behaviours (Genders and Player, 1995; Lees *et al.*, 2004; Warren *et al.*, 2004). For example, some individuals with 'personality disorders' gain understanding of the reasons for their impulsive behaviours and learn ways to manage anger more effectively (Warren *et al.*, 2004). This is achieved through the provision of opportunities for residents to reflect on, and gain insights from, events that occur in the day to day life of the therapeutic community, including incidents involving the expression of anger. In addition, therapeutic communities provide residents with opportunities to try out new ways of relating to others, and of safely expressing anger and other feelings. Practical ways in which this is achieved are described in Bree *et al.* (2003), Byrt (2006), Kelly *et al.* (2004) and Norton (2004).

For some individuals, gains related to understanding and expressing anger safely and assertively are related to prevention of reoffending (Rawlings, 2005; Warren *et al.*, 2004). In general, non-secure NHS therapeutic communities and Grendon Prison have been found to decrease rates of recidivism in individuals who complete treatment (Norton and Warren, 2004; Rawlings, 2005).

However, other studies have found that therapeutic communities in secure hospitals result in no changes in reoffending (McMurran *et al.*, 1998; Reiss *et al.*, 1996, cited in Byrt, 2006). A prison run as a therapeutic community increased recidivism in individuals who scored high on measures of psychopathy on Hare's psychopathy checklist (Harris *et al.*, 1994).

Alternative crisis services

Several writers have described alternatives to acute admission wards, such as crisis houses and other residential accommodation, which emphasise the importance of beneficial social milieux, usually based on therapeutic community principles (Department of Health, 2003; Mental Health Foundation and Sainsbury Centre for Mental Health, 2002; Rose, 2001). Residential crisis houses aim to provide refuge and opportunities to discover strengths and explore problems in a healing and homely environment, often without the use of antipsychotic or other medication (Berke, 2003; Paget and White, 2004; Mental Health Foundation and Sainsbury Centre for Mental Health, 2002). Other crisis services offer telephone lines and centres providing support in the evening (Mental Health Foundation and Sainsbury Centre for Mental Health, 2002). All these facilities offer individuals opportunities to talk to someone who is accessible and available to listen. Some service users express a preference for these types of crisis service, partly because they enable the individual to deal autonomously with acute problems, with recognition of clients' strengths, rather than focusing mainly on their mental illness (Mental Health Foundation and Sainsbury Centre for Mental Health, 2002, citing Augarde 1999; Mental Health Foundation, 2001). Crises are considered in relation to the individual's perspective and are often seen as a means to her/his development of positive coping strategies. Respect for the individual is emphasised, including sensitivity in relation to her/his culture, ethnic group and gender (Department of Health, 2003; Mental Health Foundation and Sainsbury Centre for Mental Health, 2002).

Crisis services do not cater for all individuals, e.g. those who are compulsorily admitted. People with aggressive behaviours are not precluded from some crisis services, with a philosophy that relaxing environments where people are respected will reduce the likelihood of violence (Mental Health Foundation and Sainsbury Centre for Mental Health, 2002). The role of crisis services in relation to individuals with offending histories does not appear to have been widely documented.

Some crisis houses have been commissioned and/or funded by statutory health and social services; and many have been founded by service users and/or voluntary organisations (Mental Health Foundation and Sainsbury Centre for Mental Health, 2002; Rose, 2001). These facilities include houses run according to Mosher's Soteria model (Barker, 2005); by the Arbours Association (Berke, 2003; see Box 4.1); and by Community Housing and Therapy (Paget and White, 2004; Tucker, 2000). One American house, run on Soteria principles, was found to be equally effective as an acute admission unit, and resulted in higher client satisfaction and lower costs (Barker, 2005, citing Fenton *et al.*, 1998). A study of a Swiss Soteria house found 'that roughly two thirds of newly diagnosed persons with schizophrenia recover, with little or no drug treatment, in two to twelve weeks' (Barker, 2005, p. 14, citing Ciopmi, 2004).

Box 4.1 The Arbours Crisis Centre (quoted from Berke, 2003, p. 116).

The Arbours... Crisis Centre... is a unique community because... the 'resident therapists'... live at the house on a full time basis. It is their home. People come not as patients, but as guests...

The term 'guest' conveys hospitality, and the idea of a 'treat', something warm and enjoyable, as opposed to a 'treatment', which is often impersonal and disagreeable.... Our aim is to help them to shed, or never take on, the learned role of mental patient or institutionalised other. Moreover, we want them to achieve a position of respect and dignity, as well as the relief of whatever pain brought them to the Centre...

Psychosocial interventions

Psychosocial interventions also have implications for beneficial social environments in the community and in acute and secure mental health services, including those for individuals with histories of offending. In relation to individuals with mental health problems, the term *psychosocial interventions* usually refers to a variety of therapeutic approaches, particularly cognitive behavioural therapies and psychoeducation (education about mental illness) (Baguley and Dulson, 2004; Gamble with Curthoys, 2004). These approaches aim to enable the active participation of the client and, with his/her agreement, that of family, partner and other people involved in his/her care at home. All psychosocial interventions aim to reduce or relieve the following (Baguley and Dulson, 2004; Birchwood *et al.*, 2000; Keen, 2003; Gamble with Curthoys, 2004; McKeown and McCann, 2000):

- Stress associated with the precipitation and exacerbation (i.e. worsening) of symptoms of mental illness.
- The distress that individuals often experience in relation to these symptoms. Examples of potentially distressing symptoms include persistent and persecutory voices telling the individual that he or she is useless; finding it difficult to concentrate on or enjoy any activities; and intrusive and unwelcome thoughts.
- Distressing problems and symptoms, with the development of positive problem solving and coping strategies.
- For some individuals, this relates to violence and aggression and offending behaviours associated with individuals' stress, distress and various problems and symptoms.
- Prevention of relapse or an exacerbation of symptoms.

Psychosocial interventions are usually combined with antipsychotic medication (Gillam, 2002; Gournay, 1999; Turner, 2003). The National Institute for Health and Clinical Excellence (2002) states that research suggests that most individuals with schizophrenia have better outcomes from a combination of these two treatments. However, one study found that some individuals with schizophrenia made good recoveries without medication, but with the provision of a low expressed emotion environment (Raguram *et al.*, 2002).

Psychosocial interventions are informed by stress vulnerability models which postulate, based on research findings, that in certain people with a genetic and biochemical predisposition, episodes of mental illness can be triggered by both internal stressors (e.g. distressing delusions or the ingestion of certain drugs) and external stressful events (Baguley and Dulson, 2004, citing Zubin and Spring, 1997; Fahy and Dudley, 2000). Research has found that sources of external stress include aspects of the individual's social environment, both at home with family members and partners and within mental health services (Harris *et al.*, 2002). For example, some individuals with schizophrenia experience symptoms of post-traumatic stress disorder as a result of: (a) distressing experiences of symptoms of schizophrenia; and (b) adverse experiences of mental health services (Watkins, 1996). There is evidence that the provision of non-stressful and beneficial family and ward environments can reduce the deleterious effects of distressing symptoms. For this reason, psychosocial interventions include ways of reducing stress in both the client's family or other domestic environment and mental health service settings (Baguley and Dulson, 2004; Gamble with Curthoys, 2004; Harris *et al.*, 2002; Keen, 2003). These approaches are based on research findings that certain social environments are either beneficial or harmful to individuals with mental health problems. Much of this research is concerned with optimum environments for individuals with schizophrenia (Timko and Moos, 2004), including those with histories of offending (Cross and Kirby, 2002; Ewers and Ikin, 2002; McKeown and McCann, 2000).

Relevant research findings include the following:

- 'Significantly greater relapse rates' are associated with high expressed emotion (e.g. considerable hostility, criticism and over-involvement) in the patient's family and amongst staff in inpatient and residential mental health services (Fahy and Dudley, 2000, p. 239, citing Kavanagh, 1992). This has particular relevance for nursing patients with histories of offending when the latter is associated with specific symptoms of mental illness (McKeown and McCann, 2000).
- Institutionalisation and under-stimulation and a lack of activity can worsen some schizophrenic symptoms (Brennan *et al.*, 2000). One of the first authors to note this was Barton (1966), in a book ('Institutional Neurosis') which still has some relevance. Kelly *et al.* (2001, p. 139) found '... a weak, but statistically significant correlation... between involvement in activities and self-reported quality of life...'.
- Research has found that some people with schizophrenia have difficulties with processing information and experience sensory overload, feeling bombarded by external sensory stimuli, e.g. noises, and by their own thoughts and hallucinations. They sometimes find it difficult to concentrate, and to distinguish between, for example, an important conversation and other stimuli (Fahy and Dudley, 2000). Assessment needs to be made of environmental factors that may act as stressors, and appropriate action taken to reduce these. For example, some patients who suffer from sensory overload may be especially stressed by periods of excessive activity, such as meal times, or by noise from loud music or a blaring television. The use of quiet space and the moderation of excessive noise may reduce the stress of these individuals (Fahy and Dudley, 2000; Whittington, 2000).

- Watkins (1996) outlines research findings suggesting that many individuals with schizophrenia have a particular need for quiet space. He argues that some people with this diagnosis become withdrawn and apparently lacking in motivation because they need time to be by themselves, as part of recovery from acute symptoms of schizophrenia. Part of the individual's sensory overload may relate to frightening hallucinations and delusions (Watkins, 1996). (An example of this ('Alan Amber') is given later in this chapter).

Measuring and changing mental health service environments: the Ward Atmosphere Scale

Rudolf Moos devised a Ward Atmosphere Scale to measure the social environments of mental health wards (Moos, 1974, 1989, cited in Middelboe *et al.*, 2001; Timko and Moos, 2004). Moos and other researchers also devised similar scales to measure social environments of day centres and other services (Timko and Moos, 2004).

The Ward Atmosphere Scale consists of 10 subscales, measuring different aspects of the social environment (Middelboe *et al.*, 2001, p. 214; Timko and Moos, 2004, p. 146):

1. **Involvement**: Patients' activity and energy in the service's programme.
2. **Support**: This subscale measures patients' mutual support and help and support provided by staff.
3. **Spontaneity**: The extent that there is 'open expression of feelings by patients and staff' (Timko and Moos, 2004, p. 146).
4. **Autonomy**: The degree of patients' independence and self-sufficiency in decision making.
5. **Practical orientation**: How far patients acquire practical skills to enable them to live effectively in the community.
6. **Personal problem orientation**: This subscale measures patients' searches 'to understand their feelings and personal problems' (Timko and Moos, 2004, p. 146).
7. **Anger and aggression**: A measure of the incidence of patient arguments, aggression and overt anger within the ward.
8. **Order and organisation**: The perceived importance of these features in the ward's programme.
9. **Programme clarity**: How far patients are aware of what will happen in the daily life of the service, and the extent that 'rules and procedures' (Moos, 2004, p. 146) are explicit.
10. **Staff control**: The extent that staff ensure essential controls in patient care.

Ideal ward environments for individuals with schizophrenia

Findings of studies suggest, in relation to the Ward Atmosphere Scale, that wards are most likely to meet the needs of individuals with schizophrenia if they have certain characteristics (Baker,

2000; McKeown *et al.*, 2002; Middelboe *et al.*, 2001; Timko and Moos, 2004). This will now be considered in relation to expressed emotion and ward structure and activities.

The literature, including service user accounts, suggests that many individuals with schizophrenia benefit from an environment which, amongst other features, has an absence of sensory overload, a clear structure, and low expressed emotion (absence of hostility, criticism and emotional over-involvement: Timko and Moos, 2004; Watkins, 1996).

> Patricia Ruocchio has given a graphic description of how she used withdrawal to provide herself with a 'safety shield' which helped to protect her from the extreme and unendurable anxiety and distress she experienced as a result of contact with others and the world:
> ... 'If I cannot actively make people around me disappear, I try to disappear myself... I tend to withdraw... sometimes feeling myself melt into an inanimate object, actually becoming a chair or a wall.... There are many times I feel so vulnerable, I need to pull away from the rest of the world...' (Ruocchio, 1991, p. 359, quoted in Watkins, 1996, p. 15f)

Mills *et al.* (2006) refer to the importance of professionals' self-awareness and endeavouring to understand, and base their interventions on, the individual's experience. For example, apparently limited motivation may be a strategy to enable the individual to manage distressing symptoms (including those associated with offending behaviours) and enable recovery. Over-ambitious programmes of activities, with which the individual cannot cope, may increase her/his stress and feelings of being pressured (Mills *et al.*, 2006). This has implications for the type of social environment with which the individual feels most comfortable, as in the following example.

'Mr Alan Amber': an example of the importance of the environment of a mental health service.

This example is based on the nursing experience of the writer. However, to ensure confidentiality and anonymity, the individual and low secure unit described are fictitious.

'Mr Alan Amber' is 27 years old. He is a skilled gardener, and a keen supporter of his local Premiership football team, sometimes watching their matches on television. He keeps sporadic contact with his parents and a friend, but generally prefers his own company. When Alan can concentrate, he enjoys reading science fiction and listening to some types of music, particularly Atomic Kitten CDs, which he finds relaxing.

Alan's first episode of schizophrenia occurred when he was 17, and since then he had rarely been free of symptoms of this illness. He often experienced intrusive, persistent auditory hallucinations (voices), which called him 'wimp' and other abusive names, and accused him of various misdemeanours. Alan also had persecutory delusions associated with the hallucinations, believing that other people were responsible for them. He experienced considerable distress in relation to his voices and his associated delusional beliefs.

One evening, Alan assaulted a man who had, he said, accused him of being a wimp. When Alan appeared before the local Magistrates' Court, he was remanded to hospital for assessment, under Section 38, and later, for treatment, under Section 37 of the Mental

Health Act 1983 (Powell and Dolan, 2000). Alan was admitted to 'Oaks', a low secure unit for patients receiving assessment, care and treatment by a local forensic mental health multidisciplinary team. In his early days at Oaks, Alan made frequent threats to hit people, and occasionally did so. At these times Alan appeared particularly distressed, and often mentioned that the people he threatened were calling him by derogatory names.

The antipsychotic medication that Alan was taking at the time of his admission was reviewed by his consultant psychiatrist, who discussed this with him and with members of the multidisciplinary clinical team. Alan agreed to the prescription of Clozapine, an antipsychotic which has been found to be effective for individuals whose schizophrenic symptoms have not been alleviated by other medication (Forchuk and Jensen, 2003). Although some critics have outlined the harmful effects of many drugs used to treat mental illness (Lehmann, 2001; Rogers and Pilgrim, 2003; Romme and Escher, 2000), some service users have reported that antipsychotics relieve the distress associated with auditory hallucinations and other symptoms. To monitor any possible serious side effects of Clozapine, such as agranulocytosis (reduced white blood cell count), Alan's blood levels of this drug were regularly monitored, as is always the case when it is prescribed (Keen, 2003).

In addition, with the informed consent and participation of Alan, his named nurse and a clinical psychologist devised a programme which was incorporated into his multidisciplinary care plan. As part of the application of psychosocial interventions, cognitive behavioural therapy (CBT) was used. This included an initial assessment of the number of threats and violent incidents precipitated by Alan, with observations of factors (antecedents), which seemed to precede, or be associated with, his violence and aggression. These factors included: agitation and other signs of distress and stress that he appeared to be experiencing at the time; persecutory voices and other distressing symptoms; and environmental variables. When Alan felt able to participate, he was asked to identify these factors. Initially, Alan was asked to record the number of times he experienced his persecutory auditory hallucinations and beliefs, and to rate, on a scale of 1 to 10, the degree of distress that he experienced in response to his voices at particular times.

The effects of aspects of the social environment of Oaks were assessed. Alan reported, and the nurses observed, that he became very distressed (and on one occasion was violent) when staff tried to persuade him to leave his room and engage in activities in communal areas. In line with research findings on sensory overload (Gamble and Brennan, 2006), it was also observed that Alan's hallucinations and associated distress became more frequent when the ward environment and the communal dining area were noisy or crowded. Alan said that, when his voices were particularly persistent, he generally felt more relaxed and less aggressive if he could stay in his room, undisturbed, either listening to his Atomic Kitten CDs or reading science fiction.

As a result of the initial assessment, Alan's care plan included the areas listed below. The plan included the provision of a beneficial social environment, with the aims of ensuring the safety of Alan and other patients and staff, and reducing his distress. Interventions included opportunities to talk with staff and the provision of private space, with reduced sensory overload from the presence of other people, excessive noise and the demands or expectations that Alan found hard to cope with.

It was agreed that:

- Staff would maintain discreet, but regular and recorded, observations to ensure the safety and well-being of Alan and other people.
- Alan would inform a member of his primary nursing team if his voices or other symptoms were particularly distressing, and if he felt like threatening or hitting someone.
- He would be offered an opportunity to talk to a member of nursing staff in a quiet room – but in adjoining areas where other staff were present, so that the nurse who was with Alan was not vulnerable to assault. Nurses would *actively listen*, endeavour to understand Alan's experiences and distress, and enable him to ventilate feelings, with the intention of *reducing anxiety*.
- Alan would have the choice to withdraw from communal areas and activities so that he could listen to his music or read. The latter served as distractions from his symptoms and the associated distress.
- A nurse arranged sessions with Alan to teach *specific relaxation techniques* to enable him to reduce anxiety associated with his voices and other symptoms.
- Staff would not make excessive demands on Alan, such as persuading him to come out of his room (unless this was necessary for safety reasons). It was agreed, also, that Alan would not be expected to participate in any activities with other people that he found extremely stressful.
- This included the communal dining area. To reduce Alan's sensory overload and associated stress, it was agreed that he could eat meals in a quiet area of the unit.
- In the multidisciplinary care plan, there was particular emphasis on measuring the effects of each intervention on:
  - The *frequency* of Alan's persecutory delusions and hallucinations and other *distressing symptoms*.
  - The *intensity of distress* experienced by Alan, which he continued to rate on a scale of 1 to 10.

Over time, Alan was gradually enabled to feel more comfortable with other people, and to increase his skills in interacting with them. Alan was encouraged to use relaxation techniques before meeting others; and, as part of cognitive behavioural therapy, to use graded exposure (Gega, 2004). This involved Alan in spending a gradually increased amount of time with one or two individuals with whom he felt reasonably comfortable, in a quiet and non-threatening environment. Once he found such interactions relatively stress-free, Alan found it possible to spend less time in his room. Gradually, he found other people less threatening, and began to sometimes enjoy their company. His level of reported distress dropped from an average of 9 at the start of the graded exposure to around 3 six months later. At this time, Alan reported a lessening in the frequency and intensity of accusatory voices and related delusional beliefs, which appeared to be related, at least in part, to the effects of the Clozapine.

At an appropriate time, psycho-education sessions were arranged for Alan and, with his agreement, his family. Receiving information about schizophrenia helped Alan to further maintain control over his distressing symptoms, and increased his family's understanding (Gillam, 2001; McKeown *et al.*, 2002). The psycho-education also enabled Oaks' staff to increase their understanding of the experiences and perspectives of Alan and his family (Gamble with Curthoys, 2004).

Besides aiming to reduce Alan's distress and improve his quality of life, the psychosocial interventions were also intended to reduce the risk of reoffending, with the provision of positive coping strategies that Alan could apply to situations where he believed people were talking in a derogatory way about him. Strategies included withdrawing from situations that were socially stressful and, when Alan was eventually discharged home, contacting a member of his community forensic mental health team if he was experiencing a relapse signature (Birchwood *et al.*, 2000; see Chapter 17) or felt suspicious about others.

Gradually, over several months, Alan reported reductions in both the frequency of his voices, and an increased ability to reduce their distressing effects through using the strategies on his multidisciplinary care plan. The number of threats and violent incidents reduced, with none occurring in the period six to twelve months after the introduction of psychosocial interventions and Clozapine.

Low expressed emotion (EE) in staff

In interventions with Alan Amber, staff ensured low expressed emotion through non-judgemental listening, without criticism; and avoidance of demands which would expose Alan to excessive demands or noise with which he could not cope (e.g. in participation in group activities or meals in a communal dining area). Research findings suggest the importance of low expressed emotion (EE) for acute and secure forensic service environments. Studies have found that nursing and other staff vary in their levels of EE. In one study, 'low EE staff were found to appear more supportive, dwelt less on negative feelings and elicited more self-affirmation from their clients...' (McKeown *et al.*, 2002, p. 223, citing Moore and Kuipers, 1992). McKeown *et al.* (2002) commented, in relation to staff over-involvement, on the importance of professionals not making decisions or performing tasks for clients that they could manage themselves.

In a study concerned with community accommodation for mental health clients: '... Higher [staff] EE ratings were associated with poorer results on a residents' quality of life measure, and with greater hostility and suspiciousness on the part of residents...' (McKeown *et al.*, 2002, p. 223, citing Snyder *et al.*, 1994). (This finding has some similarities with research findings of Morrison (1992) that high levels of authoritarianism in staff were strongly associated with aggressive behaviours in some mental health patients). Conversely, Kirby (1997), from measurements of ward atmosphere on two wards in a medium secure unit, concluded that nurses did not need to exert custodial control, but used their relationships with patients, and a relaxed ward environment, to prevent and reduce aggression. A poem by Watters (1996) is a very vivid example of high EE in a nurse.

Planting one polyanthus: attempts to provide a low expressed emotion environment on Pennine Ward

Pennine is an assessment and admission ward in Arnold Lodge medium secure unit, Leicester. A social and physical environment is provided to carefully assess and reduce risk. Besides clear policies related to physical security, this includes avoidance of making demands on patients that they find difficult to cope with, in relation to recognition of the distress caused by auditory hallucinations, delusions, intrusive thoughts and other stressful symptoms. For example, patients faced with these symptoms can eat meals on the ward in a relatively quiet environment, rather than in a noisier communal dining area, and have some choice in decisions about their waking times in the morning. A low-key community meeting is available for patients to express views and ideas concerning the ward. This meeting is optional, as it is recognised that many patients find even small groups stressful, so there are also opportunities for patients to express views individually to the independent patients' advocate, as well as to managers and staff. Nurses are readily available for patients to talk to.

Activities are individually tailored to each individual's needs and preferences, without imposing expectations for participation that would be stressful to patients. Amongst many low-key activities is a ward-based gardening group. This was facilitated by the author in response to patients' requests, and with the support of managers and staff. The ward garden is a safe and secure extension of the ward, to which patients (with rare exceptions for safety reasons) have free and open access at all times during the day.

The value of activities that 'connect with the natural environment' (Paget and White, 2004, p. 79) has been described, and is emphasised by Thrive (2006), a voluntary organisation that provides horticultural opportunities for people with mental health problems and other specific needs. Pennine's gardening group is a 'low expressed emotion' activity, in that it gives individuals an opportunity to decide whether or not to be involved, and to participate in any way that they wish. They are free to choose to come and go from the garden as they wish. Participation includes observing other people gardening, planting one polyanthus, and, if people wish, sustained activity for half an hour or more. Two patients have recently expended considerable energy and time in redesigning the garden.

The gardening group enables people to express their talents and abilities, with an opportunity to obtain satisfaction from nurturing plants and see them grow (Paget and White, 2004). Whilst the relative lack of autonomy, for safety reasons, of patients in a medium secure unit should not be denied (Mason and Mercer, 1998), the gardening group gives people an opportunity to make decisions, even though these are limited (e.g. about what to grow and ways to develop the garden).

Patients' expressed emotion

Some research on mental health patients' views suggests that they find high levels of aggression (an aspect of high expressed emotion) in other patients particularly stressful (Bowers *et al.*, 1999); and prefer services which score low on levels of 'Anger and Aggression' (Timko and Moos, 2004, p. 146), as measured on Ward Atmosphere and other scales (Rossberg and Friis, 2004). Research suggests that environmental factors in acute service settings are often important in contributing to, or triggering, violence and aggression (Baguley and Dowson, 2004; Collins and Munroe, 2004).

Amounts of structure and activities

Studies indicate that individuals with schizophrenia benefit from 'high levels... [of] support, practical orientation, order and organisation and programme clarity' (Middelboe *et al.*, 2001, p. 217) – as measured by Ward Atmosphere and related scales.

Research on stressors suggests that the extent and nature of activities should be individually tailored to the specific needs of individuals with schizophrenia, based on an assessment of particular stressors which may precipitate or worsen symptoms. For example, as with the example of 'Mr Alan Amber' (described earlier in this chapter), staff's making excessive demands on an individual to participate in several group activities may be experienced by her/him as particularly stressful if she/he is experiencing abusive voices and paranoid beliefs about other people. However, conversely, an absence of structure or any activities may result in under-stimulation, and a possible worsening of negative symptoms of schizophrenia, such as apathy and withdrawal (Mills *et al.*, 2006).

Siddle and Everitt (2002) comment on the importance of flexibility in activities for people with negative symptoms and inactivity. For example (p. 125):

> ... Setting short-term achievable goals allows for the client to develop a sense of achievement regarding the day's activities and will enhance engagement. Care is clearly needed to ensure the person is not overloaded and that a number of purely pleasurable activities are included for each day or activity period...

'Treatment environments and in [patient] programme outcomes'

Timko and Moos (2004), citing Moos (1997), found that, in inpatient and community services, patient satisfaction was associated with professional interventions that stressed patient autonomy and opportunities to learn vocational and social skills and to increase understanding of self. When these interventions supported clients, and were organised effectively, individuals gained in interpersonal skills and were less likely to be aggressive: a finding which has implications for clients with histories of offending. In contrast, excessive control by staff was found to be 'associated with low patient morale and self-confidence' (Timko and Moos, 2004, p. 151). Patients' effective functioning in the community, following discharge, was associated with programmes with good organisation that enabled clients' effective problem solving, autonomy and personal development (Timko and Moos, 2004, p. 152, citing Moos, 1997).

In summary, research findings suggest that the most beneficial social environments for individuals with schizophrenia include staff who are non-judgemental, non-authoritarian, and endeavour to empathise with individuals' experiences of distressing symptoms. Other beneficial aspects of service environment include an avoidance of an over-stimulating, over-structured regime, and ensuring an avoidance of excessive noise and too many stressful demands (e.g. unreasonable expectations that clients participate in group or other activities) which they find anxiety-provoking. On the other hand, research findings suggest that it is important to ensure that there is sufficient structure to avoid the effects of boredom and institutionalisation (i.e. becoming apathetic and unmotivated as a result of a stay in a ward or other mental health service) (McKeown and McCann, 2000; Whittington, 2000). These findings appear to reduce individuals' distress and the risk of reoffending (McKeown and McCann, 2000).

Conclusion

In this chapter, aspects of the ward environment have been considered, for example in relation to planning the patients' day, activities and the setting aside of 'therapeutic time' to be with patients. Therapeutic community principles and psychosocial interventions are outlined as therapeutic frameworks which can inform beneficial social environments which reduce patients' stress, and aim to reduce the risk of reoffending. Some service users have expressed a preference for crisis services, including residential facilities run as therapeutic communities.

Research findings suggest that services users benefit from opportunities for communication with nursing staff, wards with low expressed emotion, structured, meaningful activity and avoidance of an over-stimulating environment and sensory overload.

References

Baguley, I. and Dulson, J. (2005) Psychosocial Interventions. In: *Acute Mental Health Nursing: From Acute Concerns to the Capable Practitioner* (eds. M. Harrison, D. Howard and D. Mitchell), Chapter 10. Sage, London.

Baker, J. A. (2000) Developing psychosocial care for acute psychiatric wards. *Journal of Psychiatric and Mental Health Nursing*, **7**, 95–100.

Barker, P. (2005) Putting acute care in its place. *Mental Health Nursing*, **23**(1), 12–15.

Barton, R. (1966) *Institutional Neurosis*, 2nd edn. John Wright, Bristol.

Berke, J. (2003) Who's in charge here? Projective processes, of course! *Therapeutic Communities*, **24**(2), 115–26.

Birchwood, M., Fowler, D. and Jackson, C. (eds.) (2000) *Early Intervention in Psychosis: A Guide to Concepts, Evidence and Interventions*. Wiley, Chichester.

Bowers, L., Jarrett, M. and Clark, N. (1999) Absconding. Part 1. Why patients leave. *Journal of Psychiatric and Mental Health Nursing*, **6**(3), 199–205.

Bree, A., Campling, P. and Liderth, S. (2003) Empowerment in mental health: the therapeutic community model. In: *Empowerment and the Health Service User* (eds. J. Dooher and R. Byrt), Chapter 10. Quay, Salisbury.

Byrt, R. (1999) Nursing: the psychosocial environment. In: *Therapeutic Communities: Past, Present and Future* (eds. P. Campling and R. Haigh), Chapter 5. Jessica Kingsley, London.

Byrt, R. (2006) Nursing interventions in therapeutic communities. In: *Forensic Mental Health Nursing: Interventions with People with 'Personality Disorder'* (ed. National Forensic Nurses' Research and Development Group), Chapter 14. Quay, London.

Byrt, R., Wray, C. and 'Tom' (2005) Towards hope and inclusion: nursing interventions in a medium secure service for men with 'personality disorders'. *Mental Health Practice*, **8**(8), 38–43.

Collins, M. and Munroe, P. (2004) Preventing and managing violence and aggression in in-patient settings. In: *From Toxic Institutions to Therapeutic Environments: Residential Settings in Mental Health Services* (eds. P. Campling, S. Davies and G. Farquharson), Chapter 13. Gaskell, London.

Crockford, H. A., Brunton, J. and Surgenor, T. E. (2003) Clinical effectiveness of an acute psychiatric day hospital run on therapeutic community lines. *Therapeutic Communities*, **24**(1), 37–54.

Cross, D. and Kirby, S. (2002) Using psychoeducational interventions within an integrated psychological approach to forensic mental health and social care. In: *Therapeutic Interventions for Forensic Mental Health Nurses* (eds. A. M. Kettles, P. Woods and M. Collins), Chapter 5. Jessica Kingsley, London.

Davies, S. (2004) Secure psychiatric services. In: *From Toxic Institutions to Therapeutic Environments: Residential Settings in Mental Health Services* (eds. P. Campling, S. Davies and G. Farquharson), Chapter 23. Gaskell, London.

Davies, S., Bennion, L., McPhee, D., Osgerby, C. and Wylie, B. (2005) Cedars Community: using a therapeutic community approach in a high security hospital. *Therapeutic Communities*, **26**(2), 139–49.

Department of Health (2003) *Mainstreaming Gender and Women's Mental Health: Implementation Guidance*. Department of Health, London.

Dodds, P. and Bowles, N. (2001) Dismantling formal observation and refocusing nursing activity in acute psychiatry: a case study. *Journal of Psychiatric and Mental Health Nursing*, **8**(2), 183–8.

Doyle, M., Aiyegbusi, A. and Burbery, P. (2006) Personality disorder: specialist psychological approaches. In: *Forensic Mental Health Nursing: Interventions with People with 'Personality Disorder'* (ed. National Forensic Nurses' Research and Development Group), Chapter 15. Quay, London.

Ewers, P. and Ikin, P. (2002) Nursing interventions and future directions with the severely mentally ill. In: *Therapeutic Interventions for Forensic Mental Health Nurses* (eds. A. M. Kettles, P. Woods and M. Collins), Chapter 6. Jessica Kingsley, London.

Fahy, K. and Dudley, M. (2000) An introduction to psychosocial interventions. In: *Lyttle's Mental Health and Disorder* (eds. T. Thompson and P. Mathias), Chapter 9. Baillière Tindall/Royal College of Nursing, Edinburgh.

Firth, W. (2004) Acute psychiatric wards: an overview. In: *From Toxic Institutions to Therapeutic Environments: Residential Settings in Mental Health Services* (eds. P. Campling, S. Davies and G. Farquharson), Chapter 17. Gaskell, London.

Forchuk, C. and Jensen, E. (2003) The person who hears disturbing voices. In: *Psychiatric and Mental Health Nursing: The Craft of Caring* (ed. P. Barker), Chapter 30. Arnold, London.

Gale, J. and Sanchez, B. (2005) Reflections on the treatment of psychosis in therapeutic communities. *Therapeutic Communities*, **26**(4), 485–94.

Gamble, C. and Brennan, W. (eds.) (2006) *Working with Serious Mental Illness*, 2nd edn. Baillière Tindall, Edinburgh.

Gamble, C. with Curthoys, J. (2004) Psychosocial interventions. In: *The Art and Science of Mental Health Nursing: a Textbook of Principles and Practice* (eds. I. Norman and I. Ryrie), Chapter 14. Open University Press, Maidenhead.

Gega, L. (2004) Behavioural techniques. In: *The Art and Science of Mental Health Nursing: a Textbook of Principles and Practice* (eds. I. Norman and I. Ryrie), Chapter 24. Open University Press, Maidenhead.

Genders, E. and Player, E. (1995) *Grendon: a Study of a Therapeutic Prison*. Clarendon Press, Oxford.

Gillam, T. (2001) Listening to what Simon says. *Mental Health and Learning Disability Care*, **4**(7), 237–9.

Gillam, T. (2002) Treating schizophrenia: how psychosocial interventions can complement medication. *Mental Health Practice*, **6**(4), 28–32.

Gilligan, J. (2001) *Preventing Violence*. Thames and Hudson, London.

Gournay, K. (1999) Management of schizophrenia. *Mental Health Practice*, **2**(9), 33–8.

Harris, G. T., Rice, M. E. and Cormier, C. A. (1994) Psychopaths: is a therapeutic community therapeutic? *Therapeutic Communities*, **15**(4), 283–99.

Harris, N., Williams, S. and Bradshaw, T. (eds.) (2002) *Psychosocial Interventions for People with Schizophrenia: a Practical Guide for Mental Health Workers*. Palgrave Macmillan, Basingstoke.

Hartman, D. and Smith, L. (2002) Developing community groupwork on a locked psychiatric intensive care unit. *Therapeutic Communities*, **23**(1), 5–16.

Holmes, J. (2004) What can psychotherapy contribute to improving the culture on acute wards? In: *From Toxic Institutions to Therapeutic Environments: Residential Settings in Mental Health Services* (eds. P. Campling, S. Davies and G. Farquharson), Chapter 20. Gaskell, London.

Keen, T. (2003) The person with schizophrenia. In: *Psychiatric and Mental Health Nursing: The Craft of Caring* (ed. P. Barker), Chapter 32. Arnold, London.

Kelly, S., McKenna, H. and Parahoo, K. (2001) The relationship between involvement in activities and quality of life for people with severe and enduring mental illness. *Journal of Psychiatric and Mental Health Nursing*, **8**, 139–46.

Kelly, S., Hill, J., Boardman, H. and Overton, I. (2004) Therapeutic communities. In: *From Toxic Institutions to Therapeutic Environments: Residential Settings in Mental Health Services* (eds. P. Campling, S. Davies and G. Farquharson), Chapter 25. Gaskell, London.

Kennard, D. (1998) *An Introduction to Therapeutic Communities*. Jessica Kingsley, London.

Kent, M. (2005) My mental health. *Mental Health Practice*, **8**(8), 22.

Kettles, A. M., Woods, P. and Collins, M. (eds.) (2002) *Therapeutic Interventions for Forensic Mental Health Nurses*. Jessica Kingsley, London.

Kirby, S. (1997) Ward atmosphere on a medium secure long-stay ward. *Journal of Forensic Psychiatry*, **8**(2), 336–47.

Lees, J., Manning, N. and Rawlings, B. (2004) Therapeutic community research: an overview and meta-analysis. In: *A Culture of Enquiry: Research Evidence and the Therapeutic Community* (eds. J. Lees, N. Manning, D. Menzies and N. Morant), Chapter 2. Jessica Kingsley, London.

Lehmann, P. (2001) Coming off neuroleptics. In: *This is Madness Too: Critical Perspectives on Mental Health Services* (eds. C. Newnes *et al.*), Chapter 8. PCCS Books, Ross-on-Wye.

Liderth, S. (2003) Untitled section. In: Empowerment in mental health: the therapeutic community model (A. Bree, P. Campling and S. Liderth) in: *Empowerment and the Health Service User* (eds. J. Dooher and R. Byrt), Chapter 10. Quay, Salisbury.

Mason, T. and Mercer, D. (eds.) (1998) *Critical Perspectives in Forensic Care: Inside Out*. Macmillan, Basingstoke.

McKeown, M. and McCann, G. (2000) Psychosocial interventions. In: *Forensic Mental Health Nursing: Current Approaches* (eds. C. Chaloner and M. Coffey), Chapter 12. Blackwell Science, Oxford.

McKeown, M. *et al.* (2002) PSIs in institutional settings. In: *Psychosocial Interventions for People with Schizophrenia: a Practical Guide for Mental Health Workers* (eds. N. Harris, S. Williams and T. Bradshaw), Chapter 16. Palgrave Macmillan, Basingstoke.

McKenzie, B. M. (2001) Psychological approaches to longer-term patients presenting with challenging behaviours. In: *Psychiatric Intensive Care* (eds. M. D. Beer, S. M. Pereira and C. Paton), Chapter 6B. Greenwich Medical Media, London.

McMillan, I. (2006) Wards improved when changes embraced. *Mental Health Practice*, **9**(6), 4.

McMurran, M., Egan, V. and Ahmadi, S. (1998) A retrospective evaluation of a therapeutic community for mentally disordered offenders. *Journal of Forensic Psychiatry*, **9**,103–13.

Meehan, T., McIntosh, W. and Bergen, H. (2006) Aggressive behavior in high-secure settings: the perceptions of patients. *Journal of Psychiatric and Mental Health Nursing*, **13**(1), 19–25.

Mental Health Foundation and Sainsbury Centre for Mental Health (2002) *Being There in a Crisis: a Report of the Learning from Eight Mental Health Crisis Services*. Mental Health Foundation and Sainsbury Centre for Mental Health, London.

Middelboe, T., Schjødt, T., Byrsting, K. and Gjerris, A. (2001) Ward atmosphere in acute psychiatric in-patient care: patients' perceptions, ideals and satisfaction. *Acta Psychiatrica Scandinavica*, **103**, 212–19.

Mills, J., Kerr, S. and Goldspink, S. (2006) Dealing with blankness and deadness. In: *Working with Serious Mental Illness*, 2nd edn (eds. C. Gamble and W. Brennan), Chapter 12. Baillière Tindall, Edinburgh.

Modernisation Agency Clinical Governance Support Team (2005) *Case Study. Finding the Ways to a Service User-Centred Mental Health Service. Improving In-Patient Services at North Essex Mental Health Partnership NHS Trust*. Accessed 18 September 2005 through: `http://www.cgsupport.nhs.uk/`.

Morrison, E. (1992) A coercive interactional style as an antecedent to aggression in psychiatric patients. *Research in Nursing and Health*, **15**(6), 421–31.

National Institute for Health and Clinical Excellence (NICE) (2002) *Core Interventions in the Treatment and Management of Schizophrenia in Primary and Secondary Care*. NICE, London.

Norton, K. (2004) The therapeutic milieu. In: *The Art and Science of Mental Health Nursing: A Textbook of Principles and Practice* (eds. I. Norman and I. Ryrie), Chapter 9. Open University Press, Maidenhead.

Norton, K. and Warren, F. (2004) Assessing outcome at Henderson Hospital. In: *A Culture of Enquiry: Research Evidence and the Therapeutic Community* (eds. J. Lees, N. Manning, D. Menzies and N. Morant), Chapter 14. Jessica Kingsley, London.

Paget, S. and White, T. (2004) Connecting with the natural environment. In: *From Toxic Institutions to Therapeutic Environments: Residential Settings in Mental Health Services* (eds. P. Campling, S. Davies and G. Farquharson), Chapter 8. Gaskell, London.

Raguram, R. *et al.* (2002) Traditional and community resources for mental health: a report of temple healing from India. *British Medical Journal*, **325**(7354), 38.

Rawlings, B. (2005) Researching therapeutic communities in secure settings. *Therapeutic Communities*, **26**(4), 465–83.

Reiss, D., Grubin, D. and Meux, C. (1996) Young 'psychopaths' in special hospital: treatment outcome. *British Journal of Psychiatry*, **168**(1), 99–104.

Riordan, S. (2005) Multidisciplinary statutory follow-up of conditionally discharged patients. In: *Multidisciplinary Working in Forensic Mental Health Care* (eds. S. Wix and M. Humphreys), Chapter 6C. Elsevier Churchill Livingstone, Edinburgh.

Rogers, A. and Pilgrim, D. (2003) *Mental Health and Inequality*. Palgrave Macmillan, Basingstoke.

Romme, M. and Esher, S. (2000) *Making Sense of Voices: the Mental Health Professional's Guide to Work with Voice Hearers*. Mind, London.

Rose, D. (2001) *Users' Voices: The Perspectives of Mental Health Service Users on Community and Hospital Care*. The Sainsbury Centre for Mental Health, London.

Rossberg, J. I. and Friis, S. (2004) Patients' and staff's perceptions of the psychiatric ward environment. *Psychiatric Services*, **55**(7), 798–803.

Ruocchio, P. (1991) First person account: the schizophrenia inside. *Schizophrenia Bulletin*, **17**(2), 359. Quoted in Watkins, J. (1996) *Living with Schizophrenia: and Holistic Approach to Understanding, Preventing and Recovering from Negative Symptoms*. Hill of Content, Melbourne.

Sainsbury Centre for Mental Health (2006) *The Search for Acute Solutions. Improving the Quality of Care in Acute Psychiatric Wards*. Sainsbury Centre for Mental Health, London.

Siddle, R. and Everitt, J. (2002) Identifying and overcoming negative symptoms. In: *Psychosocial Interventions for People with Schizophrenia: a Practical Guide for Mental Health Workers* (eds. N. Harris, S. Williams and T. Bradshaw), Chapter 9. Palgrave Macmillan, Basingstoke.

Thrive (2006) Website home page. http://www.thrive.org.uk/. Accessed 14 April 2006.

Timko, C. and Moos, R. H. (2004) Measuring the therapeutic environment. In: *From Toxic Institutions to Therapeutic Environments: Residential Settings in Mental Health Services* (eds. P. Campling, S. Davies and G. Farquharson), Chapter 14. Gaskell, London.

Tucker, S. (ed.) (2000) *A Therapeutic Community Approach to Care in the Community: Dialogue and Dwelling*. Jessica Kingsley, London.

Turner, T. (2003) *Your Questions Answered. Schizophrenia*. Churchill Livingstone, Edinburgh.

Warren, F., Evans, C., Dolan, B. and Norton, K. (2004) Impulsivity and self-damaging behaviour in severe personality disorder: the impact of democratic therapeutic community treatment. *Therapeutic Communities*, **25**(1), 55–72.

Watkins, J. (1996) *Living with Schizophrenia: an Holistic Approach to Understanding, Preventing and Recovering from Negative Symptoms*. Hill of Content, Melbourne.

Watters, S. (1996) A patient's life in the day of a psychiatric nurse. Poem. In: *Sweet, Sour and Serious: Illustrated Anthology* (Survivors' Poetry, Scotland), p. 26. Survivors' Press, Glasgow.

Whittington, R. (2000) Changing the environment in the management of aggression. In: *Forensic Mental Health Care: a Case Study Approach* (eds. D. Mercer, T. Mason, M. McKeown and G. McCann). Churchill Livingstone, Edinburgh.

CHAPTER 5

Preventing and reducing violence and aggression

Richard Byrt and Mike Doyle

This chapter considers the meaning of aggression and violence, their causes and triggers and relevant nursing/multidisciplinary interventions.

Basic values and principles

Firstly, it is proposed that all assessment and interventions to prevent and reduce violence and aggression need to be informed by values and principles in the following list. This is based on the authors' nursing practice, much of the relevant literature, and several recent reports on violence and aggression (National Institute for Clinical Excellence (NICE), 2005; National Institute for Mental Health in England (NIMHE), 2004; Blofeld, 2003; Royal College of Psychiatrists Audit Team, 2005; Turnbull and Paterson, 1999a). It is proposed that the following are crucial:

- Valuing and respecting the client and her/his individuality, uniqueness, diversity and dignity.
- Ensuring safety and minimising risk (i.e. the likelihood of harm) to the client, other service users, visitors, staff, students and members of the public.
- Ensuring that all interventions follow the Nursing and Midwifery Council (NMC) Code of Professional Conduct, are legal and respect clients' rights (e.g. under the Human Rights Act 1998, the Children Acts of 1989 and 2004 (in relation to children and young people) and the Mental Health Acts for the various countries of the UK).
- Ensuring that all interventions involve the least amount of restrictions necessary to ensure the safety and health of the client and others.
- Ensuring non-verbal and verbal communication that conveys respect and an appreciation of the client's perspective, experiences and feelings.
- Providing holistic assessments and nursing/multidisciplinary interventions which take account of the individual's varied needs and problems (biological, psychological, social, spiritual, cultural, psychosexual, economic, legal) and their influence on violence and aggression.
- Ensuring that assessment and interventions:
  - Enable the client's participation and views, as much as possible.

  - Are sensitive to her/his culture, ethnic group, religion, gender, age, sexual orientation, gender identity, specific problems, and level of intellectual, cognitive, physical and sensory ability.
- Ensuring recognition of distress that may underlie, or contribute to, violence and aggression, with interventions to relieve this distress.
- Providing interventions within a therapeutic framework to inform both short-term and long-term interventions.
- This therapeutic framework, and all nursing and multidisciplinary assessments and interventions should be:
  - Acceptable, as far as possible, to clients and their carers, and incorporate their views.
  - Based on the experiences of clients, carers and professionals in relation to what works in practice.
  - Based on valid and reliable risk assessments.
  - Based on evidence, from research and audit findings, of what works.
  - Delivered by staff who have high-quality clinical supervision, support and education to enable self-awareness, positive attitudes and reflection in, and on, their practice.

Box 5.1 Points for consideration/discussion

- To what extent do you agree or disagree with each of the 'basic values and principles' on the above list?
- Are there any other values and principles that you would add to this list?

Definitions of aggression and violence

Some authors do not define aggression or violence, or use the two terms interchangeably (Rippon, 2000). However, several authors distinguish between:

- **Aggression** as the *intention* to cause harm.
- **Violence** as *actual* harm (physical harm; some definitions also include verbal abuse) caused by an individual (NICE, 2005; Turnbull and Paterson, 1999b)

> ... If the perpetrator had intended to cause harm to the other person, these actions could be described as aggressive, whether or not the victim suffered injury.... Where physical injury is suffered and the perpetrator intends to inflict this harm, this would be construed as violence... (Turnbull and Paterson, 1999b, pp. 2–3).

In addition, definitions of violence often include reference to the illegal use of force (Mason and Chandley, 1999, p. 6; NICE, 2005, p. 5) and the illegitimate use of power, including 'threats and intimidation... neglect and all types of physical, sexual and psychological abuse' (World Health Organization, 2002, p. 5). Some definitions of violence also include verbal abuse, including discriminatory language, in addition to physical assaults. Research suggests that, for some staff, verbal abuse may cause as much distress as physical injury (Health Services Advisory Committee, 1997, p. 2; Royal College of Nursing, 1998).

Box 5.2 indicates reasons why it is important to clearly define and measure incidents of violence and aggression, in relation to the care of forensic patients in acute mental health services.

Box 5.2 Why it is important to clearly define and measure incidents of aggression and violence in acute mental health services (Rippon, 2000; Rogers et *al.*, 1999)

- Clear, standard definitions and categorisations of incidents enable accurate measurement of the extent to which different types of aggression and violence occur in various health settings.
- Accurate estimates enable managers, staff, the Department of Health, professional associations and trade unions to have accurate information on which to base decisions for further resources (e g, increases in staffing and measures to ensure safety and staff support and training).
- These increased resources may have positive impacts on:
- The care and safety of patients and visitors.
- The safety, morale and retention of staff.
- Health and Safety at Work and related legislation requires that incidents are accurately recorded and monitored, with subsequent action to prevent staff injuries from violence and aggression.
- Department of Health, and local policy require the recording of incidents in the event of litigation or insurance claims.

Ways of expressing anger

Anger has been defined as an emotion subjectively experienced by the individual, accompanied by physiological changes. The latter are normally experienced as unpleasant by the individual. The individual, and others observing him/her usually perceive that he/she is 'angry' (Sookoo, 2004).

Various authors have distinguished between assertive, passive and aggressive anger (Duxbury, 2000; Tschudin and Schober, 1998). However, statements about assertive behaviours in the literature sometimes appear to be unsupported by research findings and often fail to consider the cultural context. What is seen as assertive in one social or cultural group may be viewed as aggressive or passive in another (Arnold, 2003b).

The relevance of assertive and other expressions of anger to nursing and multidisciplinary interventions

Research suggests that violence and aggression can be successfully prevented and achieved when practitioners are assertive (e.g. setting clear limits to ensure safety where necessary, but doing so calmly, politely and respecting the patient, client or visitor and his/her rights as an individual (McDougall, 1998; Turnbull and Paterson, 1999a). In contrast, studies have found that both staff aggression in the form of authoritarian (unnecessarily restrictive) attitudes (Morrison, 1992) and failure to make safe limits and structure clear (Whittington, 2000), can contribute to, or worsen, violence and aggression.

Patients who are assertive have sometimes been pathologised (Goffman, 1968; Pilgrim and Rogers, 2005) and labelled by practitioners as aggressive, 'difficult' or 'unpopular'. Patients seen as 'difficult' include those who complain, are justifiably assertive or have health choices that differ from those of professionals (Duxbury, 2000; Stockwell, 1972). In contrast, the value of mental health patients' creative anger has been outlined (Hopton, 1995):

> Nurses must accept that successful programmes are likely to lead patients to question nursing interventions.... Conflicts can arise between patients and.... staff, who may wrongly attribute patients' assertiveness to 'non-compliance', rather than seeing it as a reflection of growing independence.... Unless these misunderstandings are resolved, patients can become increasingly frustrated, lose control and become verbally or even physically aggressive... (Warner, 1992, p. 46).

A proposed model to consider factors causing/contributing to violence and aggression and related interventions

It is proposed that effective interventions to prevent and reduce violence and aggression need to consider the factors identified in Figure 5.1:

- All aspects of mental health nursing and multi-professional assessment and interventions are relevant to ensuring the safety of patients, visitors, students and staff – including the interventions outlined in this chapter.
- Ensuring safety of the individual patient and others is the basis of all nursing and multidisciplinary interventions with forensic mental health patients (Dale and Gardner, 2001; Doyle and Duffy, 2006; West and Abolins, 2003).

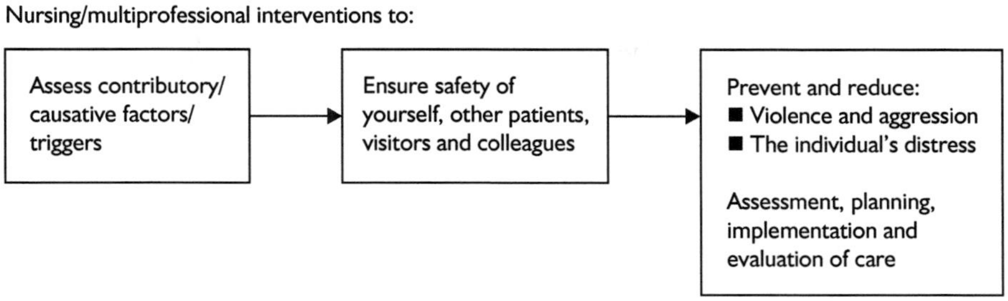

Figure 5.1 A proposed model to consider factors causing/contributing to violence and aggression and related interventions

Causative and contributory factors and triggers

A distinction can be made between causative factors, contributory factors and triggers.

Causative factors

Causative or aetiological factors directly result in violence or aggression, e.g:

- A young man who is diabetic, and who becomes (uncharacteristically) aggressive as a result of hyperglycaemia (high blood sugar).
- A woman who is violent only in response to persecutory auditory hallucinations which cause her considerable distress.

It is not intended, from the above examples, to suggest that most individuals with diabetes or mental illness are violent and aggressive. (See Appleby *et al.* (2001) and Rogers and Pilgrim (2003) for reviews of research findings that there is little or no association between most mental health problems and violence. Exceptions relate to individuals with antisocial personality disorder, or with certain types of paranoid delusion; and people with problematic use of alcohol and other drugs: Doyle and Duffy (2006), Rogers and Pilgrim (2003)).

Contributory factors

In some individuals, there appear to be clear causative factors, as in the above examples. However, in many instances, it is difficult to isolate these. A variety of contributory factors, rather than specific causes, is sometimes found to be associated with the aggressive or violent behaviours of some patients (Whittington, 2000).

Triggers

Triggers are factors that precipitate an episode of aggression or violence (Paterson and Leadbetter, 1999). In some cases, triggers are 'the last straw that broke the camel's back'. An example would be an anxious visitor ('Mr Brown') who has been kept waiting for his partner's Primary Nurse to discuss his queries. He has had an hour's wait, in a dingy room, with no explanation or apology, and no access to a drink, increasing the dry mouth resulting from his anxiety. He also has no access to a telephone to explain to his boss that he has been delayed. The trigger ('last straw') precipitating aggression could be an abrupt, off-hand response from the nurse when they eventually meet.

The NICE (2005, p. 17) Guideline comments:

> Efforts should be made to ascertain the service user's own views about their trigger factors, early warning signs of... violent behaviour and other vulnerabilities, and the management of these. Sensitive and timely feedback should complete this process.

Explanatory models: separate or integrated?

Various models have been produced to explain causative/contributory factors and triggers of violence and aggression, and to inform associated interventions. These models relate to one or more of the following factors:

- Biological
- Psychiatric
- Psychological/interpersonal
- Cultural
- Issues of diversity and discrimination
- Spiritual
- Social (organisational)
- Demographic
- Societal
- Sociological

Recently, it has been argued that, in the prevention and reduction of violence and aggression, it is necessary to consider a wide variety of the above factors (Crichton, 1995; NICE, 2005).

For convenience, the factors listed above will now be considered separately. However, clearly (as with the example of 'Mr Brown', the anxious visitor described above), there are often a variety of different factors that contribute to a particular incident of violent or aggressive behaviour.

Biological models

Biological models include consideration of neurological, hormonal, genetic and physiological factors. Biological models examine, for example, ways in which violence and aggression may be caused by physical illnesses; biochemical and other changes in mental illness; and alcohol and other drugs (Turnbull, 1999).

Parts of the brain concerned with violent and aggressive feelings and behaviours include (Wilson, 2003):

- The amygdala in the temporal lobe
- The pre-frontal cortex in the frontal lobe
- The hypothalamus at the base of the cerebrum

Violence and aggression can result when these areas are damaged. Damage to the frontal lobe can affect violent and aggressive feelings and behaviours, particularly if the individual's judgement, including interpretation of others' intentions, is affected (Wilson, 2003). Amongst forensic mental health patients, there may occasionally be damage to the amygdala, pre-frontal cortex and hypothalamus. This can be caused by, for example, by (Wilson, 2003):

- Cerebral tumours in these areas
- Head injury from severe road traffic accidents, gunshot wounds, birth injury and other factors
- Strokes
- Types of dementia
- Some forms of epilepsy (e.g. 'complex partial seizures' (previously called 'temporal lobe epilepsy'): (Turnbull, 1999, pp. 32ff)

Low levels of the neurotransmitter serotonin, but high levels of the neurotransmitters norepinephrine and dopamine, have been found to be linked with high levels of aggression (Wilson, 2003, p. 390). A neurotransmitter is 'a chemical message passing from one neuron (nerve cell) to another' (Gray and Bressington, 2004, quoted in Byrt and Woods, 2006, p. 4). Excessive amounts of dopamine have been found in individuals with schizophrenia. Antipsychotic medication which reduces dopamine may result in diminished violence and aggression in the minority of clients with schizophrenia with such behaviours. This is partly because of the effects of antipsychotics in reducing symptoms, such as delusions and hallucinations, which may result in violence or aggression (Gelder *et al.*, 2001).

A large number of physical health problems are occasionally associated with violence and aggression. These include:

- The effects of alcohol and other drugs, and withdrawal from these substances: factors which considerably increases the risk of violence and aggression (Kettles, 2006).
- Delirium (acute confusional state), with many causes: e.g. following a severe infection in an individual who was severely under-nourished (Shepherd, 2001).
- Hyperglycaemia (raised blood sugar) in individuals with diabetes (Shepherd, 2001).

Psychiatric models

Biological models of violence and aggression include some psychiatric models which explain violence and aggression largely in relation to the individual's health problems, including physical illness; personality disorder; biochemical and other changes in mental illness; and problematic use of alcohol and other drugs (Gilligan, 2001; Turnbull, 1999).

Psychological models

Some psychological models are concerned with the influence of personality on propensities to be violent and aggressive (Smith *et al.*, 2003; Turnbull, 1999). Other psychological models include the following:

- **Frustration**: discomfort from the individual's failure to attain a desired goal (Turnbull, 1999; Whittington, 2000).
- Models based on **social learning theory** and behaviourism postulate that violence and aggression are learnt behaviours: e.g. the individual discovers that they bring rewards or fail to result in sanctions (Turnbull, 1999; Whittington, 2000).
- The **cognitive behavioural** model is concerned with 'how the interaction of external events, internal process [e.g. thoughts] and emotions combines to produce behaviour' (Turnbull, 1999, p. 47). This model has implications for cognitive behavioural therapies to enable people to manage and express their anger creatively, avoiding harm to themselves and others (Byrt *et al.*, 2005; Doyle *et al.*, 2006).
- **Interpersonal** and **social psychological** models are concerned with relationships and modes of communication and their influence on violence and aggression. The literature suggests that certain aspects of non-verbal and verbal communication can prevent or reduce (de-escalate) violence and aggression (Paterson and Leadbetter, 1999).
- **Psychodynamic** models postulate the existence of an unconscious part of the mind. This is outside the individual's conscious awareness, but has an effect on his/her behaviour. According to these models, violence and aggression are influenced by unconscious and unresolved conflicts concerning parents and other people significant in the individual's life (Braithwaite, 2001). Sigmund Freud and his followers are the main proponents of this model.
- **Attachment** models, which reflect psychodynamic theory, postulate that violence and aggression are a way of communicating distress, caused, at least in part, by a lack of 'attachments' with parents or other adults in parental roles. Some individuals with 'personality disorder' have a lack of attachment in early childhood, often with multiple neglect and abuse (Jeffcote and Watson, 2004). Where such experiences are associated with antisocial personality disorder, there is a propensity for increased violence and aggression (National Forensic Nurses' Research and Development Group, 2006).

Cultural and diversity models

Models involving cultural factors and issues concerning diversity and discrimination are partly concerned with anger in response to oppression and discriminatory practices in wider society and within health services (Dooher and Byrt, 2003). Some recent reports on violence and aggression have emphasised the need to consider cultural factors in nursing/multi-professional assessments and interventions (Blofeld, 2003; NICE, 2005; NIMHE, 2004; Royal College of Psychiatrists Audit Team, 2005).

Models concerned with spirituality

Models concerned with spirituality are concerned to make sense of individuals' violence and aggression, in part, by understanding the meaning that violence and aggression has for them (Addo, 2006; Swinton, 2002). For example, the need to present as tough and 'not to be messed with' might be crucial for survival and provide a sense of identity for individuals who have experienced violence in their families or in prisons/young offenders' institutions (Meehan *et al.*, 2006).

Social models

Social (sometimes called ecological, environmental and organisational) models are concerned with aspects of social and physical environments and their influence on violence and aggression, both within health services and in wider society. Researchers in this area have examined, for example:

- Social factors such as too little or too much activity, waiting times and staff–client/patient communication, attitudes, roles and relationships.
- The effects of noise, décor, temperature, crowding and other physical variables (Whittington, 2000).

Demographic and societal models

Demographic models examine the influence on violence and aggression of such factors as individuals' age, gender, ethnic group and social class (Turnbull, 1999).

Societal models are concerned with the influence of social factors on violence and aggression, including poverty, housing, educational achievement and work opportunities and unemployment (Gilligan, 2001; World Health Organization, 2002).

Sociological models

Sociological models examine the influence of people in wider society on individuals' perceived violence and aggression. Some 'sociologists of deviance' are concerned with why and how certain people, and not others, are construed as 'violent' (e.g. why are some behaviours described in this way, but others, causing as much harm, are socially accepted?) (Pilgrim and Rogers, 2005).

Sociologists are also concerned with ways in which people's apparently violent behaviours are a response to others' labelling or stigmatising them in various ways (Pilgrim and Rogers, 2005).

Box 5.3 Questions for consideration/discussion

1. What models do: (a) clients and (b) staff use mainly to explain violence and aggression in your area of practice?
2. Do you think any other of the models outlined in this chapter would be useful in understanding forensic patients' violence and aggression in acute mental health settings?

Aspects of nursing and multidisciplinary interventions in preventing and reducing (de-escalating) violence and aggression

Nursing and multidisciplinary interventions in preventing and reducing (de-escalating) violence and aggression all aim to both:

- Ensure the safety of the individual with violent or aggressive behaviours, other clients, carers, staff and students
- Reduce the distress of the individual with violent or aggressive behaviours
  The rest of this chapter will consider particular interventions.

Ensuring safety

Underpinning all interventions to prevent and reduce violence and aggression, is the need to ensure safety, at all times, of (Willis and Gillett, 2003):

- The individual displaying violence or aggression
- Yourself

- Other patients/visitors
- Staff and students

Whilst the NMC (2004) Code of Professional Conduct does not mention violence and aggression explicitly, it indicates that Registered Nurses have a duty of care, both to the client with violent or aggressive behaviours and to other clients to 'act to identify and minimise the risk to patients and clients' (NMC, 2004, Clauses 1.4, and 8, pp. 4 and 11).

The following principles to ensure safety are based on the authors' nursing practice experience and the literature (NHS Security Management Service, 2005a; Turnbull and Paterson, 1999; Willis and Gillett, 2003):

- Of relevance in ensuring safety are all aspects of communication and other good nursing practice, and all of the principles and values outlined at the beginning of the chapter and in the literature (NHS Security Management Service, 2005a).
- Avoid isolating yourself with patients (e.g. in rooms distant from colleagues), particularly if it is assessed that the individual is likely to become violent or aggressive.
- A minimum of three staff, with appropriate skills, need to be available for nursing interventions with clients likely to be physically violent.
- The appropriate manager should be informed if there are staff shortages in such circumstances.
- Patients who are likely to be violent or aggressive should be cared for in areas where they can be easily observed and engaged with.
- When working with patients in general, but particularly with those likely to be violent or aggressive:
  - Place yourself in a position where you can easily leave via the nearest exit.
  - Avoid having your back to the patient.
  - Do not put yourself in positions where you could easily be backed into a corner or against a wall.
  - See patients/visitors likely to be violent or aggressive with at least one colleague – with other colleagues near at hand, if needed.

Provision of safe and otherwise beneficial ward environments

Violence and aggression can be reduced by ensuring that acute mental health environments have the following (Bowers *et al.*, 2002; National Institute for Health and Clinical Excellence, 2005; Royal College of Psychiatrists Audit Team, 2005):

- Wards designed to facilitate observation, with:
  - Safe furnishings and fixtures
  - Attractive, culturally appropriate décor and furnishings
- Provision of rooms for quiet and reduction of arousal and sensory overload (see Chapter 4)
- Seclusion rooms that enable observation and have levels of ventilation, humidity and temperature, and safe lavatories and wash basins, in accordance with Department of Health requirements

- Opportunities for clients to:
  - Express feelings and concerns safely
  - Engage in meaningful activities (This is particularly emphasised in NICE, 2005)
  - Exercise choice, within the parameters of safety

Risk assessment and risk management

Frequent, valid and reliable **risk assessment** helps to ensure safety. Risk assessment can be defined as evaluation of the extent to which patients are likely to put themselves or others in danger: e.g. through self-harm or neglect of self or through violence and aggression towards others (Doyle and Duffy, 2006). Risk assessment includes observation with engagement (Jones and Jackson, 2004; Kettles and Woodally, 2006); and, with other assessments, can be used to inform the planning, implementation and evaluation of care to address factors associated with violence and aggression and their **risk management** (Doyle and Duffy, 2006). The latter term refers to all interventions to reduce behaviours that result in harm to self or others (Doyle and Duffy, 2006; Morgan and Wetherell, 2004).

Risk assessment aims to both:

- Evaluate, as accurately as possible, the extent that the individual is likely to be violent and/or aggressive. (This involves the use of valid and reliable measures of risk: see p. 000 for definitions of validity and reliability).
- Ensure that the individual is not stigmatised or labelled as 'dangerous' or 'always violent' (Morgan and Wetherell, 2004).

In relation to the second point, high-quality risk assessment and risk management include the recognition that the individual's level of risk of violence or aggression will change over time (Doyle and Duffy, 2006), with the aim of empowering the individual to use positive coping strategies to relieve distressing symptoms or problems associated with increased risk. The aims of interventions are to reduce not only the risk to others and to the patient, but to reduce his/her distress, and to provide holistic care, based on respect for the individual and his/her various needs, including those related to diversity.

Specific aspects of violence risk assessment

It is not surprising that institutional violence has increasingly been the focus of research interest. Key factors identified in the literature as showing associations with institutional violence include: young age (James *et al.*, 1990; Kennedy *et al.*, 1995; Beauford *et al.*, 1997; Hoptman *et al.*, 1999); a previous history of violence and/or criminality (Krakowski *et al.*, 1989; Palmstierna and Wistedt, 1989; Walker and Seifert, 1994; Kennedy *et al.*, 1995; Soliman and Reza, 2001) and a history of threatening behaviour immediately preceding admission to hospital (McNiel *et al.*, 1988;

McNiel and Binder, 1989; Beauford *et al.*, 1997; Hoptman *et al.*, 1999). Although substance abuse has been shown to be associated with violence in a number of studies (Palmstierna and Wistedt, 1989; Hoptman *et al.*, 1999; Young *et al.*, 1999; Soliman and Reza, 2001), it remains unclear which substances exert the most notable effect. It is now recognised that psychopathy (Doyle *et al.*, 2002; Hill *et al.*, 1996; Young *et al.*, 1999) and personality disorder in general (Soliman and Reza, 2001) also show significant associations with violence, while childhood sexual abuse has also been found to be significant (Hoptman *et al.*, 1999).

From a psychopathological perspective, institutional violence has also been found to be associated with positive symptoms of psychosis, such as paranoid and threat-control override symptoms (Lowenstein *et al.*, 1990; Hoptman *et al.*, 1999; Link *et al.*, 1999) and general disturbances in mental state (Lowenstein *et al.*, 1990; McNiel and Binder, 1994) including confusion, irritability, threats of violence and verbal abuse (Noble and Rodger, 1989; Linaker and Busch-Iverson, 1995; Whittingham and Patterson, 1996). Research suggests that assessment tools, such as the six-item Broset Violence Checklist (Linaker and Busch-Iverson, 1995), that focus on the latter psychopathological and behavioural associations indicate reasonable predictive accuracy for violence 24 hours after assessment (Almvik and Woods, 1998). Anger and hostility, as factors influencing violent behaviour, have received relatively little attention in the literature, despite evidence that patients with high anger ratings are significantly more assaultative in institutions (Novaco, 1994; Novaco, 2003) than those with low anger ratings.

However, there are a number of methodological concerns that limit our ability to draw firm conclusions from the current literature. Studies vary considerably in terms of setting, patient sampling and characteristics, period covered, choice of putative predictors, scales used, methods of analysis, competence of other methods of care and level of detail provided (Royal College of Psychiatrists, 1998). Also, it is clear that, as a result of risk management measures, the rate of inpatient violence tends to diminish the longer the person remains in hospital (Heilbrun *et al.*, 1998). Although research aimed at identifying risk factors for violence in inpatient populations is warranted, there is also a pressing need to investigate and understand the theoretical basis of violence, with a view to identifying potential management interventions, given that clinicians are more concerned with risk management than risk prediction (Heilbrun, 1997, 2002; Hart, 1998).

The risks of labelling

An individual can become labelled if one episode of aggression results in other people seeing him/her solely as someone who is 'dangerous', without appreciating his/her other qualities. This may culminate in the transformation of the person's identity as a 'violent' individual. According to labelling theory, this may reinforce or contribute to his/her propensity to behave violently, and the latter is said to be present, partly or wholly, in response to other people's expectations: a self-fulfilling prophecy (Pilgrim and Rogers, 2005). Labelling can occur also in 'moral panics', in which there are widespread negative, often stigmatising, attitudes in society towards people with mental health problems, all of whom are seen as having propensities to violence. This is relevant to preventing and reducing violence and aggression, partly because of the need to ensure that nurses' attitudes to particular clients/patients are not adversely affected by 'moral panics' and widespread attitudes in wider society (Byrt and Dooher, 2006; Byrt *et al.*, 2006).

Box 5.4 An example from nursing practice: Mr Clive Crimson and the relevance of labelling theory

Details have been changed, here and later in this chapter, to ensure confidentiality and the anonymity of the individual described. Examples are based on the experience of one of the authors.

I worked as an agency staff nurse on an acute admission ward, and was employed to work solely with Mr Clive Crimson. In my initial handover, staff regaled me with several stories about Clive's violence. He had assaulted several nurses, and was described as 'interfering with other patients' and a 'trouble maker'. Clive had gained a reputation for being the most violent patient on the ward, and was awaiting transfer to a medium secure unit.

In receiving this information, it was important that I recognised three things in relation to labelling theory:

- Labels can sometimes arise as a result of an individual's behaviour, rather than the reverse (Pilgrim and Rogers, 2005). It was important that I used the information in the handover to inform my assessment of the risk that Mr Crimson posed to other patients and to staff, including myself.
- I also needed to recognise the stress that Clive's behaviour had caused staff, and their need to ventilate realistic and understandable feelings and concerns about his aggression and violence (albeit in a way that did not label or stigmatise Clive).
- Whilst I needed to base my nursing interventions on an assessment of the risk Clive posed to others and to himself, I determined that I was not going to label him. I decided that I would try to ensure that my communications and relationship with Clive, and my nursing interventions, were not negatively influenced by assumptions that he would inevitably be violent – and that nothing could be done to prevent this.
- My decision to try to avoid labelling was based on awareness of the possibility that Clive's violence might influence negative attitudes of staff (including myself) which might lead to further violence: a self-fulfilling prophecy (Pilgrim and Rogers, 2005).
- Attempts to avoid labelling also made it easier for me to establish a nurse–patient relationship which included an active interest and willingness to listen to Clive and what he had to say about his writing and other interests.

Physical and psychological arousal in violence and aggression

Arousal refers to the combination of a subjective experience of a particular feeling (e.g. anger) with marked accompanying physiological changes (Smith *et al*., 2003; Wilson, 2003). The latter are often known as 'the fight or flight reaction' (Paterson and Leadbetter, 1999, p. 100). They result when, in response to an external event, neurotransmitters (chemical messages) are sent from the hypothalamus at the base of the cerebrum to the 'sympathetic nervous system, adrenal medulla, adrenal cortex [and] pituitary gland' (Smith *et al.*, 2003). The stimulation of the sympathetic nervous system and the release of 'stress hormones' results in physiological changes, which may be experienced as unpleasant. These may include (Smith *et al.*, 2003):

- Increases in:
  - Heart and pulse rate and blood pressure
  - Respiration
  - Muscle tension
  - Sweating
  - Peristalsis in stomach and intestines ('butterflies' in the stomach)
  - Urgent desire to pass urine
- Decreases in:
  - Salivation, leading to dry mouth
  - Appetite

Signs of impending violence and aggression vary according to the individual, and can be established through careful risk assessment and observation (Willis and Gillett, 2003). The individual may, for example, stare in a hostile way, pace restlessly, clench fists, raise his/her voice (Paterson and Leadbetter, 1999) and have 'facial expressions [that are] tense and angry' (NICE, 2005, p. 18). Importantly, risk assessment may reveal that the individual shows similar behaviours before each occurrence of violence (NICE, 2005), and in forensic patients this may mirror behaviours that occurred prior to offences. Where the latter is the case, this is known as **analogue behaviour**.

Patients who are aggressive or violent may also be experiencing anxiety and other unpleasant feelings, with any of the accompanying uncomfortable physical sensations, as outlined above. Nurses should bear this in mind during their interventions (Turnbull and Paterson, 1999a).

Nursing interventions to reduce physiological and psychological arousal

In responding to patients' violence and aggression, the nurse needs to be aware of:

- Her/his own state of physiological and psychological arousal (e.g. as a result of understandable anxiety).
- The state of physiological and psychological arousal of the violent or aggressive individual (Paterson and Leadbetter, 1999; Whittington, 2000).

Part of the nurse's self-awareness includes recognition of factors which are likely to reduce or increase the individual's level of arousal and escalation of violence or aggression. Triggers may increase arousal: for example, inappropriate eye contact or condescending remarks, such as 'there's no need to get angry' (Paterson and Leadbetter, 1999, p. 103).

Attention to the individual's physical, as well as psychological, needs may help to reduce arousal. The physiological concomitants of aggression are likely to be experienced as physical discomfort, which will probably be increased if there is underlying anxiety or other unpleasant feelings, as is often the case. Bearing this in mind, arousal (and consequently, violence or aggression) may be reduced in the following ways (Turnbull and Paterson, 1999a):

- Providing an opportunity to sit down, with the nurse also doing so (if this is safe).
- Providing an opportunity for the individual to talk, and be listened to (provided this is safe). In some (though not all) circumstances, this may help the individual to 'get things off his/her chest', with a consequent reduction in physical, as well as psychological, tension.
- Use of non-verbal and verbal communication skills.
- Offering a hot or cold drink. (The individual is likely to have a dry mouth. In addition to alleviating this, the drink can indicate the practitioner's caring.)
- In some circumstances, making food available, particularly if the individual has not eaten for a while and has a low blood sugar level.
- Bearing in mind health considerations, some individuals' arousal may be reduced if they have opportunities to smoke. For example, research suggests that nicotine reduces arousal from distressing symptoms in individuals with schizophrenia; McChargue *et al*., 2002). Certainly, clinical experience suggests that refusal to allow an individual to smoke could escalate violence or aggression.
- Providing diversion, channelling and safe means to communicate feelings.

De-escalation: reducing violence and aggression

The term *de-escalation* refers to the use of 'verbal and non-verbal [communication] skills' which are used to decrease the individual's violence or aggression. De-escalation has also been used to refer to 'the role of the organisation, including its culture, organisation, policies and procedures' (Paterson and Leadbetter, 1999, p. 95).

The following list is not comprehensive, but includes skills often mentioned in the literature and based on the author's clinical experience. However, research evidence for the effectiveness of some these skills appears to be limited.

1. Maintain and convey respect for the individual. This includes ability '... to convey interest in, and respect for, a person's individuality and an active involvement in their situation...' (Garnham, 2001, p. 40).
2. Demonstrate commitment to service users' rights and appreciation of their perspectives (NICE, 2005).
3. Maintain authenticity: awareness of your own feelings and reactions (Burnard, 1999).
4. Maintain active listening: conveying, through non-verbal and verbal communication, interest in what the individual is saying, avoiding interruptions or lack of interest (Arnold, 2003a).
5. Ensure careful timing of interventions. For example, if a client is aggressive, it is important not to say something which could increase this.
6. Talk quietly, but clearly. Avoid shouting or talking loudly, as this may increase violence or aggression (Leadbetter and Paterson, 1999).

7. Maintain a non-threatening body posture. (Avoid aggressive postures: e.g. standing with arms folded or hands on hips like a cowboy in a Western!)
8. Maintain appropriate, non-threatening eye contact.
9. Suggest you both sit down (provided this is safe) (Leadbetter and Paterson, 1999).
10. Ensure that the way you sit or stand does not invade the individual's personal space. (People who are aggressive may require more space than usual (Whittington, 2000). Some individuals may require varying amounts of space for cultural reasons (Arnold, 2003b)).
11. Acknowledge reasons for anger, taking care not to assume that the individual's anger is pathological or unjustified (Warner, 1992).
12. Indicate that you treat the individual, what he/she says, and the reasons for his/her anger seriously, and are prepared to help if you can (Evans and Byrt, 2003).
13. Maintain genuineness: '... respond in an open... manner which avoids stereotypes and... 'over-professional' responses' (Garnham, 2001, p. 40).
14. Try to develop empathy, with understanding of the individual's perspectives and feelings, communicating this to him/her and taking appropriate action (Garnham, 2001, p. 40; Kunyk and Olson, 2001).
15. Ensure that the individual has the right amount of information that they want – in understandable language (Arnold and Boggs, 2003; Lugton, 2002).
16. Take appropriate action in response to complaints.
17. Offer apologies and explanation, as necessary (Evans and Byrt, 2002).
18. Be aware of other feelings which may be expressed through aggression: e.g. grief, fear, anxiety (Lugton, 2002).
19. If it is safe to do so, encourage ventilation of feelings, if the individual wishes, through active listening, indication of interest and empathy, and offering support (Arnold and Boggs, 2003).
20. Monitor carefully whether this ventilation of feelings is safe. (In some cases, it may trigger further aggression; Paterson and Leadbetter, 1999).
21. Avoid remarks which may appear patronising or provocative: e.g. 'calm down', 'don't be silly' (Paterson and Leadbetter, 1999, p. 107).
22. Avoid being argumentative, challenging or discriminatory.
23. If possible, try to come up with safe solutions, acceptable to the individual, which enable him/her to maintain self-respect, without 'loss of face'. Use negotiation rather than confrontation, with attempts, as much as is practicable, to work in partnership with the client (Lowe, 1992; McDougall, 2002).
24. In both the short term and the long term, an important aim is to engender trust, and eventually establish a therapeutic alliance (Kirby and Cross, 2002).

Service users' views, rights and preferences

The literature refers to the importance of considering service users' views, rights and preferences in relation to interventions to prevent and reduce violence and aggression (Duxbury and Whittington, 2005; O'Hagan, 2004; National Institute for Health and Clinical Excellence, 2005; Royal College of Psychiatrists Audit Team, 2005). Proposals include:

- Treating all service users 'with dignity and respect' (National Institute for Health and Clinical Excellence, 2005, p. 26).
- Using the least coercive and restrictive measures in response to incidents (Meehan *et al.*, 2006; O'Hagan, 2004; Secker *et al.*, 2004).
- Information, including explanation of rights under the Mental Health Act 1983 (or of other mental health legislation outside England and Wales); complaints procedures; the availability of independent advocates; and interventions that will be used in the event of violence and aggression (National Institute for Health and Clinical Excellence, 2005).
- Giving patients the chance to write advance directives, outlining their preferences regarding 'intervention(s) they would and would not wish to receive... These should be recorded in the service user's plan and healthcare record' (National Institute for Health and Clinical Excellence, 2005, p26).
- Actively involving patients in identifying triggers and causative factors related to violence and aggression, and in interventions (National Institute for Health and Clinical Excellence, 2005).
- 'The service user should be given a copy of their care plan, and subject to their agreement, a copy should be given to their carer' (National Institute for Health and Clinical Excellence, 2005, p. 26).

Several recent reviews of violence and aggression have involved the active participation of service users and/or carers (Blofeld, 2003; National Institute for Health and Clinical Excellence; Royal College of Psychiatrists Audit Team, 2005).

Patients' individual needs and diversity

Violence and aggression can be prevented by ensuring that all patients and their visitors are treated with respect, with freedom from discrimination and harassment, in relation to privacy and dignity, within the parameters of safety; and the provision of a culturally sensitive and culturally competent service (Andrews and Boyle, 2003). The latter relates to the individual's culture religion, gender, sexual orientation, gender identity, age, disability, and specific illness and problems. Several studies have found that patients' satisfaction with mental health services is partly related to professionals' sensitivity to, and attempts to meet, needs related to these aspects of diversity (Addo, 2006; Aiyegbusi and Byrt, 2006). Dissatisfaction with services, which fail to be sensitive to the individual's needs, may be associated with assertive or aggressive anger.

The National Institute for Health and Clinical Excellence (2005) Guideline on Violence states that there should be policies for interventions with patients with disabilities. The Guideline stresses, also, that professionals should listen to the perspectives of individuals from a variety of ethnic and other backgrounds, and provide particular help to patients who have adverse experiences of services. National Institute for Health and Clinical Excellence (2005, p. 29) also comments that members of Trust Boards must have 'specific responsibility for all matters relating to equality and diversity', including relevant training, collection of data on the ethnicity of users of services and 'consultation with local Black and minority ethnic groups'.

The 'Independent inquiry into the death of David Bennett' considered factors concerning the death of Mr Bennett in a medium secure unit whilst he was being restrained following a violent incident. The inquiry concluded that, although Mr Bennett was 'treated kindly... there... was insufficient attention paid to his cultural, social and religious needs' (Blofeld, 2003, p. 24). The inquiry team found evidence of institutionalised racism in previous services used by Mr Bennett and concluded that no action was taken by staff in response to his complaints about another patient's racism toward him.

Patients' physical health needs associated with violence and aggression

In relation to physical health problems associated with violence and aggression, nursing and multi-professional interventions include assessing, and then treating or alleviating, the cause. The National Institute for Health and Clinical Excellence (2005) Guideline on Violence emphasises the importance of assessing and meeting patients' physical health needs from admission.

An example of meeting an individual's physical health needs, based on one of the authors' clinical experience, is given in Box 5.5.

Safe access to fresh air and exercise may prevent and reduce violence and aggression (National Institute for Health and Clinical Excellence, 2005). Sporting activities can be used to channel and creatively express aggressive and other forms of anger. Research '... shows that after exercise, there is a decrease in irritability, tension and anxiety, fewer psychotic features, a more positive mood through the increased output of endorphins and active seeking of physical and cognitive diversions to cope with thoughts' (Adams 2002, p. 124).

Box 5.5 'Mr Clive Crimson's' physical needs

Thirst, hunger, low blood sugar and lack of sleep may all contribute to irritability, and in some instances, to aggression or violence; and this needs to be considered in the planning and implementation of care for forensic and other mental health patients, as in the following example.

Mr Crimson found it hard to find time to drink, eat or sleep because of overactivity during a hypomanic episode of a recurring bipolar mental illness. A flexible approach helped. Clive's Primary Nurse, in liaison with the dietician, ensured that drinks and nutritious snacks were readily available on the ward, thus obviating the need to go to an overstimulating dining area. Pillows and blankets were made available in a quiet room to enable Clive to catch up on sleep in the day. However, in such a situation, thought needs to be given to possible disadvantages: e.g. whether this would prevent sleep at night and result in reversals of sleep patterns.

The social environment

Chapters 3 and 4 refer to the features of 'social environment' in mental health services. Research suggests that these features are sometimes related to some individuals' violent and aggressive behaviours and to the prevention or de-escalation of the latter. In particular, there is evidence that the following factors are crucial (Meehan *et al.*, 2006; NICE, 2005; Royal College of Psychiatrists Audit Team, 2005; Secker *et al.*, 2004):

- Meaningful activities and structure to the patients' day, and avoidance of both over- and under-stimulation. Reduced sensory overload, with spaces (within the parameters of safety) for privacy and quiet. (An example of the therapeutic use of activities to channel aggression is given in the next section).
- A low expressed emotion environment, with avoidance of authoritarian, critical and other attitudes; and of demands that the individual finds hard to meet.
- Opportunities for patients to communicate with approachable non-judgemental nursing and other staff.
- Clear managerial leadership

The use of diversion and channelling: an example from practice: 'Mr Clive Crimson'

In the author's experience, diversion and channelling can be used to prevent violence in the nursing care of individuals experiencing the hypomanic phase of bipolar mental illness. Like other individuals with this condition, Mr Clive Crimson experienced pressure of thought, with dozens of ideas occurring to him in rapid succession. He talked rapidly, and felt the need for intense activity. Huge amounts of paper were filled with drafts of poems and sketches, which he often scattered round the activity room.

In view of Clive's recent violence, it was imperative that its prevention was a priority. Most of his physical violence had been preceded by arguments with other patients who had taken exception to his comments.

Clive sometimes told the author that he wanted to see another patient to 'settle a score', adding comments such as 'I'm not going to let him get away with remarks like that'. However (as is often the case with people with hypomania; Gelder *et al.*, 2001), these thoughts were usually very fleeting, and succeeded by other thoughts related to quite different topics. It was usually possible to prevent a possibly violent situation by using diversion to respond to Clive's intention to 'settle a score'. For example: 'I understand Dave doesn't want to be disturbed just now. But you said you wanted to read me your latest poem. What about doing that now?'.

In addition to diversion, the use of writing and drawing also provided Clive with a safe and creative way of channelling his anger, and therefore he had access to a room with considerable supplies of paper and other materials. Here the term 'channelling' is used to refer to ways of expressing feelings creatively and in an enjoyable way, without harming self or others (Duxbury, 2000). The use of the arts in enabling people to express and channel feelings has been described (Green and Tones, 2003; Solanki and Byrt, 2003).

The physical environment

Recent audits and reviews of the literature on violence and aggression suggest that: 'facilities should have adequate means of controlling light, temperature, ventilation and noise' (National Institute for Health and Clinical Excellence, 2005, p. 14). Attractive, culturally appropriate décor and furnishings and avoidance of overcrowding have also been suggested (Royal College of Psychiatrists Audit Team, 2005; Whittington, 2000).

Therapeutic frameworks to prevent and reduce violence and aggression

Certain therapeutic frameworks can prevent and reduce violence and aggression, particularly in the longer term, and thus manage risk. These include the following, which are outlined in more detail in Chapters 4 and 17:

- **Cognitive behavioural therapy** can be used to measure the extent of violent and aggressive behaviours and reduce their incidence. Anger management principles are used to enable individuals to express anger assertively and creatively and to reduce violence and aggression (Byrt *et al.*, 2005; Tennant *et al.*, 2000).
- **Therapeutic community principles** have been used to help people understand the reasons for violence and aggression, learn about themselves and try out new ways of behaving and relating to others (Byrt, 2006; Kelly *et al.*, 2004).
- **Psychosocial interventions** include therapeutic uses of ward and home environments, especially for individuals with schizophrenia (Gamble and Brennan, 2006; McKeown and McCann, 2000).

Responding to crises: legal aspects and the registered nurse's responsibility

This section of the chapter considers situations of crisis where, sadly, the nurse's communication and other skills are ineffective in de-escalating violence and aggression. Ethical problems relate, in part, to ensuring both:

- The safety of the individual who is, or may be, violent and aggressive – and the safety of other patients and other people
- The autonomy, choice, privacy and dignity of the individual with violent or aggressive behaviours.

In situations of violence, where de-escalation techniques are ineffective, 'reasonable' force (e.g. in the use of control and restraint and seclusion) can legally be used to prevent serious injury to the nurse, patients, visitors and colleagues, in accordance (in England and Wales) with the Code of Practice of the Mental Health Act Commission (Department of Health and Welsh Office, 1999; National Institute for Health and Clinical Excellence, 2005):

> Reasonableness means, first, that the force used should be:
>
> - 'No more than is necessary to accomplish the object for which it is allowed...'
> - 'The reaction must be in proportion to the harm that is threatened' (Dimond, 2005, p. 302).

Unsafe techniques were used in the control and restraint of David Bennett, who died after being restrained in the prone position for about ten minutes (Blofeld, 2003). The NMC (2004) Code of Conduct (Clause 6.2, p. 9) states:

> To practise competently, you must possess the knowledge, skills and abilities required for lawful, safe and effective practice without direct supervision. You must acknowledge the limits of your professional competence and only undertake practice and accept responsibilities for those activities in which you are competent.

Alternatives to control and restraint and seclusion

There have been criticisms of an over-concentration on physical methods, such as control and restraint and seclusion, in response to violence, instead of using non-aversive methods, such as communication skills, which seek to minimise discomfort and avoid pain to clients (Duxbury and Whittington, 2002; Meehan *et al.*, 2006; NIMHE, 2004, p. 31). Despite nurses' intentions to avoid pain when using control and restraint, this may unfortunately result if, for example, a client persistently struggles. NIMHE (2004) highlight the considerable ethical issues related to this, including those concerning the Human Rights Act 1998: e.g. Article 3 (the right to be free from torture or inhuman or degrading treatment or punishment) (HM Government, 1998, cited in National Institute for Health and Clinical Excellence, 2005, p. 10). NIMHE (2004) refers to Royal College of Nursing (1998) and the Mental Health Act Commission (Department of Health and Welsh Office, 1999) who both state that 'physical interventions should not rely on the infliction of pain':

> Pain or discomfort should be avoided wherever possible. However, there may be extraordinary situations where pain or discomfort is unavoidable for both staff and service users, i.e. need to breakaway from an attacker or its use is deemed the only way to safely resolve an emergency where alternative interventions have been considered, and proven, ineffective.

> In such circumstances, the member of staff involved must report and record such action through established reporting systems. The decision and action taken needs to be justified as being the minimum use of force, which is appropriate to the risk associated with that particular set of circumstances (NIMHE, 2004, p. 31).

O'Hagan (2004) reviews mental health service users' views of control and restraint and seclusion, with suggestions for practical alternatives.

The needs of nurses

Finally, some authors suggest that managers' awareness and meeting of staff needs is essential to the prevention and reduction of violence and aggression, with nurses and other professionals having opportunities for the following (NHS Security Management Service, 2005b; NICE, 2005; Watson and Kettles, 2006):

- Managerial commitment to ensuring a safe environment, in line with health and safety legislation.
- Education and training on a wide range of non-aversive interventions, as provided by the NHS Security Management Service (2005b).
- Debriefing as soon as possible after incidents.
- Clinical supervision and other opportunities to reflect on practice.
- Support provided by managers and colleagues, including support, especially following incidents of staff assault.
- Opportunities for staff to evaluate their interventions.

Conclusion

This chapter has considered the meaning of violence and aggression, factors associated with their occurrence, and nursing/multidisciplinary interventions used in prevention and de-escalation. In conclusion, it can be argued that all aspects of assessment, care and treatment are relevant. Interventions which respect the individual and his/her uniqueness and diversity, and which reduce distress, are also likely to reduce risk and the propensity for violence and aggression.

Acknowledgements

Thanks to Minal Sikotra and Kate Williams.

References

Adams, L. (2002) Nursing interventions and future directions for exercise therapy. In: *Therapeutic Interventions for Forensic Mental Health Nurses* (eds. A. M. Kettles, P. Woods and M. Collins), Chapter 8. Jessica Kingsley, London.

Addo, M. (2006) Culture, spirituality and ethical issues in caring for clients with personality disorder. In: *Forensic Mental Health Nursing: Interventions with People with 'Personality Disorder'* (ed. National Forensic Nurses' Research and Development Group), Chapter 5. Quay, London.

Aiyegbusi, A. and Byrt, R. (2006) Gender and sexuality. In: *Forensic Mental Health Nursing: Interventions with People with 'Personality Disorder'* (ed. National Forensic Nurses' Research and Development Group), Chapter 8. Quay, London.

Almvik, R. and Woods, P. (1998) The Broset Violence Checklist (BVC) and the prediction of inpatient violence: some preliminary results. *Psychiatric Care*, **5** (6), 208–11.

Andrews, M. M. and Boyle, J. S. (eds.) (2003) *Transcultural Concepts in Nursing Care*. Lippincott, Williams and Wilkins, Philadelphia.

Appleby, L., Shaw, J., Sherratt, J. *et al.* (2001) *Safety First: Five-Year Report of the National Confidential Inquiry into Suicide and Homicide by People with Mental Illness*. Department of Health, London.

Arnold, E. (2003a) Developing therapeutic communication skills in the nurse–patient relationship. In: *Interpersonal Relationships*, 4th edn (eds. E. Arnold and K. U. Boggs), Chapter 10. Saunders, St Louis.

Arnold, E. (2003b) Intercultural communication. In: *Interpersonal Relationships*, 4th edn (eds. E. Arnold and K. U. Boggs), Chapter 11. Saunders, St Louis.

Arnold, E. and Boggs, K. U. (eds.) (2003) *Interpersonal Relationships*, 4th edn. Saunders, St Louis.

Beauford, J., McNiel, D. and Binder, R. (1997) Utility of the therapeutic alliance in evaluating psychiatric patients' risk of violence. *American Journal of Psychiatry*, **154**(9), 1272–6.

Blofeld, J. (2003) *Independent Inquiry into the Death of David Bennett*. An independent inquiry set up under HSG (94) 27. Department of Health, London.

Bowers, L.., Crowhurst, N., Alexander, J., Callaghan, P., Eales, S., Guy, S., McCann, E. and Ryan, C. (2002) Safety and security policies on psychiatry acute admission wards: results from a London-wide survey. *Journal of Psychiatric and Mental Health Nursing*, **9**, 427–33.

Braithwaite, R. (2001) *Managing Aggression*. Routledge/Community Care, London.

Burnard, P. (1999) *Counselling Skills for Nurses and Health Care Professionals*. Stanley Thornes, Cheltenham.

Byrt, R. (2006) Nursing interventions in therapeutic communities. In: *Forensic Mental Health Nursing: Interventions with People with 'Personality Disorder'* (ed. National Forensic Nurses' Research and Development Group), Chapter 14. Quay, London.

Byrt, R. and Dooher, J. (2006) The social consequences of a 'personality disorder' diagnosis. In: *Forensic Mental Health Nursing: Interventions with People with 'Personality Disorder'* (ed. National Forensic Nurses' Research and Development Group), Chapter 3. Quay, London.

Byrt, R., Wray, C. and 'Tom' (2005) Towards hope and inclusion: nursing interventions in a medium secure service for men with 'personality disorders'. *Mental Health Practice*, **8**(8), 38–43.

Byrt, R., Graley-Wetherell, R., 'R', Studley, R., D'Silva, K., James, L. and Pocock, T. (2006) Service user experiences and professional attitudes. In: *Forensic Mental Health Nursing: Interventions with People with 'Personality Disorder'* (ed. National Forensic Nurses' Research and Development Group), Chapter 4. Quay, London.

Crichton, J. (1995) *Psychiatric Patient Violence: Risk and Response*. Duckworth, London.

Dale, C. and Gardner, J. (2001) Security in forensic environments: strategic and operational issues. In: *Forensic Mental Health: Issues in Practice* (eds. C. Dale, T. Thompson and P. Woods), Chapter 23. Baillière Tindall/Royal College of Nursing, Edinburgh.

Department of Health and Welsh Office (1999) *Mental Health Act 1983 Code of Practice*. Stationery Office, London.

Dimond, B. (2005) *Legal Aspects of Nursing*, 4th edn. Pearson Longman, Harlow.

Dooher, J. and Byrt, R. (eds.) (2003*) Empowerment and the Health Service User*. Quay, Salisbury.

Doyle, M. and Duffy, S. (2006) Assessing and managing risk to self and others. In: *Forensic Mental Health Nursing: Interventions with People with 'Personality Disorder'* (ed. National Forensic Nurses' Research and Development Group), Chapter 10. Quay, London.

Doyle M., Dolan, M. C. and McGovern, J. (2002) The validity of North American risk assessment tools in predicting inpatient violent behaviour in England. *Legal and Criminological Psychology*, **7**(2), 141–54.

Doyle, M., Aiyegbusi, A. and Burbery, P. (2006) Personality disorder: specialist psychological approaches. In: *Forensic Mental Health Nursing: Interventions with People with 'Personality Disorder'* (ed. National Forensic Nurses' Research and Development Group), Chapter 5. Quay, London.

Duxbury, J. (2000) *Difficult Patients*. Butterworth-Heinemann, Oxford.

Duxbury, J. and Whittington, R. (2005) Causes and management of patient aggression and violence: staff and patient perspectives. *Journal of Advanced Nursing*, **50**(5), 469–78.

Evans, S. and Byrt, R. (2003) The right to complain? In: *Empowerment and the Health Service User* (eds. J. Dooher and R. Byrt), Chapter 15. Quay, Salisbury.

Gamble, C. and Brennan, W. (eds.) (2006) *Working with Serious Mental Illness*, 2nd edn. Baillière Tindall/ Elsevier, Edinburgh.

Garnham, P. (2001) Understanding and dealing with anger, aggression and violence. *Nursing Standard*, **24**(16), 37–42.

Gelder, M., Mayou, R. and Cowen, P. (eds.) (2001) *Shorter Oxford Textbook of Psychiatry*. Oxford University Press, Oxford.

Gilligan, J. (2001) *Preventing Violence*. Thames and Hudson, London.

Goffman, E. (1968) *Asylums: Essays on the Social Situation on Mental Patients and Other Inmates*. Penguin, Harmondsworth.

Gray, R. and Bressington, D. (2004) Pharmacological interventions and electro-convulsive therapy. In: *The Art and Science of Mental Health Nursing: a Textbook of Principles and Practice* (eds. I. Norman and I. Ryrie), Chapter 11. Open University Press, Maidenhead. Cited in: Byrt, R. and Woods, P. (2006) Introduction. In: *Forensic Mental Health Nursing: Interventions with People with 'Personality Disorder'* (ed. National Forensic Nurses' Research and Development Group), Chapter 1. Quay, London.

Green, J. and Tones, K. (2003) The creative arts and empowerment. In: *Empowerment and the Health Service User* (eds. J. Dooher and R. Byrt), Chapter 19. Quay, Salisbury.

Hart, S. D. (1998) The role of psychopathy in assessing risk for violence: conceptual and methodological issues. *Legal and Criminological Psychology*, **3**, 121–37.

Health Services Advisory Committee (1997) *Violence and Aggression to Staff in Health Services: Guidance on Assessment and Management*. HSE Books, Sudbury.

Heilbrun, K. (1997) Prediction versus management models relevant to risk assessment: the importance of legal decision-making context. *Law and Human Behavior*, **21**(4), 347–59.

Heilbrun, K. (2002) Violence risk: from prediction to risk management. In: *Handbook of Psychology in Legal Contexts*, 2nd edn (eds. D. Carson and R. Bull). John Wiley & Sons, Chichester.

Heilbrun, K., Hart, S. D., Hare, R. D., Gustaffson, D., Nunez, C. and White, A. J. (1998) Inpatient and post discharge aggression in mentally disordered offenders: the role of psychopathy. *Journal of Interpersonal Violence*, **13**, 514–27.

Hill, C. D., Rogers, R. and Bickford, M. E. (1996) Predicting aggressive and socially disruptive behaviour in a maximum-security forensic hospital. *Journal of Forensic Sciences*, **41**, 56–9.

Hoptman, M., Yates, K., Patalinjug, M., Wack, R. and Convit, A. (1999) Clinical prediction of assaultative behavior among male psychiatric patients at a maximum-security forensic facility. *Psychiatric Services*, **50**(11), 1461–6.

Hopton, J. (1995) The application of ideas of Frantz Fanon to the practice of mental health nursing. *Journal of Advanced Nursing*, **21**(4), 723–8.

James, D. V., Fineberg, N. A., Shah, A. K. and Priest, R. G. (1990) An increase in violence in an acute psychiatric ward. *British Journal of Psychiatry*, **156**, 846–52.

Jeffcote, N. and Watson, T. (eds.) (2004) *Working Therapeutically with Women in Secure Mental Health Settings*. Jessica Kingsley, London.

Jones, J. and Jackson, A. (2004) Observation. In: *Acute Mental Health Nursing: From Acute Concerns to the Capable Practitioner* (eds. M. Harrison, D. Howard and D. Mitchell), Chapter 8. Sage, London.

Kelly, S., Hill, J., Boardman, H. and Overton, I. (2004) Therapeutic Communities. In: *From Toxic Institutions to Therapeutic Environments: Residential Settings in Mental Health Services* (eds. P. Campling, S. Davies and G. Farquharson). Gaskell, London.

Kennedy, J., Harrison, J., Hillis, T. and Bluglass, R. (1995) Analysis of violent incidents in a regional secure unit. *Medicine, Science and the Law*, **35**(3), 255–60.

Kettles, A. M. (2006) Dual diagnosis of personality disorder and substance misuse. In: *Forensic Mental Health Nursing: Interventions with People with 'Personality Disorder'* (eds. National Forensic Nurses' Research and Development Group), Chapter 13. Quay, London.

Kettles, A. M. and Woodally, J. (2006) Observation and engagement with people with personality disorder. In: *Forensic Mental Health Nursing: Interventions with People with 'Personality Disorder'* (ed. National Forensic Nurses' Research and Development Group), Chapter 12. Quay, London.

Kirby, S. D. and Cross, D. (2002) Socially constructed narrative interventions: a foundation for therapeutic alliances. In: *Therapeutic Interventions for Forensic Mental Health Nurses* (eds. A. M. Kettles, P. Woods and M. Collins), Chapter 12. Jessica Kingsley, London.

Krakowski, M., Czobor, P. and Chou, J. C. (1999) Course of violence in patients with schizophrenia: relationship to clinical symptoms. *Schizophrenia Bulletin*, **25**, 505–17.

Kunyk, D. and Olson, J. K. (2001) Clarification of conceptualisations of empathy. *Journal of Advanced Nursing*, **35**(3), 317–25.

Linaker, O. M. and Busch-Iverson, H. (1995) Predictors of imminent violence in psychiatric inpatients. *Acta Psychiatrica Scandinavica*, **92**(4), 250–4.

Link, B., Monahan, J., Stueve, A. and Cullen, F. T. (1999) Real in their consequences: a sociological approach to understanding the association between psychotic symptoms and violence. *American Sociological Review*, **64**, 316–22.

Lowe, T. (1992) Characteristics of effective nursing interventions in the management of challenging behaviour. *Journal of Advanced Nursing*, **17**, 1226–32.

Lowenstein, M., Binder, R. L. and McNiel, D. E. (1990) The relationship between admission symptoms and hospital assaults. *Hospital and Community Psychiatry*, **41**, 311–13.

Lugton, J. (2002) *Communicating with Dying People and their Relatives*. Radcliffe Medical Press, Abingdon.

Mason, T. and Chandley, M. (1999) *Managing Violence and Aggression: a Manual for Nurses and Health Care Workers*. Churchill Livingstone, Edinburgh.

McChargue, D. E., Gulliver, S. B. and Hitsman, B. (2002) Would smokers with schizophrenia benefit from a more flexible approach to smoking treatment? *Addiction*, **97**, 785–93.

McDougall, T. (2000) Violent incidents in a forensic adolescent unit. *NT Research*, **5**(5), 346–62.

McKeown, M. and McCann, G. (2000) Psychosocial interventions. In: *Forensic Mental Health Nursing: Current Approaches* (eds. C. Chaloner and M. Coffey), Chapter 12. Blackwell Science, Oxford.

McNiel, D. E. and Binder, R. L. (1989) Relationship between preadmission threats and later violent behaviour by acute psychiatric inpatients. *Hospital & Community Psychiatry*, **40**, 605–8.

McNiel, D. E. and Binder, R. L. (1994) The relationship between acute psychiatric symptoms, diagnosis and short-term risk of violence. *Hospital & Community Psychiatry*, **45**, 133–7.

McNiel, D. E., Binder, R. L. and Greenfield, T. (1988) Predictors of violence in civilly committed acute psychiatric patients. *American Journal of Psychiatry*, **145**, 965–70.

Meehan, T., McIntosh, W. and Bergen, H. (2006) Aggressive behavior in high-secure settings: the perceptions of patients. *Journal of Psychiatric and Mental Health Nursing*, **13**(1), 19–25.

Morgan, S. and Wetherell, A. (2004) Assessing and managing risk. In: *The Art and Science of Mental Health Nursing: a Textbook of Principles and Practice* (eds. I. Norman and I. Ryrie), Chapter 8. Open University Press, Maidenhead.

Morrison, E. F. (1992) A coercive interactional style as an antecedent to aggression in psychiatric patients. *Research in Nursing and Health*, **15**, 421–31.

National Forensic Nurses' Research and Development Group (ed.) (2006) *Forensic Mental Health Nursing: Interventions with People with 'Personality Disorder'*. Quay, London.

National Institute for Health and Clinical Excellence (NICE) (2005) *Violence Guideline*. NICE, London. Available on: http://www.nice.org.uk/.

National Institute for Mental Health in England (NIMHE) (2004) *Developing Positive Practice to Support the Safe and Therapeutic Management of Aggression and Violence in Mental Health In-patient Settings*. NIMHE, London.

NHS Security Management Service (2005a) *Not Alone: A Guide for the Protection of the Workers in the NHS*. NHS Security Management Service, London.

NHS Security Management Service (2005b) *Promoting Safer and Therapeutic Services: Implementing the National Syllabus in Mental Health and Learning Disability Services*. NHS Security Management Service, London.

Noble, P. and Rodger, S. (1989) Violence by psychiatric in-patients. *British Journal of Psychiatry*, **155**, 384–90.

Novaco, R. (1994) Anger as a risk factor for violence among the mentally disordered. In: *Violence and Mental Disorder: Development in Risk Assessment* (eds. J. Monahan and H. Steadman). University of Chicago Press, Chicago.

Novaco, R. W. (2003) *The Novaco Anger scale and Provocation Inventory (NAS-PI)*. Western Psychological Services, Los Angeles.

Nursing and Midwifery Council (2004) *Code of Professional Conduct for the Nurse, Midwife and Health Visitor*. Nursing and Midwifery Council, London.

O'Hagan, M. (2004) Force in mental health services: international user and survivor perspectives. Parts 1 and 2. *Mental Health Practice*, **7**(5), 12–17.

Palmstierna, T. and Wistedt, B. (1995) Changes in the pattern of aggressive behaviour among inpatients with changed ward organisation. *Acta Psychiatrica Scandinavica*, **91**(1), 32–5.

Paterson, B. and Leadbetter, D. (1999) De-escalation in the management of aggression and violence. In: *Aggression and Violence: Approaches to Effective Management* (eds. J. Turnbull and B. Paterson), Chapter 6. Macmillan, Basingstoke.

Pilgrim, D. and Rogers, A. (2005) *The Sociology of Mental Health and Illness*, 3rd edn. Open University Press, Maidenhead.

Rippon, T. J. (2000) Aggression and violence in health care professions. *Journal of Advanced Nursing*, **31**(2), 452–60.

Rogers, A. and Pilgrim, D. (2003) *Mental Health and Inequality*. Macmillan, Basingstoke.

Rogers, R., Salvage, J. and Cowell, R. (eds.) (1999) *Nurses at Risk: A Guide to Health and Safety at Work*, 2nd edn. Macmillan, Basingstoke.

Royal College of Nursing (1998) *Dealing with Violence against Nursing Staff: an RCN Guide for Nurses and Managers*. Royal College of Nursing, London.

Royal College of Psychiatrists (1998) *Management of Imminent Violence: Clinical Practice Guidelines to Support Mental Health Services*. OP41, March.

Royal College of Psychiatrists Audit Team (2005) *The Health Care Commission National Audit of Violence, 2003–2005*. Royal College of Psychiatrists, London.

Secker, J., Benson, A., Balfe, E., Lipsedge, M., Robinson, S. and Walker, J. (2004) Understanding the social context of violent and aggressive incidents on an inpatient unit. *Journal of Psychiatric and Mental Health Nursing*, **11**(2), 172–8.

Shepherd, J. (2001) *Violence in Healthcare: Understanding, Preventing and Surviving Violence: a Practical Guide for Professionals*, 2nd edn. Oxford University Press, Oxford.

Smith, E. E., Nolen-Hoeksema, S., Frederickson, B. and Loftus, G. R. (eds.) (2003) *Hilgard's Introduction to Psychology*, 14th edn. Harcourt College Publishers, Fort Worth.

Solanki, M. and Byrt, R. (2003) Finding a voice: writing and empowerment. In: *Empowerment and the Health Service User* (eds. J. Dooher and R. Byrt), Chapter 20. Quay, Salisbury.

Soliman, A. and Reza, H. (2001) Risk factors and correlates of violence among acutely ill adult psychiatric patients. *Psychiatric Services*, **52**(1), 75–80.

Sookoo, S. (2004) Therapeutic management of aggression and violence. In: *The Art and Science of Mental Health Nursing: a Textbook of Principles and Practice* (eds. I. Norman and I. Ryrie), Chapter 27. Open University Press, Maidenhead.

Stockwell, F. (1972) *The Unpopular Patient*. Royal College of Nursing, London.

Swinton, J. (2002) Spiritual care in forensic nursing: spiritual interventions and future directions for care. In: *Therapeutic Interventions for Forensic Mental Health Nurses* (eds. A. M. Kettles, P. Woods and M. Collins), Chapter 13. Jessica Kingsley, London.

Tennant, A., Davies, C. and Tennant, I. (2000) Working with the personality disordered offender. In: *Forensic Mental Health Nursing: Current Approaches* (eds. C. Chaloner and M. Coffey) Blackwell Science, Oxford.

Tschudin, V. and Schober, J. (1998) *Managing Yourself*. Macmillan, Basingstoke.

Turnbull, C. (1999) Theoretical approaches to violence and aggression. In: *Aggression and Violence: Approaches to Effective Management* (eds. J. Turnbull and B. Paterson), Chapter 3. Macmillan, Basingstoke.

Turnbull, J. and Paterson, B. (eds.) (1999a) *Aggression and Violence: Approaches to Effective Management*. Macmillan, Basingstoke.

Turnbull, J. and Paterson, B. (1999b) Introduction. In: Turnbull, J., Paterson, B. (eds.) *Aggression and Violence: Approaches to Effective Management* (Chapter 1). Macmillan, Basingstoke.

Walker, Z. and Seifert, R. (1994) Violent incidents in a psychiatric intensive care unit. *British Journal of Psychiatry*, **164**, 826–8.

Warner, C. (1992) Responding to aggression. *Nursing Times*, **88**(30), 46–7.

Watson, C. and Kettles, A. M. (2006) Education, training and support for staff working with clients with a diagnosis of personality disorder: some thoughts. In: *Forensic Mental Health Nursing: Interventions with People with 'Personality Disorder'* (ed. National Forensic Nurses' Research and Development Group), Chapter 7. Quay Books, London.

West, M. and Abolins, D. (2001) Dealing with hostility. In: *Forensic Nursing and Mental Disorder in Clinical Practice* (eds. N. McClelland, M. Humphreys, L. Conlon and T. Hillis), Chapter 4. Butterworth-Heinemann, Oxford.

Whittington, R. (2000) Changing the environment in the management of aggression. In: *Forensic Mental Health Care: a Case Study Approach* (eds. D. Mercer, T. Mason, M. McKeown and G. McCann). Churchill Livingstone, Edinburgh.

Willis, B. and Gillett, J. (2003) *Maintaining Control: An Introduction to the Effective Management of Violence and Aggression*. Arnold, London.

Wilson, J. F. (2003) *Biological Foundations of Human Behaviour*. Thomson Wadsworth, Belmont, CA.

World Health Organization (2002) *World Report on Violence and Health*. World Health Organization, Geneva.

Young, M., Justice, J. and Erdberg, P. (1999) Risk factors for violent behavior among incarcerated male psychiatric patients: a multimethod approach. *Assessment*, **6**(3), 243–58.

CHAPTER 6

Forensic aspects of acute inpatient assessment

Mike Doyle and Michael Coffey

Introduction

This chapter aims to help you explore and analyse assessment practice related to forensic issues within the field of acute mental health care. Mental health assessment is highly topical in terms of central government policy agendas. Assessment is, of course, the mainstay of all clinical practice, and we can claim that without assessment there is no practice, or at least, no professional and considered practice.

One of the first things we have to consider with any assessment is its prime purpose. What are we being asked to do in an assessment? Is the assessment to offer treatment advice to a third party? Is it to establish the presence of identified problems for which we must select from a repertoire of interventions in response? Is it to assess for treatability, for effects of treatment or for the presence of a range of health needs? The simplest categorisation of assessment is whether it is a global assessment to establish the breadth of issues to be addressed in the future, or whether it is specific to one particular proposed intervention or identified problem.

It is a simple and linear relationship, but nevertheless a useful one, to consider that, in an ideal world, we might wish to start with broad assessments and then focus to more specific assessments of individual factors or problems as they become identified. Simple, because that's not how it often happens in practice, as we may be asked to make snap assessments of individuals in crisis in which a broad assessment would be too time-consuming and not appropriate. An example would be determining the level of risk of someone who is contemplating self-harm. In relation to people with acute mental health problems with an associated forensic element, the main focus of concern may, at first glance, appear to be offending behaviour and risk of further offending behaviours. We say at first glance, because to focus on these aspects alone is to miss the relationship between other aspects of the person's situation and the behaviour which gives rise to concern. Examples that will be covered in this chapter include assessment of need and symptom assessment, as these can directly relate to the types of behaviour that attract the forensic label. This chapter will also address the important task of assessment of risk behaviours.

A starting point

Before considering assessment practice specifically, we must determine the principles and values that should underpin assessment procedures in mental health care. Some examples of these are that assessments are collaborative, aware of gender and ethnicity issues, person-centred, based upon the person's experience, non-maleficent and evidence-based. Values are an important feature of any intervention, and an understanding that a twin approach of values-based and evidence-based practice should underpin our assessment practice is a useful starting point (Woodbridge and Fulford, 2004). An important and central value to mental health nursing is that people in receipt of services should be involved, as much as possible, in determining priorities that are meaningful to them. Forming a trusting, compassionate therapeutic relationship as the basis for future work is a crucial element in assessment and will help to forge true collaborative working with the person (Edwards, 2005).

We have to also consider the emphasis of assessment: is it a problem-based assessment, a needs-based assessment or a strengths-based assessment? Each approach will have relative benefits and limitations and the situation before us may provide an indication of what will prove most helpful. It may be necessary to have a short-term problem focus to address initial issues, but in the longer term, we must try to see the person as having a range of social, psychological, physical and spiritual needs.

Values-based assessment

The process of assessment in any clinical situation gives rise to a number of conceptual issues that should be explicitly acknowledged by the person conducting the assessment.

All assessments are conducted with some intent. The mental health nurse's intent in assessing is to provide treatment or to deny it. The person's intent may be to convince the nurse of their need or to deny access to their problems; for instance, someone intent on suicide may present a façade of happiness or indifference to the point of trying to convince the nurse that they are not at risk of attempting this behaviour.

Assessment necessarily will have a particular and prescribed scope in determining what will be addressed, how it will be conducted and from what perspective. For example, standardised structured assessments may adopt a positivist perspective, the assessment assuming some claim to be able to objectify the world of the person it is assessing. Mental health nurses, rather than being in thrall to the supposed power of standardised assessment, should develop critical awareness of its benefits and limitations and ask themselves: how sure can we be that this assessment procedure does what it claims, and how can we check? This type of assessment is often based upon the professionals' view of the world: see, for example, Sullivan's (2003) paper discussing alternative views on quality of life measurement. Structured and standardised assessments have a role in the assessment of a range of mental health problems, but they remain only part of the process of assessment and should not be used as a substitute or proxy for a complete and thorough attempt to understand what is going on for the person.

One aspect of a values-based view of mental health nursing practice is the realisation that it is not a pick-and-mix affair. It should permeate all aspects of interaction with others in professional practice. In assessment, one example is ownership. We should ask ourselves: who owns the assessment? Can it be shared? And who are the stakeholders in the outcomes of the assessment? For instance, service users have indicated a desire to be better informed and involved in professionals' assessments of the risk behaviours they sometimes present (Langan and Lindow, 2004). Involving people in assessments is not only useful in contributing to a more comprehensive picture of the current situation, but also fits with the values of collaboration and partnership that move beyond mere rhetoric (Edwards, 2005).

There is an undeniable power relationship in assessment interviews. The nurse, as the assessor, in many ways holds the means to provide the person with the services that they want or need, or to deny them these should this be judged to be appropriate. Assessments can directly and indirectly determine issues related to the person's liberty: for instance, when giving advice in regard to Mental Health Act assessments, recall to hospital, section 25, and section 117 (H. M. Government, 1983), or indeed in relation to the criminal justice system and suitability for transfer for mental health care. This should be recognised by the nurse and assessment handled with the sensitivity and professionalism that such a responsibility entails.

To this end, the process of assessment itself is an important signifier of what people can expect from services and what they can expect of mental health nurses. The ways in which the nurse conducts herself/himself and the assessment interview, the genuine attempts at engagement with the person, the feedback offered to them about the assessment and the nurse's skilful approach are all of key importance in successful assessment. This can often be the first point of contact for the person with mental health services and the seeds of successful and helpful therapeutic relationships are sown here. Analysis of these process issues and the development of reflexive ability will help both deepen understanding of assessment in practice and improve the ability to offer assessments that are equitable, fair and just. These ethical and moral considerations of assessment form part and parcel of the values base for contemporary mental health practice. These concerns have significant relevance to health needs and the distribution of resources, but we must also consider the conduct of the assessment, its theoretical and cultural emphasis and its ability to do harm.

Practical issues

Within the context of what we have already covered, there are also very real issues associated with actually doing assessments in practice. Practical issues related to training, experience of specific and general assessment procedures, awareness of the limitations of various instruments or approaches, opportunities to conduct assessments, theoretical approaches to assessment, and skills as an interviewer and in engagement with people with mental health problems will all play a part in mental health assessment. For many mental health nurses, the ideal scenario is to observe expert assessment practice of colleagues being demonstrated a number of times, then to conduct assessments, under the supervision of an expert colleague, before eventually conducting assessments alone, but accessing expert clinical supervision on the process following completion of the assessment. This model of supervised practice will equip mental health nurses to conduct assessments expertly and to continue to learn from the experience of doing so.

Box 6.1 Goals of assessment (Rogers and Curran, 2004)

- Detailed and precise description of problems
- A clear description of current symptoms
- A comprehensive risk assessment
- A description of the social, occupational and domestic circumstances
- Supports available to the person
- Family/carer perspectives
- A management care plan
- A treatment plan
- Methods of evaluation

Rogers and Curran (2004) outline what they see as the main goals of assessment in acute mental health care (see Box 6.1). This emphasises the need to consider a clear and structured approach to assessment in its broadest sense. It also usefully encourages mental health nurses to look beyond the assessment process towards the outcomes of assessment and the eventual delivery of good-quality evidence and values-based care.

Guidance from the government in the form of requirements for the Care Programme Approach (Welsh Assembly Government, 2003), and the recent reviews of mental health nursing in England and Wales (Department of Health, 2006) and Scotland (Scottish Executive Health Department, 2006) articulate the need for mental health professionals to provide a range of good-quality assessment practices. Ultimately, for the nurse, assessment must inform a care plan and for this to be meaningful, the person being assessed should be involved. When working with people with mental health problems and a history of offending, care planning must address the range of complexity often inherent in this area of practice (Coffey, 2005). To achieve this, assessment must be comprehensive, and specific aspects of this are outlined below.

Mental health needs assessment

Mental health services are frequently directed to provide needs-led services. The question of what constitutes a health need and who gets to decide this is a difficult one to resolve (Doyal and Gough, 1991). Separating out the differences between needs, demands and wants can be almost impossible. One criticism of some approaches to needs assessments is that they often take the normative view based upon what professionals understand to be the range of needs, derived from some types of empirical data. This approach can ignore the expressed need of individuals themselves and can lead to different views of need and the priority that they should be given. Essentially, if professionals and service users fail to have a shared sense of what the assessed needs are, this will inevitably lead to fractures in the therapeutic relationship, with consequent difficulties in securing improvements in outcomes.

Slade (2003) provides a very useful and accessible overview of this topic and outlines a range of standardised measures that seek to redress the balance in favour of a service user evaluation of their health needs. One example of such an assessment of need, designed specifically for working with people with forensic histories, is the Camberwell Assessment of Need – Forensic Version (CANFOR) (Thomas *et al.*, 2003). CANFOR covers a broad range of health, social, clinical and function needs of people with mental health problems with forensic histories. It does so by seeking the person's assessment of their needs in tandem with a professional and, in some cases, the views of carers as well. This allows the completion of a needs assessment with multiple perspectives and provides the mental health team with the opportunity to highlight differences in opinion for further discussion and negotiation. It is a first step approach to identifying need, and does not explore need in detail. In this regard, areas that are highlighted will require further examination and, perhaps, more detailed specialist assessment.

Mental health symptom assessment

Clearly articulated mental health symptom assessment of people with forensic mental health problems is a necessary basis for establishing the role of symptoms, or otherwise, in the behaviours causing concern. A very useful mental health assessment for exploring symptoms from the person's point of view is the KGV assessment (Krawiecka *et al.*, 1977). This assessment (named after the first initials of the surnames of its developers) provides a comprehensive and structured assessment of symptoms. It is possible to score individual sections or parts of the assessment, but it is perhaps most useful in enabling the practitioner to record clear descriptions of symptoms from the point of view of the person experiencing them. It allows nurses to gather information about what the person is saying and doing within a known framework and to arrive at a formulation and plan to help deal with these.

The KGV assesses the person's experience of symptoms, with subscales on anxiety, depression, suicidality, elevated mood, hallucinations and thoughts and beliefs, using standardised questions and supplemental questions of a Socratic nature. It further provides for assessment of symptoms that can be observed during the course of the assessment interview. Skilled use of this mental health symptom assessment requires training and supervised practice, but is well within the capabilities of mental health nurses.

The collaborative assessment of needs and symptoms for people with mental health problems and criminal offending behaviours is a useful first step in determining the scope of depth of nurse involvement. It also contributes to both the care plan and wider multidisciplinary discussions with the person about what interventions are best suited to them and their situation. Risk assessment and its management, however, remain an important focus when working in forensic mental health, and we will now turn to this in more detail.

Risk assessment

Assessing and managing the risk to self and others has long been a key task for clinicians working in mental health services. People with mental health problems are at much greater risk of harming themselves than of harming others (Department of Health, 2001) and, in comparison with the general population, this risk of self injury is very significant, as it has been noted that severe mental illness increases this type of risk by as much as ten times (Allebeck and Allgulander, 1990). Although the majority of users of mental health services are not violent, it is clear that a small yet significant minority are violent in inpatient settings and the community (Swanson *et al.*, 1990; Monahan, 1992; Hiday, 1997). It is important that mental health nurses have a clear structured approach to risk assessment. This is because clinical decisions on risk are made at all stages of the clinical care process and prioritising treatment need, and predicting subsequent outcome of any therapeutic approach will rely heavily upon the level of risk (Department of Health, 2000).

Role of mental health nurses in risk assessment and management

Risk assessment is an inexact science. Ultimately, the decision on the level of risk is based on clinical judgement. Ideally, in practice, a multidisciplinary team, involving all the clinicians involved in the care, treatment and management of the individual being assessed, should make decisions on risk. Mental health nurses play a pivotal role in the assessment and management of risk.

Mental health nurses are a major source of clinical information that needs to be considered by the nurse and the team as a whole when assessing risks. Mental health nurses in inpatient settings have access to 24-hour observation of behaviour and have greater opportunities than other professionals to develop relationships with service users and their family/carers (Allen, 1997). Mental health nurses are constantly making decisions based on the level of risk to and/or from service users in these environments: for example, managing crises as they arise, controlling freedom of movement within and outside the mental health facility and maintaining safe levels of supervision and observation. This unique position makes the role of the mental health nurse crucial to the process of assessing and managing risk.

Mental health nurses are often highly skilled practitioners. They may have advanced competencies in psychosocial interventions employing behavioural and cognitive therapies, counselling, psychodynamic therapies and family therapy. Clearly, the knowledge, skills and experience that mental health nurses possess are crucial to clinical interventions involved in the process of assessing and managing risk. In summary, it is clear that the role of the mental health nurse is pivotal in the assessment and management of risk. However, it is far from clear how mental health nurses assess and manage risks.

The multidisciplinary approach to risk assessment and management

The stages of clinical risk assessment and management may be conceptualised as an ongoing process. This has been described as a *Risk Management Cycle* (Doyle, 1998) and is usually implicit in the provision of good quality health care and integrated into the Care Programme Approach. The basis of any assessment relies on the accumulation of reliable information and consideration of risk factors. Doyle (1996) found that community mental health nurses used a variety of sources to assess the risk of violence from patients. Those used included interviews, observation, record reviews, liaison with others (clinicians, other agencies, family, significant others), via the therapeutic relationship, physical examinations and intuition. Psychometric tests and rating scales based on actuarial or 'objective' information are also increasingly used to assess risk (e.g. the Historical Clinical Risk Management 20 Items (HCR-20); Webster *et al.*, 1997). These can prove very useful and efficient, although they should be used only by people trained in their use or under supervision by somebody with such training (e.g. a clinical psychologist or clinical nurse specialist).

Assessing the risk of self-harm and suicide

Problems with definition

The term *self-harm* is subject to much debate. Behaviour intended to takes one's own life and non-lethal self-harming behaviour are not necessarily considered to be the same phenomenon. There is evidence to suggest that individuals with these behaviours constitute largely different populations, but there is also data to suggest considerable overlap (MacLeod *et al.*, 1992). Self-mutilation and self-injurious behaviour is a very common problem in forensic services and a significant proportion of persons who self-injure are at a greatly increased risk of committing suicide at some later date (Doyle and Duffy, 2006). While accepting that it can be very difficult to distinguish between self-harming behaviour on the basis of ultimate intention, this section will focus on assessing and managing the risk of self-harm which is likely to result in life threatening injury or death.

Suicide

Suicide is legally defined as '... the intentional act of self destruction committed by someone knowing what he/she is doing and knowing the probable consequences of his/her action' (Bluglass and Bowden, 1990). Suicide is a major cause of death in Britain, accounting for 1% of all deaths annually. It is likely that the rate of suicide is even higher, as many suicides may have been recorded as undetermined deaths (Health Advisory Service, 1994, p. 9). People with mental health problems are at much greater risk of harming themselves than of harming others (Department of Health, 2001) and, in comparison with the general population, this risk is very significant. All service users must be assessed for the risk of self-harm, ranging from initial screening to more detailed assessment.

Risk factors

As with all risk assessments, there is a need to identify factors that are associated with an increased risk. Extensive data exist on demographic and biological correlates of risk of self-harm and suicide (Health Advisory Service, 1994, p. 10; University of Manchester, 1996, p. 53). These correlates are useful in describing groups of people at risk and possible trends, but they have limited utility in clinical settings. If an initial screening indicates that there is a risk of self-harm, further risk factors must be considered.

Current presentation

In order to assess the risk, it is advisable that the following areas are covered through careful questioning:

- Hopes that things will turn out well
- Gets pleasure out of life
- Feels hopeful from day to day
- Feels able to face each day
- Sees a point to it all
- Ever despairs about things
- Feels that it is impossible to face the next day
- Feels life to be a burden
- Wishes it would all end
- Knows why he or she feels this way (e.g. wants to be with a dead person)
- Has thoughts of ending life; if so, how persistently?
- Has ever acted on any suicidal thoughts or intentions
- Feels able to resist any suicidal thoughts or intentions; and has any thoughts about what would make them disappear.

In addition, more specific factors might need to be considered as part of an overall assessment of needs and risks (see Box 6.2).

Box 6.2 Risk factors for suicide (Doyle, 1998; Hawton *et al.*, 2005)

- Current suicidal intent
- Current suicidal ideation
- Hopelessness
- Recent loss or anniversary of loss
- Substance abuse
- Fear of mental deterioration
- Past history of self-harm/suicide attempts
- Low mood
- Non-compliance with treatment
- Recent failure or rejection
- Agitation/restlessness

Current suicidal intent

Suicidal intent is the most powerful predictor of whether an individual will attempt suicide. Specific questions need to be considered and these include: (1) Is there a suicide plan? (2) Are the means for suicide/self-harm available? (3) Is there a 'contract' not to self-harm? Clinicians need to be vigilant when assessing suicidal intent, as it is not uncommon for those who are intent on committing suicide to deny and/or minimise their ultimate intentions.

Hopelessness

There is evidence that future directed thinking is in some way different in people who contemplate suicide. Studies have shown that hopelessness about the future plays a significant role in identifying people who are both depressed and have suicidal intent (Salter and Platt, 1990). The lack of rewarding short-term routines and of long-term plans and goals may be an important component of hopelessness.

Previous suicide/self-harm attempts

A history of previous attempts at self-harm/suicide is obviously significant when assessing the level of risk. When analysing past history, it is important to consider the following:

- Recency (the more recent, the higher the risk)
- Frequency (the more frequent, the higher the risk)
- Severity (the more severe, the higher the risk)
- Pattern
- Antecedents/precipitants
- Details of attempt – especially any efforts made to avoid/ensure discovery
- Consequences

Managing risk of harm to self

Attitudes

Mental health nurses, whether qualified or unqualified, should receive appropriate training and supervision to promote an understanding of the issues that may lead patients to harm themselves. The national recommendation is that such training should be undertaken at least every three years (Department of Health, 2001). A consistent, ongoing therapeutic relationship or alliance should be the foundation of any risk management plan. The development of a relationship with a named nurse or other key worker may itself be therapeutic, while the key worker who has developed an alliance will be in the ideal position to plan and monitor care across different shifts and groups of staff. Given the nature of mental health problems, developing such a relationship may be a challenge, but it is important to at least achieve some initial degree of rapport if the patient is to be encouraged to communicate and an accurate assessment of risk is to be made. By using active listening skills, the key worker is able to obtain important information from the patient about self-harming ideation, which the patient would otherwise find difficult to express to a stranger due to guilt and fear. Such rapport thus encourages the gradual development of a therapeutic relationship, helping to prevent destructive malignant alienation (Doyle and Duffy, 2006).

Care planning

The Care Programme Approach (CPA) (2000) was developed as a systematic assessment of needs and risks and systematic care planning by multidisciplinary teams. There is an emphasis on coordination by a care coordinator who ensures adherence to the agreed care plan and seeks to actively involve the patient, relatives and carers. Effective use of the CPA, with patients assessed as at risk, is a key aspect of risk management, ensuring that an individual member of staff, such as a named nurse in a ward setting, maintains an overview of the care process. CPA also ensures that the expertise of different clinicians is employed, that communication about risk is optimised, and that the care plan is implemented and reviewed appropriately. In addition, the crucial post-discharge period, when the patient is at most risk of self-harm (Department of Health, 2001), can be prepared for, for example by ensuring the person is 'in reach' of community staff before the patient returns home.

Clinical interventions

Self-harming behaviour should be seen as a symptom of other mental health problems, rather than a problem in itself, and the reasons for the behaviour should be sought and addressed. Therefore, individualised care plans should be formulated to take account of the patient's specific needs. Underlying depression should be treated with appropriate and effectively monitored medication and, in some cases, electroconvulsive therapy. This should be followed with specific interventions as part of a treatment package directed at addressing risk factors. These would include the use of problem-solving therapy, cognitive behavioural therapy, supportive counselling, and assistance with practical issues such as finance, housing or relationships and simple interventions such as sending caring letters (Comtois and Linehan, 2005).

Observation

Constant observation has always been a key part of inpatient suicide prevention, despite the fact that it is a problematic activity and unpopular with both staff and patients (Duffy, 1995; Bowers *et al*., 2000). It is noteworthy that around one fifth of inpatient suicides occurred in people who were under either constant or intermittent levels of non-routine observation (Department of Health, 2001). Constant observation can offer therapeutic benefits, as well as promote physical safety if applied by appropriately skilled staff. To this end, staff should receive appropriate skills-based training, be supported and supervised, and should not be asked to observe patients for longer than an hour at a time (Duffy, 1995). Given the potential for harm through premature reduction of observation levels, this must not take place without careful, documented risk assessment and multidisciplinary agreement (Clinical Resource and Audit Group, 2002).

Environmental safety

The development of units which offer a therapeutic ambience through the use of single bedrooms and complex layouts, while very justifiable, has meant that the observation of patients at risk has become more difficult than formerly. The main method of suicide by inpatients is by hanging, most commonly from a curtain rail, using a belt as a ligature (Department of Health, 2001), and services are now required to ensure that shower curtain rails are non-weight bearing. It is essential that likely ligature points are removed from anywhere accessible to at-risk patients and that regular audit of the clinical environment is carried out to identify potential suicide hazards, such as easily breakable windows.

Violence risk assessment and management

Throughout history, most societies have assumed a link between mental disorder and violence to others (Monahan and Steadman, 1994). 'Although the majority of users of mental health services are not violent, it is clear that a small yet significant minority are violent in inpatient settings and the community' (Doyle and Duffy, 2006, p. 135, citing Swanson *et al.* 1990; Monahan *et al.*, 2000; Hiday, 1997). In recent times, particularly following the murder of Jonathon Zito by Christopher Clunis in 1992, there has been increasing concern in the UK over law and order, specifically the risk of violence, and these issues are now high on the political agenda. Several incidents have received considerable media attention and left a strong impression of the potential dangerousness to the public of individuals with various forms of mental disorder (Ryan, 2000). There is increasing suspicion that the professionals and various institutions which are expected to manage risk in day-to-day life have not performed adequately. This has been reinforced by subsequent official inquiries, some of which reveal serious shortcomings, both in the clinical management and supervision of these individuals, and in failures in liaison and cooperation between agencies (Reed, 1997). These perceived failures can be linked in the minds of the public with the perception of inadequate service provision (for example, secure inpatient beds in the case of psychiatric services), and with the growing concern that the public are not adequately protected from dangerous individuals by current legislation (Department of Health, 1999). Regardless of whether people with mental disorder are more likely to be violent than the non-mentally disordered, it is evident that there is a significant minority of mental health service users who pose a risk to others. 'This is reinforced by the finding that nurses are the occupational group most at risk of violence... and staff working in NHS Mental Health Service Trusts are up to eight times more likely to be assaulted than staff working in non-Mental Health Trusts' (Doyle and Duffy, 2006; p. 135, citing Gallagher, 1999; NHS Executive (North West), 1999, p. 8).

Risk factors for violence

The factors that provide information about who, in a given population, is going to be violent have been termed *risk factors*, which are measurable factors that correlate with and precede the outcome of interest (Kraemer *et al*., 1997), in this case, violence. Increasing knowledge of what factors best predict challenging/aggressive behaviour could help mental health nurses to (1) recognise factors predictive/protective of violent and aggressive behaviour; (2) identify targets for intervention; and (3) equip them with knowledge and skills to reduce risk to the service user, staff and public. This should also highlight training needs and areas where improved approaches to care, treatment and management are required, as until clinicians are better informed of the factors associated with violent behaviour there is little chance of improving the accuracy of risk assessments (Monahan and Steadman, 1994).

There are many studies that have attempted to identify which factors are most closely associated with an increased risk of violence from people with mental disorder. However, the field has

Box 6.3 Warning signs that risk of violence might be escalating (quoted from National Institute for Health and Clinical Excellence, 2005, p. 18f)

- Facial expressions tense and angry.
- Increased or prolonged restlessness, body tension, pacing
- General over-arousal of body systems (increased breathing and heart rate, muscle twitching, dilating pupils)
- Increased volume of speech, erratic movements
- Prolonged eye contact
- Discontentment, refusal to communicate, withdrawal, fear, irritation
- Unclear thought processes, poor concentration
- Delusions or hallucinations with violent content
- Verbal threats or gestures
- Replicating, or behaviour similar to that which preceded earlier disturbed/violent episodes
- Reporting anger or violent feelings
- Blocking escape routes

been blighted by a number of problems and it is recognised that research in this area is flawed, with methodological shortcomings and little consistency in the research approaches (Monahan, 1984). Despite the importance of the subject area, there are few consistent studies that investigate fully the heterogeneous nature of violent behaviour in mental health services. However, a number of large multi-factorial studies have explored risk factors for inpatient violence (e.g. Royal College of Psychiatrists, 1998; Crichton, 1995; Almvik *et al.*, 1999), community violence (e.g. Monahan *et al.*, 2000; Swanson *et al.*, 1990; Klassen and O'Connor, 1988) and differences between mentally disordered and non-mentally disordered individuals, in terms of which risk factors predict violence (Bonta *et al.*, 1998). The literature is far from consistent in concluding the most valid risk factors for violence. However, there is evidence that a number of characteristics relating to past history, current functioning, protective influences and the individual's context/environment need to be taken into account when assessing violence risk. A more detailed discussion of these risk factors can be found in Chapter 5 of this book, although a summary of antecedents and warning signs for violence in acute settings is provided in Box 6.3, taken from recent national guidance (National Institute for Clinical Excellence, 2005). Consideration of some or all these factors should make the risk assessment process more systematic and transparent, while improving risk communication between clinicians as part of a multidisciplinary approach.

Managing violence risk

The management of risk to others encompasses clinical, health and safety and public protection (political) issues, which have to be balanced against the rights of the individual. Indeed, this forms one of the most vociferous debates concerning the radical changes, originally introduced in proposed reforms to the Mental Health Act (Department of Health, 1999), but later dropped (Department of Health, 2002) concerning the detention of individuals with 'dangerous and severe personality disorder' (DSPD). Despite this, under 'dangerous severe personality disorder' (DSPD) policy, individuals judged to have DSPD who are *considered to be a risk* to others can be admitted for compulsory treatment. Effective risk assessment should be part of risk management and vice versa, and as behaviour likely to cause harm to others may be symptomatic of many disorders, it is unlikely to be susceptible to any single intervention. Closely examining the factors that have contributed to past violent behaviour should prove fruitful in identifying targets for treatment that may reduce risk. For example: poor anger control – anger management; substance abuse – drug/alcohol therapy; persecutory delusions – cognitive and pharmacological interventions. In summarising the approaches to managing violence risk, Harris and Rice (1997) distinguish between several types of risk management intervention that take account of both security and therapeutic interventions. These include interventions that are:

- **Static**: involves preventing harm via such things as video monitoring, seclusion and locked doors.
- **Dynamic**: aims to prevent harm using control and restraint techniques and electronic tagging, as required.
- **Situational**: attempts to restrict access to the means of violence or potential victims; e.g. a paedophile having restricted contact with children.

- **Pharmacological**: involves using medication to alleviate symptoms or reduce arousal.
- **Interpersonal**: mainly through communication, using calming and de-escalation techniques and rapport building, with a view to developing a therapeutic relationship.
- **Self-control**: helping the service user by psychotherapeutic, psychosocial or pharmacological means to control behaviour.

In clinical practice, mental health nurses need to draw upon knowledge, skills and experience from a number of different areas. Broadly speaking, current mental health nursing practice involves applying a biopsychosocial model. Recently, in parallel with the advances in pharmacological interventions for people with serious mental illness, there has been an increasing emphasis on equipping mental health nurses with the knowledge and skills to carry out psychosocial interventions, largely as a result of the development and implementation of the *Thorn Initiative* training programme (Lancashire *et al.*, 1997). The core modules of the Thorn programme are assertive community treatment, psychological interventions (including cognitive behavioural approaches to delusions and hallucinations), and family interventions. Key elements of the courses include the use of objective assessments and adherence to the principles of evaluation, using simple, reliable measures of change (Gournay, 2000). Up until recently, the main focus of training for PSI and the implementation of the interventions has been confined to community settings, yet it is now recognised that mental health nurses working in inpatient settings have been starved of skills and require new training initiatives (Standing Nursing and Midwifery Advisory Committee, 1999). Recent reports have stated that all service users with serious mental illness should have access to psychosocial interventions as a standard part of care (Standing Nursing and Midwifery Advisory Committee, 1999; Duggen, 1997). Evidence suggests that psychosocial interventions may provide lasting benefits by reducing distress associated with positive symptoms, as well as relapse rates and the length of hospital stays, thus improving the overall functioning of service users with severe mental illness and decreasing the distress of their families (Wykes *et al.*, 1998; Drury *et al.*, 1996; Lancashire *et al.*, 1997).

In terms of risk management of violence, psychosocial interventions should be an essential part of the practice of clinicians working with service users with challenging and aggressive behaviours. The vast majority of service users who are in secure settings have serious mental illness and residual distressing positive symptoms (Ewers and Doyle, 2001). As there is often a link between violent disturbed behaviour and symptoms, any interventions that could increase the service user's self-management should play an integral part of risk assessment and management. New training programmes have been developed for mental health nurses working with forensic populations, applying the principles of psychosocial interventions (Gournay, 2000). Psychosocial interventions, and in particular, formulation-based cognitive behavioural interventions, are seen by many as the psychological treatment of choice when working with violent and forensic populations (McGuire, 1995; Wong and Gordon, 2000; Novaco, 1997; Thomson, 2000), although further rigorous treatment trials are required in this area.

Although people suffering from mental illnesses contribute little to overall violence in society, there is still a significant minority of mental health service users who pose a risk to others, usually to those who work or live with them. Therefore, there is a need for mental health nurses to assess violence risk to try to identify which service users will be violent in inpatient and community settings, and what interventions are required to prevent violence and to minimise the risk to the service user and others.

Systematic approach to assessing, formulating and managing risk in clinical practice

In a recent review of risk assessment and risk management, Doyle and Duffy (2006, pp. 145ff) conclude:

> The stages of clinical risk assessment and management may be conceptualised as an ongoing, [dynamic] process. This process has been described as a Risk Management Cycle (Doyle 1998) and is usually implicit to the provision of good quality health care and integrated into the Care Programme Approach. The basis of any assessment relies on the accumulation of reliable information and consideration of risk factors. The debate as to whether the clinical, 'subjective', or actuarial – 'statistical/objective' approach is most relevant to clinical practice is complex and beyond the scope of this chapter... The reality of clinical practice is that tests and scales can help to inform clinical judgement, not replace it, as ultimately it is people, not tests, who make decisions. There is evidence to suggest that a combination of the clinical and actuarial approach is warranted to structure clinicians' risk judgements and this may be superior to unaided clinical judgement (Borum 1996, Douglas *et al.* 1999, McNiel and Binder 1994). The *Structured Professional Judgement Approach* attempts to bridge the gap between the scientific (actuarial) approach and the clinical practice of risk assessment. This approach emphasises the need to take account of past history, objective measures, current presentation, context/environment and protective factors; and recognises the reality that the process of clinical risk assessment is a dynamic and continuous process which is mediated by changing conditions (see Doyle 2000, Dolan and Doyle 2000).

Recently, Doyle (2004) and Doyle and Duffy (2006, pp. 145ff)

> ... Proposed a sequential 5-step approach to risk management in mental health services (see Box 6.4) designed to (1) structure professional risk judgements and foster an evidence-based approach; (2) enhance understanding of origins, development and maintenance of risk behaviour; (3) involve the person being assessed; (4) identify targets for intervention; and (5) facilitate defensible decision making and positive risk taking.
>
> The first step is concerned with accumulating information about the individual, being mindful of the need for multiple assessment methods and the use of different sources of information. *Step two* involves identifying historical and current risk factors relating to the outcome of concern, e.g. self-harm, violence. *Step three* supplements step two by identifying past and present protective factors associated with a decreased risk. Protective factors could include compliance with treatment, good support from friends, family and services or restrictions on movements. *Step four* is the stage where the risk information, already collected in steps 1–3, is analysed in an attempt to gain a better understanding and formulation of the person's current risk. This stage resembles attempts to conceptualise risk behaviours for treatment purposes (for example Novaco 1994, Linehan 1993). Recently, Huessman (1998) developed a unified social information processing model which similarly linked events, schemas and emotional states to provide an information processing frame-

Box 6.4 Five-step structured professional judgement approach to risk management
Reproduced, with kind permission of Quay Books, from Doyle and Duffy (2006, p. 146)

Step 1: Case information
History, mental state, substance use

Step 2: Presence of risk factors
Historical, current, contextual

Step 3: Presence of protective factors
Historical, current, contextual

Step 4: Risk formulation
Nature, severity, imminence, likelihood, risk-reducing/enhancing

Step 5: Management plan
Treatment, management, monitoring, supervision, victim safety planning

work which explained the role of cognitions in aggression. An idiosyncratic, personalised risk formulation should inform *Step five*, where management interventions are developed into a risk management plan. The 5-step approach is meant to be broad in its applicability to different service settings. The approach is practice-based, in that it attempts both to reflect existing clinical practice while enhancing the utility of a structured evidence-based approach to risk management (Doyle and Duffy, 2006, p. 146ff).

Summary

When assessing those with mental health problems and criminal offending behaviours, nurses should recognise that a significant element of the person's needs is unlikely to differ from people more generally in contact with acute mental health services. The element of offending and concern about dangerous behaviours does, however, require specific and detailed attention. For many mental health nurses, these aspects of assessment expertise should be gained through supervised practice with more experienced practitioners. There can be significant negative outcomes arising from assessment for people with mental health problems and criminal offending behaviours. Mental health nurses should attempt to collaborate with the person during the assessment process to set a firm foundation for prioritising helpful intervention. The ultimate aim of assessment is to learn enough about the person, so that together we can build on strengths and provide the foundations for meaningful and lasting recovery.

References

Allebeck, P. and Allgulander, C. (1990) Suicide among young men: psychiatric illness, deviant behaviour and substance abuse. *Acta Psychiatrica Scandinavia*, **81**, 565–70.

Allen, J. (1997) Assessing and managing risk of violence in the mentally disordered. *Journal of Psychiatric and Mental Health Nursing*, **4**, 369–78.

Almvik, R., Woods, P. and Rasmussen, K. (1999) The Broset Violence Checklist: sensitivity, specificity and interrater reliability. *Journal of Interpersonal Violence*, **15**(12), 1284–96.

Bluglass, R. and Bowden, P. (1990) *Principles and Practice in Forensic Psychiatry*. Churchill Livingstone, Edinburgh.

Bonta, J., Law, M. and Hanson, K. (1998) The prediction of criminal and violent recidivism among mentally disordered offenders: a meta-analysis. *Psychological Bulletin*, **123**(2), 123–42.

Borum, R. (1996) Improving the clinical practice of violence risk assessment. *American Psychologist*, **51**(9), 945–56.

Bowers, L., Gournay, K. and Duffy, D. (2000) Suicide and self-harm in in-patient psychiatric units: a national survey of observation policies. *Journal of Advanced Nursing*, **32**, 437–44.

Clinical Resource and Audit Group (2002) *Engaging People: Observation of People with Acute Mental Health Problems: a Good Practice Statement*. CRAG/Scottish Executive, Edinburgh.

Coffey, M. (2005) Forensic mental health nursing. In: *Planning Care in Mental Health Nursing* (ed. R. Tummey). Palgrave, Basingstoke.

Comtois, K. A. and Linehan, M. (2006) Psychosocial treatments of suicidal behaviors: a practice-friendly review. *Journal of Clinical Psychology: In Session*, **62**, 161–70.

Crichton, J. (1995) A review of psychiatric inpatient violence. In: *Psychiatric Patient Violence: Risk and Response* (ed. J. Crichton). Duckworth, London.

Department of Health (1999) *Report of the Expert Committee: Review of the Mental Health Act 1983*. Stationery Office, London.

Department of Health (2000) *Effective Care Co-ordination in Mental Health Services: Modernising the Care Programme Approach. A Policy Booklet*. Department of Health, London.

Department of Health (2001) *Safety First: Five Year Report of the National Inquiry into Suicide and Homicide by People with Mental Illness*. Stationery Office: London.

Department of Health (2002) *Mental Health Bill. Cm 5538*. Stationery Office, London.

Department of Health (2006) *From Values to Action: the Chief Nursing Officer's Review of Mental Health Nursing*. Department of Health, London.

Dolan, M. and Doyle, M. (2000) Violence risk prediction: clinical and actuarial measures and the role of the psychopathy checklist. *British Journal of Psychiatry*, **177**, 303–11.

Douglas, K., Cox, D. and Webster, C. (1999) Violence risk assessment: science and practice. *Legal and Criminological Psychology*, **4**, 149–84.

Doyal, L. and Gough, I. (1991) *A Theory of Human Need*. Macmillan, Basingstoke.

Doyle, M. (1996) Assessing risk of violence from clients. *Mental Health Nursing*, **16**(3), 20–3.

Doyle, M. (1998) Clinical risk assessment for mental health nurses. *Nursing Times*, **94**(17), 47–9.

Doyle, M. (2000) Risk assessment and management. In: *Forensic Mental Health Nursing: Current Approaches* (eds. C. Chaloner and M. Coffey). Blackwell Science, London.

Doyle, M. (2004) Systematic approaches to assessing, formulating and managing risk. Keynote Paper Presented at Annual NW Forensic Network Conference: *Seeing Red: Current Perspectives on Violence*. Lowry Centre, Salford Quays, 25 November.

Doyle, M. and Duffy, D. (2006) Assessing and managing risk to self and others. In: *Forensic Mental Health Nursing: Interventions for People with 'Personality Disorder'* (ed. The National Forensic Nurses' Research and Development Group), Chapter 10. Quay, Salisbury.

Drury, V., Birchwood, M. and Cochrane, R. (1996) Cognitive therapy and recovery from acute psychosis: a controlled trial. II. Impact on recovery time. *British Journal of Psychiatry*, **169**, 602–7.

Duffy, D. (1995) Out of the shadows: a study of the special observation of psychiatric in-patients. *Journal of Advanced Nursing*, **21**, 944–50.

Duggen, M. (1997) *Pulling Together: Future Roles and Training for Mental Health Staff*. Sainsbury Centre for Mental Health, London.

Edwards, K. (2005) *Partnership Working in Mental Health Care: The Nursing Dimension*. Elsevier Churchill Livingstone, Edinburgh.

Ewers, P. and Doyle, M. (2001) The implementation of psychosocial interventions in a forensic mental health service. *Conference Paper Presentation at Creating Seamless Services in Forensic Psychiatry*, University of Central Lancashire, 5 June.

Gallagher, J. (1999) *Violent Times: TUC Report on Preventing Violence At Work*. Trade Union Congress Health and Safety Unit.

Gournay, K. (2000) Role of the community psychiatric nurse in the management of schizophrenia. *Advances in Psychiatric Treatment*, **6**, 243–51.

Harris, G. and Rice, M. (1997) Risk appraisal and management of violent behaviour. *Psychiatric Services*, **48**(9), 1168–76.

Hawton, K., Sutton, L., Haw, C. Sinclair, J. and Deeks, J. (2005) Schizophrenia and suicide: systematic review of risk factors. *British Journal of Psychiatry*, **187**, 9–20.

Health Advisory Service (1994) *Suicide Prevention: Mental Health Services – the Challenge Confronted*. HMSO, London.

Hiday, V. (1997) Understanding the connection between mental illness and violence. *International Journal of Law and Psychiatry*, **20**(4), 399–417.

H. M. Government (1983) *The Mental Health Act*. HMSO, London.

Huessmann, L. R. (1998) The role of social information processing and cognitive schema in the acquisition and maintenance of habitual aggressive behavior. In: *Human Aggression: Theories, Research and Implications for Social Policy* (eds. R. Geen and E. Donnerstein). Academic Press, London.

Klassen, D. and O'Connor, W. (1988) Crime, inpatient admissions and violence among male mental patients. *International Journal of Law and Psychiatry*, **11**, 305–12.

Kraemer, H., Kazdin, A., Offord, D., Kesler, R., Jensen, P. and Kupfer, D. (1997) Coming to terms with the terms of risk. *Archives of General Psychiatry*, **54**, 337–43.

Krawiecka, M., Goldberg, D. and Vaughan, M. (1977) A standardized psychiatric assessment scale for rating chronic psychotic patients. *Acta Psychiatrica Scandinavia*, **55**, 299–308.

Lancashire, S., Haddock, G., Tarrier, N., Butterworth, T. and Baguley, I. (1997) Training community psychiatric nurses in psychosocial interventions in serious mental illness: the Thorn Nurse Initiative. *The Clinician*, **12**, 45–8.

Langan, J. and Lindow, V. (2004) *Living with Risk: Mental Health Service User Involvement in Risk Assessment and Management*. Policy Press, Bristol.

Linehan, M. M. (1993) *Cognitive-Behavioral Treatment of Borderline Personality Disorder*. Academic Press, New York.

MacLeod, A., Williams, J. and Linehan, M. (1992) New developments in the understanding and treatment of suicidal behaviour. *Behavioural Psychotherapy*, **20**, 193–218.

McGuire, J. (ed.) (1995) *What Works: Reducing Reoffending: Guidelines from Research and Practice*. Wiley, Chichester.

McNiel, D. E. and Binder, R. L. (1994) Screening for risk of inpatient violence. *Law and Human Behavior*, **18**, 579–86.

Monahan, J. (1984) The prediction off violent behaviour: toward a second generation of theory and policy. *American Journal of Psychiatry*, **141**, 10–15.

Monahan, J. (1992) Mental disorder and violent behaviour: perceptions and evidence. *American Psychologist*, **47**, 511–21.

Monahan, J. and Steadman, H. (eds.) (1994) *Violence and Mental Disorder: Developments in Risk Assessment*. University of Chicago Press, Chicago.

Monahan, J., Steadman, H. J., Appelbaum, P. S., Robbins, P. C., Mulvey, E. P., Silver, E., Roth, L. H. and Grisso, T. (2000) Developing a clinically useful actuarial tool for assessing violence risk. *British Journal of Psychiatry*, **176**, 312–19.

National Institute for Clinical Excellence (2005) *Violence: The Short-term Management of Disturbed/violent Behaviour in In-patient Psychiatric Settings and Emergency Departments*. Clinical Guideline 25. Developed by the National Collaborating Centre for Nursing and Supportive Care.

NHS Executive (North West) (1999) *Campaign to Stop Violence Against Staff Working in the NHS*. Press Release. 1999/0615.

Novaco, R. (1994) Anger as a risk factor for violence among the mentally disordered. In: *Violence and Mental Disorder: Developments in Risk Assessment* (eds. J. Monahan and H. Steadman). University of Chicago Press, Chicago.

Novaco, R. (1997) Remediating anger and aggression with violent offenders. *Legal and Criminological Psychology*, **2**, 77–88.

Reed, J. (1997) Risk assessment and clinical risk management: the lessons from recent inquiries. *British Journal of Psychiatry*, **170**(suppl. 32), 4–7.

Rogers, P. and Curran, J. (2004) Acute psychiatric in-patient assessment. In: *Acute Mental Health Nursing: from Acute Concerns to the Capable Practitioner*. Sage, London.

Royal College of Psychiatrists (1998) *Management of Imminent Violence: Clinical Practice Guidelines to Support Mental Health Services*. Occasional Paper OP41. March.

Ryan, T. (2000) Exploring the risk management strategies of mental health service users. *Health, Risk and Society*, **2**(3), 267–82.

Scottish Executive Health Department (2006) *Rights, Relationships and Recovery: the Report of the National Review of Mental Health Nursing in Scotland*. Scottish Executive, Edinburgh.

Salter, D. and Platt, S. (1990) Suicidal intent, hopelessness and depression in a parasuicide population: the influence of social desirability and elapsed time. *British Journal of Clinical Psychology*, **29**, 361–71.

Slade, M. (2003) Assessing needs in community mental health care. In: *The Handbook of Community Mental Health Nursing* (eds. B. Hannigan and M. Coffey). Routledge, London.

Standing Nursing and Midwifery Advisory Committee (1999) *Practice Guidance: Safe and Supportive Observation of Patients at Risk*. Stationery Office, London.

Sullivan, M. (2003) The new subjective medicine: taking the patient's point of view on health care and health. *Social Science and Medicine*, **56**, 1595–604.

Swanson, J., Holzer, C., Ganju, V. and Jono, R. (1990) Violence and psychiatric disorder in the community: evidence from the epidemiological catchment area surveys. *Hospital and Community Psychiatry*, **41**, 762–70.

Thomas, S., Harty, M. A., Parrott, J., McCrone, P., Slade, M. and Thornicroft, G. (2003) *CANFOR: Camberwell Assessment of Need – Forensic Version*. Gaskell, London.

Thomson, L. D. (2000) Management of schizophrenia in conditions of high security. *Advances in Psychiatric Treatment*, **6**, 252–60.

University of Manchester (1996) *Learning Materials on Mental Health Risk Assessment*. School of Psychiatry and Behavioural Sciences, Manchester.

Welsh Assembly Government (WAG) (2003) *The Care Programme Approach for Mental Health Service Users: a Unified and Fair System for Assessing and Managing Care*. Welsh Assembly Government, Cardiff.

Webster, C. D., Douglas, K., Eaves, D. and Hart, S. (1997) *HCR-20: Assessing Risk for Violence – Version 2*. Simon Fraser University, British Columbia.

Wong, S. and Gordon, A. (2000) *Violence Reduction Programme: Phases of Treatment and Content Overview*. Regional Psychiatric Centre, Saskatoon, Saskatchewan.

Woodbridge, K. and Fulford, B. (2004) *Whose Values? A Workbook for Values-based Practice in Mental Health Care*. Sainsbury Centre for Mental Health, London.

Wykes, T., Tarrier, N. and Lewis, S. (1998) *Outcome and Innovation in Psychological Innovation in Schizophrenia*. Wiley, Chichester.

CHAPTER 7

Measurement of health and social functioning

Phil Woods and Alyson McGregor Kettles

Introduction

This chapter will outline an important aspect of acute mental health care – that of health and social functioning. Many patients with forensic histories who find themselves on acute mental health wards have varying health and social functioning difficulties. Many of these will be profound, perhaps based on years of problematic alcohol or drug use, and in some instances, occurring as a result of the medication they are prescribed or how enduring their disorders are. Firstly, the issues around health, mental health and social functioning will be discussed. Secondly, two particular measures that have been used to assess and determine levels of health and social functioning will be introduced. Finally, the chapter will conclude with a discussion of issues for practice.

Health, mental health and social functioning

In the widest sense, health includes mental, physical, psychological or spiritual aspects; it is worth considering what are generally known as the determinants of health. These include factors such as where we live, the state of our environment, genetics, our income and education level, and our relationships with friends and family. There is little doubt that a combination of all these factors can have a significant impact on health. According to the World Health Organization (2006), determinants of health include the social and economic environment, the physical environment, and the person's individual characteristics and behaviours.

A recent report by the World Health Organization highlighted more specific evidence relative to the social determinants of health (Wilkinson and Marmot, 2003). The authors suggest that these social determinants of health are perhaps the most challenging and complex of all, as they are concerned with living, working and lifestyle. Specifically, such issues as the social gradient, stress, a good start in early life, social exclusion, work, unemployment, social support, addiction, food and transport are highlighted as important components. Moreover, when considering acute mental health care and those who have associated forensic issues, many of these components are particularly relevant aspects of therapeutic care.

Social functioning in the widest sense is about how we go about our daily lives in society, our relationships, our work, the contributions society makes to us and those we make to society. Breaking it down to the micro level, it is heavily influenced by our social skills and levels of health; hence the strength of relationship between the two concepts of health and social functioning.

A useful quote to consider when measuring mental health and social functioning is from the World Health Organization (2003, p. 7): 'Mental health is more than the mere lack of mental disorders'. The positive dimension of mental health is stressed in WHO's definition of health, as contained in its constitution: 'Health is a state of complete physical, mental and social well-being and not merely the absence of disease or infirmity'. WHO further consider concepts of mental health to include subjective well-being, perceived self-efficacy, autonomy, competence, intergenerational dependence and recognition of the ability to realise one's intellectual and emotional potential. Mental health has also been defined as a state of well-being whereby individuals recognise their abilities, are able to cope with the normal stresses of life, work productively and fruitfully, and make a contribution to their communities.

It is perhaps appropriate to consider, at this point, the necessity for patients to 'change' in some way. When patients enter the acute clinical area they are there for some level of assessment of current mental state and because of the associated behaviour or behaviours which have brought them to inpatient care. In many cases, the person is there for the risk they present to themselves or others to be reduced, but the question must also be asked 'To what extent does making changes enhance the individual's quality of life?'. Mental health staff are looking for 'appropriate' behaviour to be established before the person is discharged from care and resumes their place in society. Negative behavior reduction has always been a part of the nurse's role, so that a person who has been violent or aggressive on admission would no longer be aggressive and would have regained some level of voluntary control over their behaviour. However, this is no longer an adequate nursing goal in itself, as the continuing evolution of care processes has now entered a new era with the advent of new models of care.

Patients are now expected to participate in their own care, so a goal of care would no longer be 'X will reduce his violent behaviour by attending anger management group, use of psychoeducation therapy and individual counseling'. Rather, the plan will be more extensive, identifying the strengths of X and using them more constructively by focusing on those strengths and what X can achieve, rather than on any weaknesses, but having an awareness of the latter, as well as including the more traditional therapies and programmes where relevant. Both the English (Department of Health, 2006) and Scottish (Scottish Executive, 2006) Mental Health Nursing Reviews have recommended that the Recovery model (Onken *et al.*, 2002) the Strengths model (Rapp and Goscha, 2006) and the Tidal model (Barker, 2002) be adopted by mental health nurses. Adoption of these models will enable a much more positive attitude and approach to care to be developed. The view exists that focusing only on areas of change is stigmatising (Dooher and Byrt, 2003). The new models of care enable and ensure that recognition of the positive aspects of individuals' lives is not only included in, but is viewed as essential to, the recovery process.

Health and social functioning scales

Over the years, many scales have developed to measure health and social functioning in mental health and forensic mental health care (more than fifty to date). Furthermore, social functioning has been given its own axis in the DSM. Whilst it is outside the scope of this chapter to discuss all of these, two measures that have been developed primarily for clinical use, but have research evaluations centred on them, will be introduced.

One of these is the Health of the Nation Outcome Scale (HoNOS) which is widely used and has a forensic adaptation. The other is the Behavioural Status Index (BEST-Index), developed for use in forensic care and widely studied in the last few years.

Health of the Nation Outcome Scale

The Health of the Nation Outcome Scale (HoNOS) was produced as a result of the UK Department of Health commissioning the Royal College of Psychiatrists' Research Unit to develop a scale to measure the health and social functioning of people with severe mental illness (Wing *et al.*, 1996). Development involved stringent testing of acceptability, usability, sensitivity, reliability and validity (Royal College of Psychiatrists, 2004). HoNOS research has resulted in many adaptations (HoNOS (Working Age Adult); HoNOS65+ (Older adults); HoNOSCA (Children and Adolescents); HoNOS-secure; HoNOS-LD (Learning Disabilities); and HoNOS-ABI (Acquired Brain Injury)) that have emerged for specific client groups. These adaptations have been the focus of considerable research in relation to health and social functioning and currently form part of the national data set for mental health in the UK.

HoNOS consists of 12 items (see Box 7.1), measured on a five-point severity scale: 0 = no problem; 1 = minor problem requiring no action; 2 = mild problem but definitely present; 3 = mod-

Box 7.1 HoNOS (Working Age Adult) items (from Wing *et al.*, 1996)

1. Overactive, aggressive, disruptive or agitated behaviour
2. Non-accidental self-injury
3. Problem drinking or drug-taking
4. Cognitive problems
5. Physical illness or disability problems
6. Problems associated with hallucinations and delusions
7. Problems with depressed mood
8. Other mental and behavioural problems
9. Problems with relationships
10. Problems with activities of daily living
11. Problems with living conditions
12. Problems with occupation and activities

Box 7.2 HoNOS-secure version 2 additional security items (from Sugarman and Walker, 2004)

A = risk of harm to adults or children
B = risk of self-harm (deliberate or accidental)
C = need for building security to prevent physical escape
D = need for a safely staffed living environment
E = need for escort on leave (beyond the secure perimeter)
F = risk to individual from others
G = need for risk management procedures

Box 7.3 From: BEST-Index risk sub-scale items

1. Family support
2. Serious violence to others without apparent trigger event
3. Serious violence to others following trigger event
4. Minor violence to others without apparent trigger event
5. Minor violence to others following trigger event
6. Serious self-harm
7. Superficial self-harm
8. Verbal aggression without apparent trigger event
9. Verbal aggression following trigger event
10. Attacks on objects without apparent trigger event
11. Attacks on objects following trigger event
12. Breaches of security
13. Disruptive episodes
14. Imitative disruption
15. Inappropriate sexual behaviours
16. Sado-masochistic behaviours
17. Macho gear and adornment
18. Obsessive-compulsive behaviours
19. Substance abuse
20. Psychiatric disturbance

erately severe problem; 4 = severe to very severe problem. A score of 9 is given to 'not known'. According to the authors, each scale should be rated in order from 1 to 12; and no information rated in an earlier item should be included in a later item except for item 10, as this is an overall rating. Raters can use any information that is available to them from any source. Ratings are usually based on the most severe problem that occurred during the preceding two-week period.

A related version relevant to the forensic patient in acute care is the HoNOS-secure version 2 (Sugarman and Walker, 2004). This adaptation was designed for use in health and social care settings such as secure psychiatric, prison health care and related forensic services, including those based in the community, owing to issues of difficult interpretation of the original HoNOS in secure settings (Royal College of Psychiatrists, 2004). HoNOS-secure has the original 12 items (see Box 7.1) with a further seven security items (see Box 7.2). For these items, severity is rated as in the original HoNOS, on a scale of 0–4 (with 4 being worst case).

For further information on both the HoNOS (Working Age Adult) and HoNOS-secure version 2, it is recommend that the Royal College of Psychiatrists' Research Unit web site (`http://www.rcpsych.ac.uk/crtu/healthofthenation.aspx`) is visited, where a comprehensive glossary of publications, information and some of the scales are available. Readers are also directed to James and Mitchell (2004), which provides a comprehensive discussion on using the HoNOS in acute mental health nursing.

Behavioural Status Index

The Behavioural Status Index (BEST-Index) (Reed and Woods, 2000; Woods *et al.*, 1999) evaluates life skills, social risk and related daily behaviours. Although developed originally as a measure of risk, the BEST-Index directly assesses many aspects of health and social functioning.

The patient is directly involved in completing the BEST-Index and is involved throughout the entire process of assessment and decision making about areas for change for however long the admission lasts. Moreover, although recent research has focused on forensic units, its use is equally applicable to acute mental health care. The BEST-Index consists of six sub-scales (social risk, insight, communication and social skills, work and recreational activities, self and family care, and empathy) which identify essential components of human social behaviour.

The social risk sub-scale contains 20 items measuring constructs commonly associated with risk in the forensic context: for example, overt and covert violence to the more generally disruptive behaviours. This scale was constructed by comparing the results of a detailed literature search with categories that emerged following concurrent discussions held with named nurses working in the forensic context (Robinson *et al.*, 1996). See Box 7.3 for a detailed list of the items.

The insight sub-scale again consists of 20 items and examines an individual's cognitive constructs of reality. An eclectic perspective is adopted which has been derived from psychodynamic, cognitive behavioural and phenomenological theories. Examples include items related to tension, anger, personal and shared situations, or treatment and problem solving. See Box 7.4 for a list of all items.

The communication and social skills sub-scale consists of 30 items. Principally examined are behaviours of the social skills type or adaptive social behaviours. The scale is also underpinned by psychometrics in the field of abnormal psychology, where the focus is on the processes by which interpersonal relationships are established. Examined are such constructs as facial expression, proxemics (appreciation and use of space), paralinguistic features, conversational interaction, potential conflict, self-presentation and interpersonal skills. See Box 7.5 for a full list of items.

The work and recreational activities sub-scale consists of 20 items. Here, paid work is not necessarily a feature and the section is concerned with those constructive activities with which a wide range of individuals could identify. These are described predominantly according to 'social skills' or cognitive behavioural theories. See Box 7.6 for a list of all items.

Box 7.4 From: BEST-Index insight sub-scale items

1. Awareness of tension
2. Description of tension
3. Tension-reducing strategies
4. Recognition of negative or angry feelings
5. Tension-producing thoughts
6. Tension-producing events
7. Personal strategy for reducing tension
8. Identifying relaxing thoughts
9. Identifying relaxing activities
10. Attributes disliked in others
11. Attributes liked in others
12. Events producing insecurity
13. Events producing security
14. Antecedent events leading to treatment
15. Ascription of responsibility
16. Self-appraisal
17. Prioritisation of problems
18. Goal-planning
19. Compliance with therapy
20. Expectations

The self and family care sub-scale consists of 30 items and measures such daily and socially important areas as, for example, personal hygiene, cooking skills and other aspects of self-care, care for other members of the family or group, and family-group relationships. See Box 7.7 for a list of all items.

The empathy sub-scale consists of 30 items and is designed to assess the capacity of patients to empathise with others, more especially with those who have been victimised. See Box 7.8 for a list of all items.

Measuring health and social functioning using the BEST-Index

All 150 items that make up the BEST-Index are scored using a stepwise approach from 1 (worst case) through 5 (best case). The logic here is that functioning is viewed within a *normative*, rather than a *sociopathic*, frame of reference; consequently a higher score indicates the achievement of a more socially adaptive or behavioural performance that would be viewed as 'socially acceptable' by others in the contexts of the patient's family, social and cultural networks. See Table 7.1 for an example item. As lower scores are indicative of poor functioning or problematic areas, these should be the main focus of concern.

Box 7.5 From: BEST-Index communication and social skills subscale items

1. Facial expression
2. Eye contact
3. Orientation to others
4. Body posture
5. Expressive gestures
6. Social distance
7. Tone of voice
8. Voice modulation
9. Verbal delivery
10. Conversational initiative
11. Amount of speech
12. Fluency
13. Turn-taking
14. Listening skills
15. Response to questions
16. Conversational topics
17. Egocentric conversation
18. Frankness
19. Expressing opinions
20. Disagreement
21. Arguments
22. Making requests
23. Assertiveness
24. Self-presentation
25. Social activities
26. Emotional control
27. Relationship with others
28. Ease of communication
29. Sociability and support
30. Deferring to others

Table 7.1 Example of BEST-Index item rating scale.

27 RELATIONSHIPS WITH OTHERS				
27.1	27.2	27.3	27.4	27.5
Unable to stay on good terms with others	Finds great difficulty in staying on good terms with others	Stays on good terms with others for half-an-hour with support	Usually stays on good terms with others spontaneously	Always stays on good terms with others

Box 7.6 From: BEST-Index work and recreational activities sub-scale items

1. Attendance
2. Timekeeping
3. Sickness absence
4. Adaptability
5. Concentration
6. Team work
7. Interest
8. Quality of work
9. Initiative
10. Responsiveness
11. Leisure pursuits
12. Leisure and relaxation
13. Planning leisure activities
14. Suitability of selection
15. Participation in leisure
16. Hobbies and interests
17. Interest in shared leisure
18. Motivation to shared leisure
19. Gender interaction
20. Potential sexual partners

Applying health and social functioning measures to practice

Any measures that are used in practice to help identify needs and problems that can direct interventions and assist in outcome measurement need to be appropriate to the task in hand and used in the way they were intended to be. HoNOS is not a clinical assessment, according to its authors, but can help identify where needs lie, measure improvement, and direct where interventions are needed. Clinical and ethical problems can arise when there are differences of opinion between the patient and staff about the assessment itself, individual assessment items, decisions about areas for change and about the interventions needed as a result of the assessment. These situations need to be handled on an individual basis in each clinical setting. However, what the BEST-Index does is to enable a much more full and frank communication between the patient and the staff about individual assessment items and the overall assessment, so that areas of difference stand a greater chance of being resolved civilly. The BEST-Index can be seen to complement HoNOS, as it is a clinical assessment that directly assesses many of the HoNOS items. It further helps to assess many forensic areas.

Box 7.7 From: BEST-Index self and family care sub-scale items

1. Nutrition
2. Cooking
3. Eating regularly
4. Preparing own meals
5. Preparing meals for others
6. Storing food
7. Stock of food
8. Personal hygiene
9. Health precautions
10. Seeking medical help
11. Dressing for weather
12. Clothing and footwear
13. Caring for clothes
14. Storing clothes
15. Household dangers
16. Managing money
17. Economy with resources
18. Caring for the home
19. Clearing-up after meals
20. Washing up
21. Making bed(s)
22. Changing bedlinen
23. Going out
24. Using public or personal transport
25. Shopping
26. Personal grooming
27. Facial care
28. Dressing for the occasion
29. Eating out
30. Behaviour at table

Box 7.8 From: BEST-Index empathy sub-scale items

1. Imagining oneself in the life-world of another person
2. Understanding the feelings of another person, distinct from those of oneself
3. Sensitivity to others
4. Expressing sympathy for the wishes and needs of another person
5. Pleased for others
6. Allows others to express themselves
7. Interest in social 'give-and-take'
8. Dealing with conflict
9. Sharing conversations
10. Curbing self-interest
11. Listening to others
12. Physical 'mirror responses'
13. Offering support
14. Avoiding abuse
15. Listening and questioning
16. Making excuses
17. Accepting ideas
18. Comforting others
19. Acknowledging the victim
20. Giving others 'breathing space'
21. The victim as a person
22. Concern for others' troubles
23. Psychological 'intrusion'
24. Sharing 'terrors'
25. Expressing consideration
26. Taking an interest
27. Asking about feelings
28. Making eye contact
29. Balancing interests
30. Doing things for others

Case history

Jeff was admitted to a mental health acute ward. He has a longstanding mental disorder, with symptoms such as delusions of grandeur and severe paranoia. He has had many admissions over the years to both acute and forensic mental health wards. His offending history has been that of violence to others. His last admission to a forensic ward was five years ago and he has been supported by his community forensic mental health nurse since his discharge. Of late, Jeff has become increasingly paranoid and has been threatening people in his surrounding neighbourhood. The clinical team responsible for him now think it is best that Jeff is admitted for a few weeks for assessment and stabilisation. The only available admission option was his local acute mental health unit. The clinical team want to avoid any potential assaults on others and consequential charges that may result.

Assessment

On admission, Jeff was observed by nursing staff for the required two weeks and then assessed using the HoNOS (Working Age Adult) scale. This assessment showed six problem areas that were in need of some form of further assessment and intervention. Two items were rated as a severe to very severe problem (item 6 – problems associated with hallucinations and delusions, and item 9 – problems with relationships). Three items were rated as a moderately severe problems (item 1 – overactive, aggressive, disruptive or agitated behaviour; item 10 – problems with activities of daily living; and item 12 – problems with occupation and activities). One item was rated as a mild problem but definitely present (item 3 – problem drinking or drug-taking).

This assessment clearly gave a picture of Jeff's problems and strengths/positive coping strategies. However, using an instrument such as the BEST-Index, we are able to further explore these issues and use the items in the care plan to help reduce or alleviate the problem areas identified through HoNOS. Although we could, and ideally would, opt for a full assessment using all sub-scales of the BEST-Index, for the purposes here, we will assume that assessment is being undertaken using four sub-scales: insight; communication and social skills; work and recreational activities; and self and family care. For illustrative purposes, the results of some items on the insight sub-scale assessment will be discussed and applied to practice.

Tension items on the insight sub-scale indicate possible intervention areas. With considerable encouragement and support, Jeff is occasionally able to express awareness of tension (insight item 1) and describe his feelings of tension reasonably clearly (insight item 2). However, he has no constructive personal strategy for relieving tension or anxiety (item 3) and is unable to articulate a strategy for preventing/reducing feeling of irritation or anger (item 7). Furthermore, he cannot identify any thoughts which are personally relaxing and pleasurable (item 8) and cannot identify any relaxing activity (item 9). He is completely unable to make a realistic appraisal of current behavioural or emotional problems (item 16); cannot decide on relative priority or urgency of problems (item 17); and finally, cannot decide on a realistic goal-planning action (item 18). However, the BEST-Index reveals what Jeff's positive coping strategies are.

Interventions

We can clearly see from our assessment, using these illustrative items from the BEST-Index insight sub-scale, that some of Jeff's ways of coping with his tension are certainly affecting his health and social functioning. This assessment has further opened up ways for us to intervene to allow Jeff to once again function back in the community. This is the whole thrust behind the BEST-Index: to allow assessment to be linked to intervention and outcome. In formulating a plan of intervention to focus on Jeff's current functioning, we could focus on some of these items on the insight sub-scale. One-to-one sessions between Jeff and his primary nurse could be an excellent vehicle for this.

Outcomes

The BEST-Index has outcome measures that relate to the assessment integrated within the item scales, thus allowing interventions and outcomes measures to be developed, alongside the assessment, that can be used to test if interventions have been successful or not. Perhaps an example would better explain this.

If we take, for example, item 3 from the insight sub-scale (tension reducing strategies) where Jeff was rated as functioning poorly, within the scale, there are five possible scores:

- score 1 (where Jeff was rated) – has no constructive personal strategy for relieving tension and anxiety;
- score 2 – aware of problem and seeks advice or attempts to develop such a strategy;
- score 3 – cooperates with therapist to develop such a strategy;
- score 4 – follows the developed strategy with encouragement and support; and finally
- score 5 (the optimal behaviour) – spontaneously follows an insightful and constructive personal strategy.

In the ideal situation, we may want Jeff to function at the score 5 behaviour, but more realistically, he may never achieve this. He was rated at the least score possible (score of 1); therefore, we may firstly focus interventions based on score 2, but always working toward score 4. The above example, albeit simplified, shows how the BEST-Index can be used as an outcome measure to focus intervention. Thus the BEST-Index scales assist outcomes to be related through reassessment of behaviours. This logically links up to the baseline measure, which initially identified areas of poor functioning.

Assessment, mental illness, personality disorder and social functioning

The issue of assessing social functioning is affected by the setting in which the assessment is made and this relates specifically to those with personality disorder and mental illness. The setting needs to be carefully thought about, as the problems in measuring personality disorder and

Table 7.2 Comparisons of mental illness with personality disorder and social functioning in terms of assessment (after Tyrer, 1990)

	Mental illness	Personality disorder	Social functioning
Mental/clinical state	Can be recorded accurately at interview	Difficult to use as diagnosis can be variable	Affected by setting in which assessment is made
Time course	May be short, medium or long term	Very long (usually since childhood/adolescence)	Short term, as behaviours change with circumstances
Source of information	Patient/significant others preferable	Patient/significant others/police/courts/social workers/others	May be any
Affected by value judgements	Low	High	High

social functioning are more difficult than in measuring mental illness alone. The setting needs to be calm, comfortable and safe for any participant, with backup measures available, and preferably, there will be no interruptions. In personality disorder assessing mental state may not be of much value, as it can vary considerably and can also 'contaminate' underlying personality. Personality 'apparently' changes during illness and there is the danger of misinterpretation. Table 7.2 illustrates some of the issues that need to be taken into account when assessing any person for mental illness, personality disorder and social functioning.

The issue of dual/triple diagnosis of mental illness and substance misuse needs to be made distinct within any assessment for personality disorder and should include specific assessment by a substance misuse specialist. Social functioning assessment for those persons suffering from a triple diagnosis of mental illness, substance misuse and personality disorder will need more time for any therapy, care and treatment resulting from assessment, as this is a long-term issue. Acute care should not only be immediate crisis care, followed by discharge, for people with personality disorders. Rather, it should be the same initial care to begin with, as for any other person suffering from a mental illness. Subsequently, care should be very carefully worked out with specialists and community practitioners to provide the best possible care for people with such complex problems.

Conclusion

Within this chapter, issues of health and social functioning have been discussed. Whilst many forensic patients may find themselves in acute mental health care, it is usually only their 'forensic' or offending histories that make them different. Therefore, whilst health and social functioning assessment should be the same as for other clients, special consideration needs to be given to the potential risk, often to others, that has been displayed in the past. Moreover, it is necessary to consider how current problems may be related to this. What we have seen is that, whilst HoNOS is a good and well tested means of assessing health and social functioning, it has limited use for more complex clients. The BEST-Index allows further exploration of problems and focuses assessment and interventions on outcome.

References

Barker, P. (2002) The Tidal Model: the healing potential of metaphor within the patient's narrative. *Journal of Psychosocial Nursing*, **40**(7), 42–50.

Department of Health (2006) *From Values to Action: the Chief Nursing Officer's Review of Mental Health Nursing*. Department of Health, London.

Dooher, J. and Byrt, R. (eds.) (2003) *Empowerment and the Health Service User*. Quay, Salisbury.

James, M. and Mitchell, D. (2004) Measuring health and social functioning using HoNOS. In: *Acute Mental Health Nursing: From Acute Concerns to the Capable Practitioner* (eds. M. Harrison, D. Howard and D. Mitchell), pp. 29–50. Sage, London.

Onken, S. J., Dumont, J. N., Ridgway, P., Dornan, D. H. and Ralph, R. O. (2002) *Mental Health Recovery: What Helps And What Hinders? A National Research Project for the Development of Recovery Facilitating System Performance Indicators*. National Association of State Mental Health Program Directors (NASMHPD) National Technical Assistance Center (NTAC), Alexandria, VA. http://www.namiscc.org/Recovery/2002/MentalHealthRecovery.htm

Rapp, C. A. and Goscha, R. J. (2006) *The Strengths Model: Case Management with People with Psychiatric Disabilities*, 2nd edn). Oxford University Press, Oxford.

Reed, V. and Woods, P. (2000) *The Behavioural Status Index: a Life Skills Assessment for Selecting and Monitoring Therapy in Mental Health Care*. Psychometric Press, UK.

Robinson, D., Reed, V. and Lange A. (1996) Developing risk assessment scales in psychiatric care. *Psychiatric Care*, **3**(4), 146–52.

Royal College of Psychiatrists (2004) *Health of the Nation Outcome Scales*. Web site: http://www.rcpsych.ac.uk/crtu/healthofthenation.aspx.

Scottish Executive (2006) *Rights, Relationships and Recovery: The Report of the National Review of Mental Health Nursing in Scotland*. Scottish Executive, Edinburgh

Sugarman, P. and Walker, L. (2004) *Health of the Nation Outcome Scale for users of secure and forensic services: HoNOS-secure (version 2)*. St Andrew's Group of Hospitals, Northampton.

Tyrer, P. (1990) Personality disorder and social functioning. In: *Measuring Human Problems* (eds. D. F. Peck and C. M. Shapiro), Chapter 6. John Wiley & Sons, Chichester.

Wilkinson, R. and Marmot, M. (2003) *Social Determinants of Health: the Solid Facts*, 2nd edn. World Health Organization, Denmark.

Wing, J. K., Curtis, R. H. and Beevor, A. S. (1996) *HoNOS: Health of the Nation Outcome Scales: Report on Research and Development July 1993–December 1995*. Royal College of Psychiatrists, London.

Woods, P., Reed, V. and Robinson, D. (1999) The Behavioural Status Index: therapeutic assessment of risk, insight and social skills. *Journal of Psychiatric and Mental Health Nursing*, **6**, 79–90.

World Health Organization (2003). *Investing in Mental Health*. World Health Organization, Geneva.

World Health Organization (2006) *The Determinants of Health*. Web site: http://www.who.int/hia/evidence/doh/en/.

CHAPTER 8

Low conflict, high therapy nursing in a psychiatric intensive care unit

Stuart Guy, Stephen Fyffe and Wendy Ifill

Background

In this chapter, we are going to describe the practical introduction of a contemporary psychiatric ward model (Bowers *et al.*, 2006; Flood *et al.*, 2006) into a Psychiatric Intensive Care Unit (PICU). The model is based on a philosophy of low conflict and high therapy mental health nursing. The chapter includes a case study, demonstrating the new way of working, and a service user contribution, reflecting on the changes to culture and practice on the PICU. The latter provides a service to the acute and low secure psychiatric wards of an NHS Trust. In 2002, the Commission for Health Improvement reported that improvements were needed in relation to the organisational culture of the PICU and the ways in which patients were managed.

The Department of Health (2002) describes the primary function of a PICU as being to provide short-term, intensive assessment and treatment for those patients who cannot safely be managed on an open acute ward. A PICU should admit patients on grounds of clinical need, safety and appropriateness for psychiatric intensive care and not on issues of security. This should be arranged after all possible strategies to effect positive change in disturbed behaviour have been tried on open acute wards. Examples of interventions in the latter include de-escalation, therapeutic activity programmes, adequate medication regimes (including rapid tranquillisation), adequate nursing support and interventions and other multidisciplinary input.

The care and management of patients with acutely disturbed behaviour poses many challenges. Patients may exhibit an array of behaviours to harm themselves or others in their immediate environment, 'be acutely confused, sexually disinhibited or prone to abscond'. Such behaviours have been termed 'patient conflict behaviours' (Bowers *et al.*, 2006, p. 165). A survey of 100 qualified psychiatric nurses identified conflict behaviours as frequently linked with reasons why nurses thought patients would benefit from a PICU environment (Bowers *et al.*, 2003).

Psychiatric Intensive Care Units are still relatively recent innovations within British psychiatry, 'with the first... unit... opening in Portsmouth in 1972' (Crowhurst and Bowers, 2003, p. 689, citing Mounsey, 1979). There is currently limited research to support their function. Besides medication,

PICU therapeutic functioning is variously influenced by 'psychoanalytical theory, neo-Freudianism and behavioural and cognitive behavioural methods' in interventions with individuals who are acutely distressed. None of these methods of intervention and management has been 'specifically evaluated within the context of PICU care' (Crowhurst and Bowers, 2003, p. 694). The latter authors make reference to a number of non pharmacological interventions, including teamwork (Brown and Wellman, 1998) reducing arousal by talking to acutely ill patients (Mills, 1997) and 'effective... observation' (Crowhurst and Bowers, 2003, p. 691, citing Saverimuttu and Lowe, 2000). Such interventions, described as non-containment behaviours (Bowers *et al.*, 2006), reflect the professional skills of the authors of this chapter, who work within such an environment.

Low conflict, high therapy nursing

Bowers *et al.* (2006) argue that variation in conflict behaviours that exist in PICUs and acute psychiatric settings may be 'because of the differences in the ways psychiatric nurses think and behave' and not anything to do with 'any obvious difference in the type of patients' (Bowers *et al.*, 2006, p. 166). In response to this hypothesis, Bowers (2002) and Bowers *et al.* (2006) have devised a working model of low conflict, high therapy psychiatric nursing (Figure 8.1).

'This model identifies three important factors in staff behaviour for the production of low conflict, high therapy psychiatric [nursing]' (Bowers *et al.*, 2006, p. 166; see also Bowers, 2002). These processes include a 'positive appreciation of patients by staff; the ability of the staff to regulate their own natural emotional reactions to patients; and the creation of effective ward structure, rules and routine...' (Bowers *et al.*, 2006, p. 166; see also Bowers, 2002). For these processes to be accomplished, the following foundations are essential (Bowers *et al.*, 2006, p. 166; Flood *et al.*, 2006, p. 260):

- 'the psychiatric philosophy of staff (how they see and understand mental illness and their role in care and treatment)' and managing risk
- 'their moral commitments' (adherence to 'professionalism, humanism, honesty') and patient centeredness
- 'their use of cognitive emotional self management methods' (use of moral and philosophical positions to manage emotional reactions and perceptions of patients)
- 'their technical mastery (in interpersonal [and engagement] skills with patients and colleagues)'
- 'teamwork skill (the achievement of cohesion, consistency and mutual support within and across disciplinary boundaries)'
- 'organisational support (provision of clinical supervision and learning opportunities'

(Quotations from Bowers et al., *2006, p. 166; see also Bowers, 2002; Flood* et al., *2006, p. 260)*

If the model is functioning correctly and the required mechanisms are in place, this results in processes being accomplished, with the demonstration of clear outcomes. The latter include positive staff attitudes, beneficial patient outcomes, high therapy, low conflict and low containment environments.

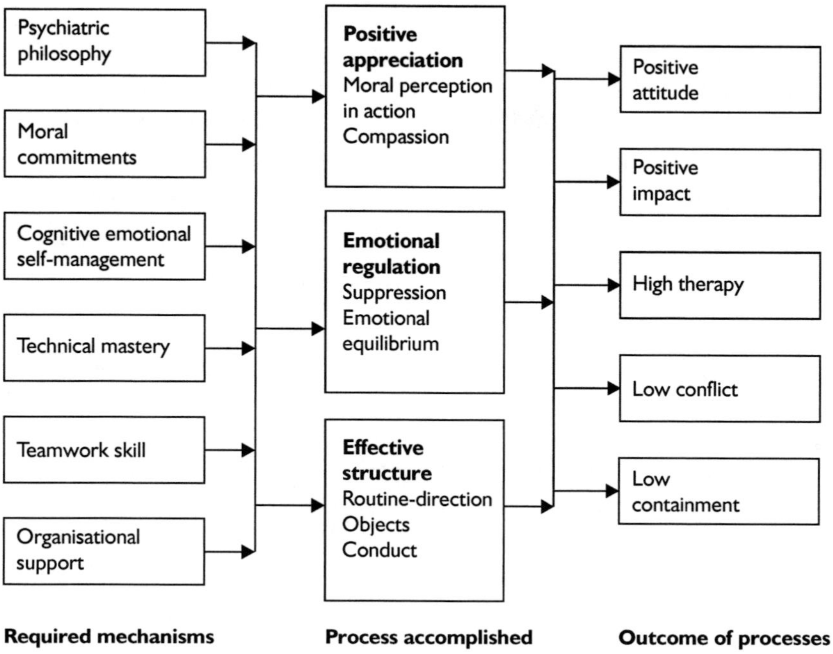

Figure 8.1 Low conflict, high therapy mental health nursing (Bowers *et al.*, 2006). (Thanks to Routledge Taylor & Francis for kind permission to reprint Figure 7.1 from Bowers, L. (2002) *Dangerous and Severe Personality Disorder Response and Role of the Psychiatric Team*, p. 144.)

Bowers (2002) describes a patient group who present with conflict behaviours will inevitably test the limits of the staff charged with caring for them. Across a spectrum of staff, this can result in the development of both positive and negative care belief systems. These competing beliefs can cause a dynamic gulf, which the patient utilises to cause numerous problems within the multidisciplinary team, interfering in the goal of providing care and treatment.

When two of the authors first started working on the PICU described in this chapter, they were confronted with the reverse of the functioning model (Bowers, 2002; Bowers *et al.*, 2006). A cultural state of negativity and pessimism was prevalent. Psychosocial treatments were considered to be ineffective. Staff demonstrated a lack of moral commitment and were, therefore, negative towards the PICU patients. They had reduced capacity for self-management skills to enable each other to cope with emotional responses to patients' violence or self-harming behaviours. Staff presented as being interpersonally unskilled, making little effort to interact with patients and deal with their conflict behaviours, spending most of the shift in the office. Teamworking lacked effective mutual support and collaboration. As a consequence, staff had lost the ability to value mentally distressed and acutely disturbed patients, rejecting and avoiding psychosocial interaction with them. Staff were unable to regulate their own emotional responses, with angry and judgemental feelings towards patients as a consistent part of their normal attitude. The PICU worked with an ineffective structure, with ambiguous roles and rules of containment, leaving staff isolated and unable to function. Staff generally showed little appetite for their work, feeling exposed and vulnerable, and were rejecting of patients and pessimistic. Opportunities for therapeutic engagement were being missed and undermined by an ineffective ward structure. Conflict between patients and between staff was frequent and intense, with a high level of seclusion being used. Recognition of these difficulties by Trust managers resulted in two of the authors being asked to develop the required mechanisms to produce a low containment, low conflict, high therapy PICU environment.

Implementing low conflict high therapy nursing on a PICU

The model aimed to address staff–patient conflicts, utilising a framework to promote positive treatment attitudes in staff caring for patients who are acutely aroused, moving the PICU away from using seclusion (Lehane and Rees, 1995) towards promoting an extra care treatment philosophy where non-confrontational nursing approaches are used, allowing for patient expression of anger and confusion (Dix and Williams, 1996). This was to be embedded in a culture of supported psychosocial engagement utilising protected therapeutic time (Kent, 2005) with patients on each shift, with the focus on reducing patient ambiguity and arousal. In line with Bowers' (2002) model, focus was given to redefining the required foundations for positive staff attitudes to start to develop.

Shift management system

The underlying principle of any PICU is to create and maintain a safe environment. This is seen as the cornerstone of building productive and therapeutic working relationships. The 'umbrella' of 'safety' includes the safety of patients, staff, visitors and the integrity of the unit environment (Beer *et al.*, 2001; Flockhart, 2002, 2004).

A structured shift management system developed by Flockhart *et al.* (2002) and Flockhart (2004) was introduced to the unit to provide the cornerstone of a safe environment, and the individual roles within the system reflected the umbrella of safety for the staff team, and visitors to the unit (see Box 8.1). The emphasis of this system was to promote patient engagement by getting staff out of the PICU office.

Direct supervision

Two of the authors worked directly with staff on shift in interventions with patients. This was in order to focus on helping staff to reduce patient and staff conflict behaviours by targeting patient arousal, thereby reducing patient ambiguity. We wanted to strengthen the model of engagement through the use of appropriate psychiatric nursing skills and medication.

Box 8.1

Coordination and coordinator role

- Shift coordination is to be carried out by qualified staff, who have the responsibility for leading that shift.
- When the shift coordinator needs to be on the unit floor and out of the office, they will nominate another member of staff to cover the office and phones.
- The shift coordinator will receive and give handover and ensure relevant information received throughout shift is accurately disseminated within the team.
- Has a responsibility for the time management of self and others via coordination and shift planner sheets.
- To maintain a safe environment (e.g. patient management and allocation of staff to patients, allocation of unit observations, 1:1 observation, medication, etc.)
- Ensure documentation and procedures are accurately and safely followed.
- Promote a safe and therapeutic environment.
- Ensure adequate staffing levels for at least two shifts in advance.
- To carry out ward management rounds as necessary.
- To coordinate/arrange/agree, any referrals, assessments, transfer (to and from PICU) with relevant parties, and to arrange practicalities of such.
- On relevant days, plan in advance/arrange staff to attend any sessions/meetings on the ward (e.g. teaching, staff meetings, case reviews etc.).
- To ensure delivery of high standards of patient care.
- Ensure items in diary are attended to.
- To ensure bank and agency are fully aware of procedures and documentation of observations (e.g. what 1:1 means and what is expected of staff whilst carrying this out (e.g. no sitting), what 15 minute observation entails.
- To give clear directions and explanations to staff in order to facilitate productive, therapeutic interventions with patients.
- To handover as per handover guidelines.
- To ensure each member of staff gets a minimum of 20 minutes break per shift.
- Ensure all incidents are dealt with in accordance with Trust policy.
- To receive feedback from the safety nurse during (but no later than) the first hour allocated as safety. (Safety person for each shift should be allocated the first hour to complete safety checks and documentation re this), and prior to handover.

Safety nurse role

The clinical team on the PICU strives to provide a safe environment for patients, staff and visitors, to the unit. It is the responsibility of the safety nurse to ensure that the unit is checked at the beginning of each shift for anything untoward that could contribute a breach of safety or become a security hazard. Particular attention should be paid to windows, doors, locks, screws and hinges. In addition, the utmost emphasis must be placed on nurses' own individual responsibility and accountability for their own personal safety and safe practice, and the safety of the unit as a whole. In order to facilitate this role, the safety nurse should (where possible) not be allocated other tasks/observations.

Unit observation role

- In order to promote and maximise a safe and proactive approach, a member of staff will be allocated 'unit observations' each hour throughout a 24 hour period.
- All patients on the PICU will be observed every 15 minutes as standard during the day. And 30 minutes during the night. This will assist in maintaining a safe and therapeutic environment and to encourage proactive interventions. There may be a need to increase this level of observation. This also helps in collecting valuable information re sleep, diet, interactions etc.
- In order to formalise and accurately document observations, the PICU observation sheets should be filled out. It is the responsibility of the individual assigned to unit observations that they fill this sheet fully and accurately.

Main roles of unit observation

- Carry out 15 minute observations on all patients, unless otherwise indicated (e.g. patient on two to one observations).
- To accurately document patient whereabouts every 15 minutes on the unit observation form.
- To handover unit observation responsibility and any issues to the next member of staff allocated for unit observation.
- Observe and monitor the general activity of the ward, including visitors, staff and the environment, inform the shift coordinator of any issues/unresolved matters.

Thanks to Pennine Care for kind permission to reprint from Flockhart, G. (2004) Cobden Operational Policy Guidelines. *Pennine Care NHS Trust, Ashton under Lyne Greater, Manchester, pp. 23, 24, 26.*

Autonomic arousal and information processing in psychosis

Initially, staff demonstrated a poor understanding of the concept of autonomic arousal and information processing deficits in patients with psychosis (Tarrier and Turpin, 1992; this is considered further in Chapters 4 and 17). This limited understanding was maintaining the office culture, as staff had difficulty engaging with patients who were aroused and presenting conflict behaviours.

The staff group were encouraged to understand in greater detail the role of autonomic arousal and information processing deficits (Marshall, 1973; Barratt, McCallum and Pocock, 1986) to the contribution of conflict behaviours with patients with psychosis and the links with high levels of seclusion. The information given was based on theories of cognitive deficits in patients with psychosis (Hemsley, 2005). In this context, information processing refers to the underlying mechanisms thought to generate psychotic phenomena. There is evidence that these mechanisms are biochemically driven, arousing other systems within the central nervous system (Hemsley and Zarwada, 1976).

The net effect of information processing is demonstrated most commonly in people with psychosis who are faced with processing complex social situations. In psychosis, the activity of the arousal system is thought not to be so controlled. In ordinary human experience, when a threat presents itself, the person's arousal system kicks in briefly, resulting in increased physiological and psychological arousal ('fight or flight') (Smith *et al.*, 2003). In psychosis, central nervous system arousal is high without this threat being present. The individual's state of arousal is influenced by hypervigilance biases, and coloured by delusional material, with the person being subjected to a stream of information, all of which demands equal attention. This causes further arousal of the central nervous system and further information processing difficulties (Tarrier and Turpin, 1992). Individuals with unaffected information processing are able to shift attention from one set of stimuli to another with relative ease. This is vital: otherwise we would be at the mercy of a bombardment of stimuli competing for attention, where our capacity for attention and processing would soon reach overload, resulting in a huge anxiety response (Hemsley and Zarwada, 1976).

In the PICU setting, this can be witnessed when a person with psychosis is both acutely unwell and aroused. Two members of staff approaching such a person for a well-intentioned therapeutic intervention may have their actions misinterpreted by the individual because of information processing deficits and increased arousal (Brezinova and Kendall, 1977; Hall *et al*, 2004), and their actions are perceived as evidence of an imminent physical attack. This will often result in a serious and untoward incident occurring, whereby staff may be assaulted and patients are secluded (Taylor, 1985).

Unfortunately, in the authors' experience, it is often common practice to target the psychosis and ignore the arousal. By targeting psychosis with neuroleptic medication, all one is doing is reducing reactivity to stress that is already there. By adding a benzodiazepine to the individual's antipsychotic medication, you are reducing stress and improving his/her information processing, reducing the likelihood of the above scenario occurring (Alexander *et al.*, 2004; Warner, 2004; International Early Psychosis Association Writing Group, 2005).

In order to address this problem, the staff team in the PICU were actively encouraged to target patient arousal proactively. The NICE Schizophrenia rapid tranquillisation guidelines (National Institute for Health and Clinical Excellence, 2002, Section 4.5, pp. 47–9) were utilised to inform this practice, and patients started to receive proactively administered, when required Lorazepam, up to 4 mg in 24 hours.

Extra care philosophy

When a patient's arousal remains problematic following appropriate medication, staff are encouraged to utilise an extra care philosophy. This involves three staff being deployed to spend time with the individual away from the wider PICU environment, where non-confrontational nursing approaches are used, allowing for patient expression of anger and confusion (Dix and Williams, 1996). This process is very patient-centred, with patients being encouraged to develop safety plans to help manage conflict behaviour and staff focus on monitoring levels of distress related to current psychotic presentation. The aim of this intervention is to minimise the requirement for use of seclusion, whilst maintaining an appropriate level of therapeutic engagement. Where patients are aroused to a degree where they pose a risk to themselves or the staff team, management and prevention of physical aggression techniques (e.g. effective communication skills) are utilised, as needed, to deal with such circumstances (see Chapter 5). These interventions have also given staff confidence in mastering the art of avoiding confrontation – knowing how to stay calm and reason with aroused patients – demonstrating a new ability to give neutral feedback about problem behaviours. This enables conflict situations to be turned into opportunities for therapeutic learning.

Patient Global Rating Scale (Guy and Hume, 1999) incorporating zoning (Ryrie et al. 1997) and Behavioural Assessment Rating Scale (Swift et al., 1998)

On each shift, patients spend a minimum of 20 minutes' protected therapeutic time (Kent 2005) with their allocated nurse. During this time, the Global Rating Scale is utilised to monitor therapeutic progress. The scale enables staff to focus on clinical, risk, criminogenic, zoning and behavioural assessment categories. The scale is scored using a three point Likert scoring system (0 = no evidence, 1 = some evidence and 2 = definite evidence; see Appendix 8.1 at the end of this chapter). Each score over 1 generates a care plan for the appropriate category. The scale, zoning and behavioural assessment ratings are used to offer structure, clarity and brevity to the nursing handover process. Information collated utilising this scale forms the main body of contribution to the weekly multidisciplinary team meeting.

Case study

The following case study represents a pathway highlighting the use of the low conflict, high therapy model. Efforts have been made to ensure confidentiality and anonymity in this example.

'Mr Ian Indigo' (a pseudonym) was 32 years old and subject to section 2 of the Mental Health Act 1983. He was admitted to the acute ward, initially for assessment. The circumstances surrounding Ian's admission involved his belief that his partner was conspiring to have him attacked. The evidence he cited for this concerned the appearance of a white van parked at the end of his street for five days in a row at the same time. Believing he was the potential attacker, Mr Indigo attempted to assault the driver and was arrested by the police and taken directly to the mental health unit. Significantly, leading up to his admission, Ian had lost his job and was experiencing money worries, with difficulty in sleeping. At the same time, his partner had got a job and was spending more time out of the house.

Days 1–2
Following Ian's admission to the acute ward, he became more aroused and less able to process information. A decision was made to transfer him to the PICU, as he was fast

becoming a psychiatric emergency. On the PICU, Ian was allocated three members of staff and nursed, utilising an extra care philosophy, in a low stimulus area, away from the rest of the patients. Because of his level of arousal and distress, he was offered two oral doses of medication. In line with Ian's first presentation, he was offered an atypical medication: 20 mg of Olanzapine dispersible, with 1 mg of Lorazepam, which he initially refused. The three staff nursing Ian spent time trying to gain his confidence and develop a therapeutic relationship. He continued to remain very aroused and suspicious of staff, believing that they were also involved in the conspiracy against him. At one point, staff had to sit next to Ian in a chair in management and prevention of physical aggression holds, as he had tried to hit one of the staff and then bang his head off the wall. Staff managed to reassure Ian that they wanted to work with him and that it would be helpful if he would consider utilising the medication that had been offered. Eventually, Ian agreed to take the medication after he had eaten lunch, as he reported that this was helping him. He stated that he knew he would have to agree to the medication, as otherwise staff would force him to take it and would not offer him lunch. (The latter was, of course, untrue.) During the remainder of the day, Ian was nursed utilising extra care, and staff monitored and recorded his blood pressure, pulse, respiration and blood oxygen levels as he was receiving Lorazepam. Staff also recorded his strength of belief and levels of distress pertaining to his belief that his wife was plotting to have him assaulted. During the remainder of that day and the next, Ian continued to accept 1 mg of Lorazepam every six hours. During his first night on the PICU he only managed to sleep for four hours. By the second night, this had increased to seven hours, with a noticeable reduction in arousal, reflected in an increased capacity to process information, as Ian's distress, related to his delusional beliefs, dropped to 50%. He continued with 20 mg of oral Olanzapine dispersible and six hourly Lorazepam 1 mg, not exceeding more than 4 mg in 24 hours. During Ian's period in extra care his wife received regular updates, although staff remained concerned that Ian could not guarantee her safety, so visits were not allowed

Days 3–5

Ian continued to make good progress, with reduced levels of arousal being noticeable. His distress around his belief conviction also continued to fall. Because of this, Ian was able to safety plan and give assurances that other patients on the unit were not involved in the conspiracy and, therefore, he was able to be nursed out of extra care. Significantly, on day 5, Ian's belief conviction had also dropped from 100% to 45%. He was starting to reflect that his life stressors and his lack of sleep might have impacted on his belief system in thinking that his wife wanted to have him assaulted. However, Ian still remained a little perturbed and cautious about dismissing this belief completely. He was able to safety plan around his wife visiting and she felt safe to visit.

See *Table 8.1 and Figure 8.2.*

Table 8.1 Global Rating Scale daily scores: 'Mr Ian Indigo'. This chart is given as an example, and is not the record of an actual patient.

Global Rating Scale daily scores					
Rating 0, 1, 2. If any rating is scored > 0 please refer to the dated entry in the risk assessment for details of the rating					
Days	**1**	**2**	**3**	**4**	**5**
		Clinical categories			
1. Hallucinations	0	0	0	0	0
2. Delusions	2	2	2	1	1
3.Negative symptoms	0	0	0	0	0
4. Low mood	0	0	0	0	0
5. Mania	1	0	0	0	0
Totals	3	2	2	1	1
		Risk categories			
1. Aggression	2	0	0	0	0
2. Threatening	2	0	0	0	0
3. Impulsivity	2	0	0	0	0
4. Orchestrating	0	0	0	0	0
5. Sexual behaviour	0	0	0	0	0
6. Self-injury behaviour	1	0	0	0	0
7. Alcohol illicit substance	0	0	0	0	0
8. Concordance with medication	0	0	0	0	0
9. Compliance with therapy	0	0	0	0	0
10. Absconding risk	0	0	0	0	0
11. Concordance with leave	0	0	0	0	0
Totals	7	0	0	0	0
		Criminogenic			
1. Index-related thoughts	N/A	N/A	N/A	N/A	N/A
2. Index-related behaviours	N/A	N/A	N/A	N/A	N/A
Totals	0	0	0	0	0
		Zoning			
1. Zoning	2	2	1	1	1
Total	2	2	1	1	1
		BARS			
1. BARS	2	1	1	0	0
Total	2	1	1	0	0
Total all	**14**	**5**	**4**	**2**	**2**

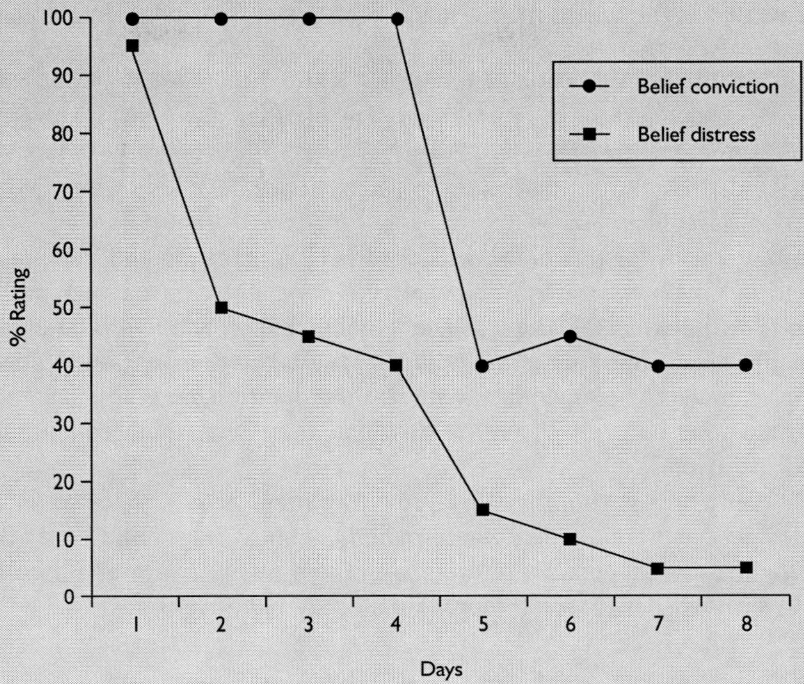

Figure 8.2 Daily recordings of strength of belief and level of distress relating to targeted positive symptom that 'Mr Ian Indigo' believed his partner was plotting to have him assaulted. This chart is given as an example, and is not the record of an actual patient.

Service user perspective by Wendy Ifill

This section includes the perspective of a service user of the PICU.

I am a 40-year-old female service user who has been in mental health services for 27 years, including adolescent, acute, forensic and secure accommodation. I have been on the PICU for five months and this is not my first stay here. I was here for 14 months, four years ago.

Comparing my current admission with my previous stay, I would say that there has been a noticeable change for the better. The atmosphere is generally a lot calmer, with fewer incidents occurring. On my previous stay, I found that some of the staff could bully patients and that if incidents occurred, there tended to be an 'act first and ask questions later' mentality. There was more use of control and restraint (which has now been replaced with other management and prevention of physical aggression techniques). Now control and restraint is rarely used. Patients are given more opportunity to be involved in planning their own care and there seems to be a lot more information available on patient advocacy services, as well as involvement from outside agencies such as a local voluntary organisation.

One of the biggest and most apparent changes for me, since my previous stay, has been the dramatic decrease in the use of seclusion. On my first stay here, I was secluded on a regular basis, sometimes for lengthy periods of time. Since being here this time, I have only been secluded for thirty minutes on one occasion. I have also witnessed a very dramatic reduction in seclusion of others.

I feel the big reason for this is the way the PICU is managed and the culture of staff, in general, to talk with the patient about effective management of their problems. This gives rise to fewer incidents, and a less heavy-handed approach, with the use of de-escalation. Probably most important is the obvious time taken to assess individual needs. As every attempt is made to help patients, with staff recognition, so problems are more often dealt with at the point before a patient may escalate their behaviour, reducing the need for restraint and seclusion.

The PICU could still be improved by providing more activities for service users and a purpose-designed extra care area where patients who were aroused could be managed away from the main ward area, therefore giving them more privacy and dignity. Lastly, I would like to see the PICU develop more female-only facilities.

Outcome of process: low conflict, high therapy nursing

The biggest difference, since the introduction of the model, has been the reduction in use of seclusion, against a background where there was little change in the incidence of recordable incidents. There were 141 incidents in the period between December 2003 and December 2004, compared with 151 between January 2005 and January 2006 (see Table 8.2). Clearly, the unit still has some way to go in achieving its goal of zero use of seclusion, but the results demonstrate the positive impact that low conflict, high therapy nursing has had in improving the care model of patients requiring Psychiatric Intensive Care.

What is of further significance is that the model has helped to reduce both conflict and containment on the unit. Previous research in the use of the model in acute psychiatry (Bowers *et al.*, 2006) demonstrated efficacy in reducing conflict on the wards it was introduced to, but with no real impact on reducing containment. The application of the model within the PICU challenges the view that containment cannot be reduced and this has got to be good news for all service users who require PICU care. This is clearly reflected in the service user contribution.

What is of further significance, is that the model has helped to reduce both conflict and containment on the unit. In previous recently published research on the use of the low conflict, high therapy model in acute psychiatry, Bowers *et al.* (2006) demonstrated efficacy in reducing conflict on wards, but no real impact on reducing containment. The application of the model within the PICU challenges the view that containment cannot be reduced, and this has got to be good news for all service users who require PICU care. The above points are clearly reflected in the service user contribution to this chapter.

Table 8.2 Effects on patients secluded in the PICU following the introduction of low conflict, high therapy nursing.

	Pre-introduction: Dec 03/Dec 04	Post-introduction: Jan 05/Jan 06	Reduction over 13 months
Total hours of patient seclusion	2469	210	92%
Single episodes of seclusion	156	62	72%
Total number of patients secluded	70	37	65%
Highest maximum hours of patient seclusion	1057.3	54.35	95%

Conclusion

The implementation of the model has helped to firmly establish a PICU Care Pathway for the Trust that manages the PICU. This has also included the development of a pre-assessment and outreach nursing role to promote low conflict, high therapy nursing within the acute ward settings.

The model supports the wider principles of the National Institute for Health and Clinical Excellence (NICE) Guidelines for both schizophrenia and violence (NICE, 2002; NICE, 2005), which emphasise optimism and recovery and getting help early. This includes the use of comprehensive assessment (medical, psychological, occupational, economic, physical and cultural) through the development of partnership working with users and carers. This involves issues of informed consent and engagement, and being aware of individuals' needs related to language and culture. Such awareness provides the basis of good information and mutual support in the caring process, in order to reduce conflict and promote high therapy.

Acknowledgements

The authors would like to acknowledge the following people in the writing of this chapter:

- Professor Len Bowers, City University
- Gary Flockhart Nurse Practitioner Pennine Care NHS Trust
- Michael McCourt Director of Service Development Pennine Care NHS Trust
- Mike Dudley Director of Link Works Sheffield Care NHS Trust
- The Director of Nursing, Service Manager and Nursing Team of the PICU described in this chapter. They are not named, in order to ensure confidentiality and anonymity.

References

Alexander, J., Tharyan, P., Adams, C., John, T., Mol, C. and Philip, J. (2004) Rapid tranquillisation of violent or agitated patients in a psychiatric emergency setting: Pragmatic randomised trial of intramuscular lorazepam *v.* haloperidol plus promethazine. *British Journal of Psychiatry*, **7**(185), 63–9.

Barrett, K., McCallum, W. C. and Pocock, P. V. (1986) Brain indicators of altered attention and information processing in schizophrenic patients. *British Journal of Psychiatry*, **4**(148), 414–20.

Beer, M. D., Pereira, S. M. and Paton, C. (eds.) (2001) *Psychiatric Intensive Care*. Greenwich Medical Media, London.

Bowers, L. (2002) *Dangerous and Severe Personality Disorder: Response and Role of the Psychiatric Nursing Team*. Routledge, London.

Bowers, L., Crowhurst, N., Alexander, J., Eales, S., Guy, S. and McCann, E. (2003) Psychiatric nurses' views on criteria for psychiatric intensive care: acute and intensive care staff compared. *International Journal of Nursing Studies*, **40**, 145–52.

Bowers, L., Brennan, G., Flood, C., Lipang, M. and Oladapo, P. (2006) Preliminary outcomes of a trial to reduce conflict and containment on acute psychiatric wards: City Nurses. *Journal of Psychiatric and Mental Health Nursing*, **13**, 165–72.

Brezinova, V. and Kendell, R. E. (1977) Smooth pursuit eye movements of schizophrenics and normal people under stress. *British Journal of Psychiatry*, **1**(130), 59–63.

Brown, K. and Wellman, N. (1998) Psychiatric Intensive Care: a developing speciality. *Nursing Standard*, **12**(29), 45–7.

Crowhurst, N. and Bowers, L. (2002) Philosphy, care and treatment on the psychiatric intensive care unit: themes, trends and future practice. *Journal of Psychiatric and Mental Health Nursing*, **9**, 689–695.

Department of Health (2002) *Mental Health Policy Implementation Guide: National Minimum Standards for General Adult Services in Psychiatric Intensive Care Units (PICU) and Low Secure Environments*. Department of Health, London.

Dix, R. and Williams, K. (1996) Psychiatric intensive care units, a design for living. *Psychiatric Bulletin*, **20**, 527–9.

Flockhart, G., Moore, S (2002). Teamwork is the key. *Nursing Standard*, **17**, 96.

Flockhart, G. (2004) *Cobden Operational Policy Guidelines*. Pennine Care NHS Trust, Ashton under Lyne, Greater Manchester.

Flood, C., Brennan, G., Bowers, L., Hamilton, R., Lipang, M. and Oladapo, P. (2006) Reflections on the process of change on acute psychiatric wards during the City Nurse Project. *Journal of Psychiatric and Mental Health Nursing*, **13**, 260–8.

Guy, S. and Hume, A. (1999) A CBT strategy for offenders with personality disorders. *Mental Health Practice*, **2**(4), 12–17.

Hall, J., Harris, J. M., Sprengelmeyer, R., Sprengelmeyer, A., Young, A. W., Santos, I. M., Eve, C., Johnstone, E. C. and Lawrie, S. M. (2004) Social cognition and face processing in schizophrenia. *British Journal of Psychiatry*, **8**(185), 169–70.

Hemsley, D. R. (2005) The schizophrenic experience: taken out of context? *Schizophrenia Bulletin*, **31**(1), 43–53.

Hemsley, D. R. and Zawada, S. L. (1976) Filtering and the cognitive deficit in schizophrenia. *British Journal of Psychiatry*, **5**(128), 456–61.

International Early Psychosis Association Writing Group (2005) International clinical practice guidelines for early psychosis. *British Journal of Psychiatry* **8**(187), s120–s124.

Kent, M. (2005) My mental health. *Mental Health Practice*, **8**(8), 22.

Lehane, M. and Rees, C. (1995) Intensive care for acute mental illness. *Nursing Standard*, **9**(36), 32–4.

Marshall, W. L. (1973) Cognitive functioning in schizophrenia: 3: The relationship between conceptual performance and information processing capacities. *British Journal of Psychiatry*, **10**(123), 428–33.

Mills, A. (1997) Incident reports in secure psychiatric units. *Nursing Standard*, **12**(6), 34–5.

Mounsey, N. (1979) Psychiatric Intensive Care. *Nursing Times*, **75**, 1811–13.

National Institute for Health and Clinical Excellence (NICE) (2002) *Guideline on Schizophrenia*. NICE, London.

National Institute for Health and Clinical Excellence (NICE) (2005) *Guideline on Violence*. NICE, London.

Ryrie, I., Hellard, L., Kearns, C., Robinson, D., Pathmanathan, I. and Sullivan, D. (1997) Zoning: a system for managing case work and targeting resources in community mental health teams. *Journal of Mental Health*, **6**(5), 515–23.

Saverimuttu, A. and Lowe, T. (2000) Aggressive incidents on a psychiatric intensive care unit. *Nursing Standard*, **14**(35), 33–6.

Smith, E. E., Nolen-Hoeksema, S., Frederickson, B. and Loftus, G. R. (eds.) (2003) *Hilgard's Introduction to Psychology*, 14th edn. Thomson Wadsworth, Belmont, CA.

Swift, R. H., Harrigan, E. P., Cappelleri, J., Kramer, D. and Chandler, L. P. (1998) *Validation of the Behavioural Assessment Rating Scale (BARS): a Novel Measure of Activity in Agitated Patients*. Collegium Internationale Neuro-Psychopharmacologium (CINP) Glasgow, Scotland, 12–16 July.

Tarrier, N. and Turpin, G. (1992) Psychosocial factors, arousal and schizophrenic relapse. The psychophysiological data. *British Journal of Psychiatry*, **7**(161), 3–11.

Taylor, P. J. (1985) Motives for offending among violent and psychotic men. *British Journal of Psychiatry*, **11**(147), 491–8.

Warner, R. (2000) *The Environment of Schizophrenia*. Brunner Routledge, London.

Appendix 8.1: Patient Shift Assessment Framework

The Global Rating Scale is to be completed each shift through meeting with your allocated patient and speaking to them and observing their behaviour during the shift (see shift assessment rating scale) for the week just gone.

Shift assessment rating tool for clinical, risk, criminogenic and zoning categories global patient rating scale

The following grid of information is to be used when making shift assessment evaluations of patients' clinical, risk and criminogenic need.

Clinical category	0: No indication	1: Some indication	2: Definite indication
1. Hallucinations: indication of patient responding or reacting to auditory, visual or somatic hallucinations in the current shift.	No indication	Evidence of auditory hallucinations is displayed infrequently to frequently, with the patient's behaviour and thinking affected to a minor degree.	Evidence of auditory hallucinations is displayed frequently to constantly, causing major disruption of thinking and behaviour, provoking verbal and behavioural responses.
2. Delusions: indications of patient responding or reacting to delusions in the current shift.	No indication	Evidence of poorly formed, unstable delusions to well-formed delusions that occasionally interfere with the patient's thinking, behaviour and social relations.	Evidence of a stable set of delusions which are systematised and numerous and which dominate the patient's life, resulting in inappropriate and irresponsible actions which jeopardise the safety of the patient and others.
3. Evidence of negative symptoms displayed in the current shift.	No indication	Evidence of a reduced range of facial and communicable gestures. Affect is flat, patient is distanced from the milieu of the ward, resisting engagement and answers questions mechanically. Thinking is rigid and repetitive.	Facial expression and communicable gestures are absent. Patient is withdrawn, and non-communicative, neglecting personal needs, with a profound lack of interest and emotional commitment.
4. Low mood: indications of negative mood, i.e. feeling bad in the current shift.	No indication	Some indication – verbally, presents feeling down, desire to or observed withdrawing contact with others.	Definite indication – acts in a depressed manner: e.g. sleep disturbed, poor dietary intake, physically isolates self, lack of social communication.

5. Mania: indications of mood becoming elevated in the current shift.	No indication	Some indication – verbally presents with pressured speech, slight grandiose ideation and increased motor activity.	Definite indication – speech very pressured and grandiose, resulting in inappropriate and irresponsible behaviour, which jeopardises the safety of the patient and others.
Risk category	**0: No indication**	**1: Some indication**	**2: Definite indication**
1. Aggression: indications of physically aggressive behaviour in the current shift.	No indication	Some indication, i.e. raised voice, increased tension, minor damage to property.	Definite physical aggression, e.g. yells, screams, hits, and major damage to property.
2. Threatening: uses threatening behaviour to staff or others in the current shift.	No indication	Some indication, e.g. uses threatening body language, intimidating behaviour.	Definite indication – threatens/acts aggressively, e.g. threats to staff, patients, bullying and intimidation.
3. Impulsivity: acts in an impulsive manner in the current shift	No indication; does not act in an impulsive manner.	Some indications – acts impulsively but shows some restraint/ consideration of alternatives.	Acts very impulsively – without consideration of consequences of alternative behaviours.
4. Orchestrating – indication of patient pushing limits and splitting the interdisciplinary team in the current shift.	No indication	Evidence of patient gently testing limits, minor attempts made to get members of the team to contradict the care plan. Indications of patient trying to incite other patients into non-compliance with their care and treatment.	Definite evidence of patient testing limits and boundaries on the ward. Wants only to speak to individual members of the clinical team. Definite evidence of patient trying to incite other patients into non-compliance with care and treatment and is intimidating and bullying other patients.
5. Sexual behaviour: acts in an inappropriate sexual manner in the current shift.	No indication	Some indication – minor overt sexual acting out or threat of acting sexually, minor preoccupation with sexual issues.	Definite behaviour – acts out in a sexual manner, e.g. sexual touching, exposure, etc. Extreme preoccupation with sexual issues.
6. Self-injurious behaviour: threatening suicide self-injury/evidence of self-injury in the last week.	No indication	Some indication – verbally threatens self-injury, possible superficial scratches noticed on skin.	Definite indications – lacerations to skin, head banging etc.

7. Alcohol and illicit substance abuse: evidence of in the current shift.	No indication	Evidence of patient requesting illicit substances/alcohol from other patients' relatives. Suspicion of the patient abusing such substances, evident by a minor change in the patient's affect, thinking and behaviour.	Definite evidence – patient observed taking/smoking illicit substances/drinking alcohol, with a major change in the patient's thinking, affect and behaviour, resulting in inappropriate and irresponsible actions which jeopardise the safety of the patient and others.
8. Compliance with medication: indications of patients' unwillingness to comply with medication in the current shift.	No indication. Fully compliant	Evidence of verbal indication from the patient that they doubt the benefit of medication that is prescribed.	Definite evidence – patient refuses medication.
9. Compliance with therapy programme: indications of patients' unwillingness to comply with the wider treatment programme in the current shift.	No indication. Fully compliant, punctual, full participation – leaves the session only when it has finished.	Evidence of verbal dissatisfaction with the programme. Also late to attend – minimal participation, leaves the session early.	Definite evidence – patient refuses to attend.
10. Absconding risk. Patients without leave trying to abscond in the current shift.	No indication	Patient verbalising a wish to leave. Evidence of patient tampering with doors and windows. Patient excessively asking to go out into the grounds without staff being present.	Definite evidence – patient attempts to abscond.
11. Compliance with leave: indication of patient's willingness to comply with the boundaries and guidelines of granted leave in the in the current shift.	No indication. Patient fully compliant. Stays within the agreed guidelines and returns on time.	Indication of patient breaching the guidelines and not returning within the agreed specified return time.	Definite evidence – patient does not return within 1 hour of their expected return time. Reports received that the patient has been observed outside of the agreed geographical parameters agreed.

Criminogenic category	**0: No indication**	**1: Some indication**	**2: Definite indication**
1. Behaviour – index related – behaves in a manner predicted by offence analysis in the current shift.			
2. Thoughts – index related – indications of thoughts identified as predicted by offence behaviour in the current shift.			
Shift category rating	**0: Score**	**1: Score**	**2: Score**
Black zone	Patients whose levels of arousal have stabilised, engaging in care, no evidence of realisation of known risk variables such as neglect, self-harm, or violence in the context of mental health problems in a given time period of 2–3 weeks; and who are ready for transfer to the Home Ward.	N/A	N/A
Green zone	Patients whose levels of arousal are reducing and becoming stable, engaging, no evidence of realisation of known risk variables such as neglect, self-harm, or violence in the context of mental health problems in a given time period of one to two weeks and are being considered for transfer to the Home Ward.	N/A	N/A

Amber zone	N/A	Patients demonstrating fluctuating levels of arousal, not in crisis, engaging, no evidence of realisation of known risk variables such as neglect, self-harm, or violence in the context of mental health problems in a 24–48 hour time period. This zone may also include patients who are unwilling to discuss their current or previous index offences. In order to move patients into the Green zone, staff will have had to be utilising the GFCBRS to support the change in risk status.	N/A
Red zone	N/A	N/A	Patients with unstable high levels of arousal and/or rapid decline in engagement and or realisation of known risk variables such as neglect, self-harm, violence or absconding in the context of mental health problems in the previous 72/24 hours. In order to move patients into the Amber zone, staff will have had to be utilising the GFCBRS to support the change in risk status.
BARS activity rating scale			
BARS rating	**Score = 0 (Consider Green or Black zone)**	**Score = 1 (Consider Amber zone)**	**Definite indication = 2 (Consider Red zone)**
	(a) asleep but responds normally to verbal or physical contact (b) quiet and awake (normal level of activity)	(c) drowsy, appears sedated (d) signs of overt (physical or verbal) activity, calms down with instructions (e) extremely or continuously active, not requiring restraint	(f) difficult or unable to rouse (g) violent, requires restraint

Global Rating Scale shift rating scores																					
Rating 0, 1, 2. If any rating is scored > 0 please refer to the dated entry in the risk assessment for details of the rating																					
Dates																					
1 Column = 1 shift																					
Clinical category																					
1. Hallucinations																					
2. Delusions																					
3. Negative symptoms																					
4. Low mood																					
5. Mania																					
Shift totals /10																					
Risk category																					
1. Aggression																					
2. Threatening																					
3. Impulsivity																					
4. Orchestrating																					
5. Sexual behaviour																					
6. Self-injury behaviour																					
7. Alcohol illicit substance																					
8. Concordance with medication																					
9. Compliance with therapy																					
10. Absconding risk																					
11. Compliance with leave																					
Shift totals /22																					
Criminogenic category																					
1. Index-related thoughts																					
2. Index-related behaviours																					
Shift totals /4																					
Zoning category																					
1. Zoning																					
Shift totals /2																					

BARS category																					
1. BARS																					
Shift totals /2																					
Shift totals all categories																					
Recording nurse sign and print																					

References to Appendix 8.1

Guy, S. *et al.* (1999) A CBT strategy for offenders with personality disorders. *Mental Health Practice*, **2**(4), 12–17.

Ryrie, I. *et al.* (1997) Zoning: a system for managing case work and targeting resources in community mental health teams. *Journal of Mental Health*, **6**(5), 515–23.

CHAPTER 9

Forensic aspects of crisis intervention team working and acute mental health care

Alyson McGregor Kettles and Paula Hall

Introduction

Crisis intervention services have a well-documented history (Mitchell, 2004) in terms of disasters and trauma. However, more recently they have developed to embrace mental health in the community, accident and emergency departments and other areas such as school crisis response teams. In specialised forensic practice, there are now designated crisis response teams in high-security areas who can respond quickly and effectively, and who have specified liaison with the police service. Crisis intervention has a foundation of both theory (Caplan, 1961, 1964, 1974; Aguilera and Messick, 1982; Marks *et al*., 1994; Roberts, 2000) and practice (Coffey, 1998).

Mental health crisis intervention (or crisis resolution or crisis response or rapid response) teams in the community are now either well established or being established across the UK (Brimblecombe *et al*., 2003; Pullen and Nisbet, 2001). There are many possible terms used, and for the purposes of this chapter teams will be referred to as crisis intervention teams.

Definitions

An emergency is an event which necessitates immediate action (Ward, 1995, p. 4), usually by others, such as health professionals and the police, whereas a crisis is any situation for which a person does not have adequate coping skills (Caplan, 1961; Marino, 1995). Therefore, *crisis* is self-defined. What is a crisis for one person may not be a crisis for another person. Crises may range from seemingly minor situations, such as not being prepared for class, to major life changes, such as moving house, death or divorce. Crisis is environmentally based. What is a crisis now may not have been a crisis before or would not be a crisis in a different setting. Crisis does not always lead to hospitalisation.

Crisis has been described as a short period of psychological stress which implies an upheaval in one's life that falls into two categories (Caplan, 1961, 1964, 1974):

1. Developmental – life stages such as retirement or leaving home.
2. Life cycle – trauma, bereavement.

Crisis is considered to have four phases (Caplan, 1961, 1964, 1974; Roberts, 2000, 2002):

1. The individual finds him/herself confronted by a problem and tries to use his/her usual problem-solving routines to restore equilibrium.
2. The usual routines fail to restore the equilibrium, which therefore creates tension and generates feelings of helplessness.
3. Anxiety levels rise and other problem-solving routines are tried.
4. All solutions fail, resulting in a breakdown of psychological resources and coping strategies due to the unresolved problem.

Stages 3 and 4 are usually when referrals are made. However, there is a recent model of crisis (Ball *et al.*, 2005) that has been developed, especially, to take account of people with severe and enduring mental illness. A grounded theory study (Ball *et al.*, 2005) was conducted in the USA and a subsequent model developed which shows the underlying vulnerability setting the scene for crisis to occur. As yet, crisis teams in the UK still tend to rely on Caplan (1961) for the stress vulnerability model of crisis that is in current use. Conducting a study in the UK would enable some comparison to be made to determine whether or not there should be a move towards the crisis model for people with severe and enduring mental illness, rather than continuing with the stress vulnerability model.

Crisis intervention teams' major role is to reduce/prevent hospitalisation and aims to alleviate the immediate problem, whilst enabling the person to remain in their own environment.

Crisis intervention attempts to deal with some of the more complex problems of the individual, which may be contributing to the immediate situation. Precipitating factors are taken into account, but these are dealt with at a more appropriate time by referring on to other services. Crisis team members need to have knowledge of all voluntary and statutory services available in the individual's area to enable specific and appropriate referrals to be made.

Crisis intervention is considered to require specific training, and the specialist learns to understand models (Caplan, 1961; Aguilera and Messick, 1982) and strategies of intervention (Roberts, 2000).

Training and education

There are training courses, but they tend to be held in America or Europe. The few training courses held in the UK appear to be run mainly by private companies and are often aimed mostly at businesses, although there are a few courses that are tailored to health and social care, such as the module run at Swansea University in their postgraduate courses. Training in mental health emergency situations, major incidents, bereavement, control and restraint, knowledge of local voluntary and statutory services are necessary components of crisis intervention education. Staff undertaking such work should have previous experience of acute and community mental health care, as this has the advantage of previous knowledge of people with enduring mental health problems. Staff require excellent communication skills to engage with individuals and or carers, especially as carers want something done immediately. The individuals themselves may have little or no insight into the situation. Engagement is the most important, and often most difficult, of all skills due to the nature of the crisis situation, and staff need to have the ability to gain quick access to other services, as necessary, when a situation arises.

Types of team

Teams come in many shapes and sizes, depending on the population, geographical, and economic factors in the Health Board or Health Authority areas in which they work. Community treatment teams or home treatment teams; crisis resolution or crisis intervention teams; and assertive out-reach or in-reach teams all use similar principles for engaging with the client in the community, no matter what the team is called. They all use assessment (Coffey, 1998; McDermott, 1998) and early intervention (Birchwood *et al.*, 1989; Sutherby and Szmuckler, 1995) to enable the client to stay in the community as long as possible. They engage with the client and carers so that warning signs of deterioration in mental state are picked up and treated as early as possible. Many are also using recovery models of care.

The relationship of crisis intervention to forensic and acute nursing practice

People are admitted to acute wards because they are either in crisis (Howard, 2004, p. 1) of one sort or another or because there has been an emergency situation requiring the person's removal to an inpatient area. In some cases the crisis intervention team may have been directly involved in arranging the admission. Bowers (2005, p. 232) states that 'acute inpatient psychiatric nurses are therefore... providing safety for the patient and others; tolerating and managing disturbed behaviour; providing personal care and managing an environment where patients can comfortably stay'.

Normal coping has been suspended and the person needs almost immediate specific help, whether admitted to inpatient areas or not. Forensic patients who have been discharged into the community, and who have community care from the forensic community psychiatric nurse, can also be seen by crisis intervention teams. There is a growing body of evidence from the UK (Marks *et al.*, 1994; Pullen and Nisbet, 2001; Brimblecombe *et al.*, 2003; Johnson *et al.*, 2005), the Americas (Langsley *et al.*, 1971; Reding and Raphelson, 1995; Mitchell, 2004) and Australasia (Reynolds *et al.*, 1990; Adesanya, 2005) that crisis intervention teams are effective at preventing readmission to inpatient services. There are some limitations to the results that have been found, even with a reduction in inpatient care. For example, no differences in clinical or social functioning (Burns *et al.*, 1993) were found in many of the studies, but patients preferred the community model and it has been shown to be cost-effective, with greater symptom improvement (Merson *et al.*, 1996).

The way a situation is handled by a crisis team can enable future situations to be managed more appropriately by the client/carer and increases the confidence of both to use the team in the future.

Howard (2004, p. 1) states very clearly that there has been a reduction in the number of inpatient beds, that people with more challenging symptoms are those who are admitted because community staff support people well in the community; and that an increased number of admissions are those of people with mental health problems complicated by substance misuse. Crisis intervention teams see people who have more challenging symptoms because they are in some form of crisis, and this crisis is often complicated by the use of substances such as drugs or alcohol or personality disorder.

Principles and models in crisis intervention

Ward (1995, p. 50) suggests that the principles of direct intervention are the keys to tackling a psychiatric emergency/crisis, with the four elements being:

- Assessment
- Intervention
- Resolution
- Support

Roberts (2002, p. 1), in contrast, prefers only three elements:

- Assessment (including triage)
- Crisis intervention
- Trauma treatment

It can be seen that some of the elements are common to all models, such as immediate assessment, including triage, whereas there are also some differences between the models. Box 9.1 shows Caplan's model of crisis intervention with the four stages he identified. Box 9.2 outlines the pattern that can be found in crisis (Crisis 211, 2006) and Box 9.3 gives the four stages of crisis according to Marino (1995). Roberts (2002) tends to take a more physiological view of crisis and considers his model in the light of the terrorist attack on the World Trade Center in New York, while Ward (1995) applies his model directly to psychiatric patient care.

Principles

Particular principles are needed to ensure that crisis management is effective. For example, even although plans are in place for dealing with any crisis that arises, some people will refuse treatment and some carers will not agree to cooperate with the reporting of relapse indicators either

Box 9.1 Caplan's four stages of crisis (1961, 1964, 1974) and Ball *et al.*'s model of the crisis experience for people with severe and enduring mental illness

Caplan (1961)	Ball *et al.* (2005)
Stage I: Mounting tension ■ Routine problem solving responses in an attempt to maintain the person's normal state	**Underlying vulnerability** Continued presence of illness symptoms Sleep disturbance Hallucinations Voices intrusive Loneliness/poverty/abuse/frustration Inability to function
Stage II: Plateau of disorganisation ■ Feeling anxious and ineffectual, 'at sea', 'chaotic' or 'going mad' ■ Repetitive unsuccessful attempts at problem solving ■ Stereotyped responses (e.g. 'hitting your head against a brick wall') ■ Increased dependence and ventilation needs	**The crisis** Being overwhelmed Lacking control Agitation, anger, aggression Feeling low Feeling anxious Euphoria
Stage III: Mobilisation of all internal and external resources ■ Maximum arousal, heightened suggestibility, increasing vulnerability to advice (good or poor) ■ Emergency methods or creative, novel solutions may be attempted, resulting in a range of potential outcomes	**Immediate responses** Getting help Managing alone
Stage IV: Adaptation or maladaptation (i) Crisis resolution: adaptation to new circumstances. Stability and steady state restored at equal or higher level (most common outcome) (ii) Maladaptation: superficial 'closure' or reactivation of past crises or recurrent medical symptoms and treatments (iii) Major disorganisation: crisis may precipitate psychotic episodes or affective disorders if vulnerable	**Crisis resolution and prevention** Crises are resolved when the individual regains a sense of control Then remaining in a controlled state is the focus for preventing crises No longer feels overwhelmed

Box 9.2 The pattern of crisis (`http://211palmbeach.org/ab_about.shtml`)

Recognition: The person realises that they are not coping.

Attempted resolution: The person struggles to find ways to solve the situation and may involve other people to try and help. Typically, the person does not perceive others as fully understanding the crisis or supporting the person in the crisis.

Emotional blockage: Not being able to solve the crisis, the person is overwhelmed by emotions. Fear, anxiety, anger, confusion, inadequacy, guilt, and grief are common.

Irrational behaviour: From the sheer intensity of the emotions, the person becomes unable to deal rationally with the situation. Usual thought processes are disrupted by feelings, and 'thinking about the problem' is not only difficult, but also frustrating and unproductive.

Loss of self-esteem: This perceived inability to deal with what is going on leads to a loss of self-esteem and reinforces the panic of emotions surrounding the situation.

Cycle formation: A vicious cycle is formed; not coping lowers the self-esteem, and the lowered self-esteem lessens the ability to cope.

Box 9.3 Marino's (1995) four stages of crisis

- A critical situation occurs in which a determination is made as to whether a person's normal coping mechanisms will suffice.
- Increased tension, anxiety and disorganisation surrounding the event escalate beyond the person's coping ability.
- A demand for additional resources, such as counselling, is needed to resolve the event.
- Referral may be required to resolve a major personality disorganisation.

for fear *of* the person themselves or *for* the person being hospitalised because of stigma or other cultural difficulty. The person him/herself should be involved at the earliest opportunity in their own symptom education and care and in designing plans for crisis intervention.

Advance statements (Mental Health Scotland Act 2003) should be used, if possible, to enable carers/team members to have a greater understanding of what the patient wants and early warning signs of deterioration.

Plans for dealing with crisis situations should be established with the person and carers in advance and be incorporated into care plans and packages. Crisis teams should have immediate access to care plans of people with enduring mental health problems/forensic history. Where possible, these can be incorporated into Integrated Care Pathways (Hall, 2004) through admission, discharge, community care and any future admissions. Box 9.4 gives the elements of an integrated care pathway. For example, the patient's journey across services and the transition from community into acute care needs to be negotiated, managed and agreed. Therapeutic and organisational arrangements need to be determined, planned and coordinated, where possible in advance. These plans should incorporate intervention strategies. Crisis plans need to include agreed action plans which include clear pathways for admission or readmission. These plans can/should include events that will probably increase stress levels, stress management skills, strategies that are known to be helpful or unhelpful when the person heads towards relapse, and information about social networks that can be used to provide support to the person and his or her carers during this crisis (Coffey and Bishop, 2000).

Early intervention

Early intervention and warning signs (Reading and Birchwood, 2005; Birchwood *et al.*, 1989, 1997) have been an established part of community care for over 25 years. Government (UK) fund-

Box 9.4 Elements of an integrated care pathway (adapted from Hall, 2004)

- Developed by multiprofessional teams in liaison with acute services, discharge planning staff and other relevant community staff, including social workers, housing staff and voluntary staff.
- Plan of anticipated clinical and social care
- Where appropriate, includes measurable outcomes
- Defines standards of care to promote consistent care and equity, despite population, geographical and economic factors
- Follows a timeline (days, hours, outcomes, stages)
- System of multi-professional recording and documentation is in place and forms all or part of the clinical record
- Designed to meet local needs and constraints, yet includes legal requirements
- Incorporates evidence-based guidelines where possible
- Uses variance tracking for day-to-day monitoring and review of performance/ability to meet set outcomes
- Crosses organisational and professional boundaries
- Is never finalised and is a continually evolving instrument

ing (Department of Health, 2000) was made available to establish early intervention teams across the country because prevention of admission is considered to be good for all concerned, as well as economically important.

Crisis team members, patients and carers need to be aware of, and taught, early warning signs and possible management of these to reduce crisis whenever possible. There are three main components to early intervention (Reading and Birchwood, 2005):

1. Early detection of psychosis – increasing the likelihood of help-seeking behaviour, including the role of relatives and carers in this.
2. Reducing treatment delay – long duration of untreated psychosis (seven days to 26 weeks) leads to poorer outcome – treat as early as possible.
3. Sustained intervention during the 'critical period' – the shorter the percentage of time with psychotic symptoms in the first two years of illness, the better the symptom scores, disability scores and overall illness scores at long-term follow-up.

Box 9.5 gives an outline of typical nursing management in early intervention for psychosis.

Early warning signs, early intervention and preparation/encouragement for independent living are, or should be, intrinsic parts of any mental health nurse's role. The crisis team may be the first point of contact for many patients and or carers. The way in which the crisis is dealt with may have both a positive or negative outcome for both, in as much that a positive outcome is dealt with promptly and to the benefit of the patient/carer. For example, trust might be instilled in a patient if she can remain in her own environment, with adequate support and follow-up. In turn, this would mean, hopefully, that the patient and her carer would feel comfortable to use the service again if necessary. With the advent of NHS 24 and other help lines available both locally and nationally, no patient should feel isolated or unable to gain quick contact and support from a professional. Negative outcomes do, and may, happen when a patient has to be detained and hospitalised under the Mental Health Act for his/her own or others' safety, and this can prevent early contact in the future.

If patients and carers are taught and are aware of their own individual early warning signs of deterioration of mental state, as well as possible management strategies, along with knowing that the crisis team is readily available to support them, they will be ensured of a satisfactory outcome and, hopefully, a reduction of future crisis.

Therefore, teaching of the patient and carer, as well as other professionals, about the role of the crisis team within the mental health system, should be a main aim of all crisis team members. All of this applies to forensic patients on the receiving end of crisis intervention.

Assessment

There are some specific forensic aspects of crisis that need more explanation in relation to acute admission of forensic patients. Risk assessment is most important for staff, carer, patient and others. For example, it should assess the extremity of the apparent crisis for the patient and the extremes that the patient may go to to achieve what he/she sees as the possible resolution of the crisis. Hostage-taking, siege situations and extreme threat, such as murder, torture and suicide,

Box 9.5 Nursing management in early intervention for psychosis

Strategies for early detection of symptoms:

- Education and training about early signs and symptoms and 'at risk' mental state for health professionals and relatives/carers
- Promotion of help-seeking behaviour
- Communication and engagement between primary and secondary care through team meetings, correspondence

Focus on therapeutic engagement:

- Use assertive outreach model of care
- Low staff to client ratio
- Flexible service to meet need/involvement of crisis team
- Client failure to meet team expectations, such as not taking medication or not attending appointments, should not lead to case closure

Assessment:

- Assessment should be comprehensive and include risk, mental state, history, vulnerabilities of all kinds
- Strengths
- Needs
- Access to resources
- Social support

Treatment in the least restrictive setting:

- Use of low dose medication
- Aim of remission of symptoms rather than adjustment to them
- Use of least restrictive and least stigmatising settings for care
- Early assessment of treatment resistance

Focus on maintenance of role and adjustment:

- Psycho education
- Strategies for symptom control education
- Use of Moos' (1982) work on uncertainty and adaptive tasks to enable coping skills
- Self-management of early signs of relapse
- Structured approach for regaining and developing life skills
- Whole person and family/carer approach to recovery

may be evident. Assessment needs to be ongoing from all previous incidents and assessments made by staff either in the community or in hospital.

Access to care plans and records of previous incidents need to be readily available. Emotional lability may be another clinical issue for acute staff, as patients who have abused substances, even up to 30 days prior to admission, may experience a sudden, unanticipated worsening of their condition. The patient may even be unaware of these emotional changes, but such emotional lability may be a safety issue for staff. The patient may suddenly become hostile or suicidal when the imminence of such behaviour was not evident before. There will be little or no warning of such behaviour, but this is one reason why crisis intervention teams may recommend hospitalisation. Therefore, it is essential that crisis intervention teams need to have up to date knowledge of patient and care plans. This can be a problem of access that the crisis intervention team encounters.

Although both ward and community staff understand what crisis intervention teams do, they need to improve their abilities in both keeping the team informed or sending copies of care plans to the team, which would enable continuation of care and permit good and effective practice.

It would be helpful, in future, if crisis intervention teams would be copied into advance statements and other appropriate documents, or have that information made available to them electronically. It is time-consuming (and time-wasting in a crisis situation) to access medical records, as teams are not usually based on the hospital or acute ward site and it is not always possible to access records from places like the Drug Prevention Service or Young People's Department. Medical records also do not have nursing care plans in them and nursing notes would often be more useful to the team. There are other issues, such as those illustrated in Box 9.6, which the nurse working in acute care or crisis intervention teams with patients with a forensic history may need to consider. There is a move in the direction of electronic records which may help to ease some of these problems.

Box 9.6 Other forensic issues in crisis situations that acute staff may need to consider

- **Spatial dimensions**: the closer the person is to the crisis or tragedy, the greater the stress they will be under (Roberts, 2002).
- **Temporal dimensions**: the greater the duration of exposure (estimated length of time exposed) the more the individual is likely to be affected (Roberts, 2002).
- **Recurrence (perceived)**: the more it is perceived that the crisis, tragedy or emergency can occur again, the greater the likelihood of intense fears which contribute to the overall crisis (Roberts).
- **Historical risk factors** such as violence (recency, frequency, severity and pattern), recent verbal threats, violent lifestyle, victim or perpetrator; Duffy *et al.*, 2004).
- **Contextual factors** such as immediate availability of a weapon, relationship and proximity to potential victim, the extent of social support and the safety of the environment (Duffy *et al.*, 2004).
- **Protective factors** such as the person's fear of their own potential for violence (Duffy *et al.*, 2004)

Intervention

Intervention by the crisis intervention team can take many forms. The team may decide that a patient requires hospitalisation or they may decide to treat the person at home. This could be by an increase in medication, with support from medical staff, enlisting carers/friends or other services, such as home care. In many areas, there are assertive outreach teams which can be accessed for almost immediate increase of care and support in the community. These teams are often multi-disciplinary, have very small caseloads and can visit the patient on a daily basis or even two or three times a day during a crisis, then reduce care as the situation becomes stabilised. Different teams use different models: some assertive outreach teams work with people who are difficult to engage; others, such as some home treatment teams, provide intensive support during a crisis to those already on their caseloads; and others, such as crisis resolution teams, provide home treatment until the person is stabilised and can be returned to the care of the Community Mental Health Team.

These teams mainly use a rehabilitative model of care which increases the patient's independence and enables the patient to remain in their own environment. McAdam and Wright (2005) identify that assertive outreach teams are a central component of the vision for mental health, with the aim of engaging clients who lose contact with traditional services and who require a more flexible approach to the provision of care. Assertive outreach nurses require sufficient training and managerial and clinical supervision to enable them to function effectively and to achieve successful outcomes for the service (Marshall and Lockwood, 1998). Personal attributes (McGrew *et al.*, 1996) as well as clinical skills and knowledge (Addis and Gamble, 2004; McAdam and Wright, 2005) are also considered to be essential for nurses to work in such a flexible environment. Competing demands, such as risk assessment versus engagement, can (and do) lead to high levels of stress and burnout (McAdam and Wright, 2005) with general mental health patients, but working with forensic patients increases stress levels (Gournay and Carson, 2001). This needs to be taken into account by staff when working with people with forensic histories and appropriate supervision needs to be made available, as well as forensic support, such as partnerships between forensic community psychiatric nurses (FCPN) and the assertive outreach or the crisis intervention teams. This will enable more effective care, backup and support systems and allows the implementation of whole systems care for the client. Box 9.7 shows the seven stages of intervention advocated by both Roberts (2002) and Ward (1995). Box 9.8 gives some 'Dos' of crisis intervention and Box 9.9 gives some 'Don'ts'.

Resolution

To get to the stage of resolution, there is the implication that intervention has had a positive effect and that the person suffering the crisis is coping with the situation. This 'post-crisis' stage indicates that the person has been able to meet their immediate needs. While there may still be some element of crisis, danger or risk, the situation is now less critical and the person can be more calm, more controlled and able to listen more effectively. At this point ongoing assessment and monitoring are required. It is therefore vital that the crisis team have an excellent liaison/communication

Box 9.7 The seven stages of intervention according to Roberts (2002) and Ward (1995)

Follow-up plan and agreement ↑

Develop and formulate action plan

Generate and explore alternatives (untapped resources and coping skills)

Explore feelings and emotions (including active listening and validation)

Identify dimensions of the presenting problem/s in the crisis (including the 'last straw' and crisis precipitators)

Establish rapport and relationship as quickly as possible

Plan and conduct crisis and other assessment/s

Box 9.8 Some 'Dos' of crisis intervention (after Ward, 1995, p. 55)

- Firstly, protect yourself. Remain safe.
- Get help by whatever means: mobile phone, shout, attract attention if necessary.
- Do something about it. You are involved, so act.
- Always give the person respect and maintain their dignity, no matter what form of intervention you choose to use.
- Use whatever intervention strategy you decide is most appropriate. Decide to do it and use the strategy. Do not stop to question your decision half way through the process.
- If what you have decided to do is wrong, you will know because it will have no effect or it will make matters worse. The situation is already bad for the person, but keep trying, as there is no single 'right' way to approach the crisis.
- Stay at arm's length from a hostile or violent person.
- Inform others where you are and organise support, help and backup wherever possible.
- Use appropriate communication and de-escalation skills, such as speaking slowly, breathing out, remaining calm, lowering your voice, adopting a non-threatening posture, careful and appropriate eye contact, and empathy. Adopt a matter-of-fact tone of voice, yet try to convey a sense of caring.

- Ward (1995) recommends trying to be unshockable. If the person sees that you are upset or embarrassed, then there may be a transfer of emotion to you and the consequence that the person may try to abuse you.
- Use time-outs and distraction techniques to give the person a rest from the emotional distress
- Admit your own limitations and get help; this recognises that you are in control of your own actions.
- You may decide to focus on the events that have precipitated the crisis to enable the person to talk about the crisis.
- Enable the person to talk about how they feel. Move to a suitable environment where possible to enable this to happen.
- Use all the principles of de-escalation primarily. If a minimum of three professionals are present, use control and restraint if other methods are unsuccessful in preventing the individual from attacking or grabbing hold of you, or otherwise becoming violent.

Box 9.9 Some 'Don'ts' in crisis intervention (after Ward, 1995, p. 57)

- Do not attempt to touch the client and certainly do not manhandle the person.
- Never retaliate against the person, no matter what the provocation may be. Never respond to personal verbal or physical hostility or abuse. It depreciates your professional credibility and reduces your own confidence in extreme and difficult situations because you have lost control. At best this shames you and at worst, is detrimental to the client.
- Do not belittle a client or be seen to be laughing at the person.
- Always make sure that your exit is clear – do not let the client stand between you and the door – you will be in danger if you cannot get out.
- Do not say anything that can be taken the wrong way – consider what you are going to say and how you are going to say it. You may only have one opportunity to say something in an emergency situation.
- Do not expect the person to be able to respond to what you are saying as their ability to use cognitive reasoning may be impaired. They may not even hear you or may carry on doing whatever they are doing.
- Modify your communication and your tone so that you may be more easily understood.
- Never leave a client who is in crisis on their own. It can be appropriate to reduce the level of contact to make the situation more tolerable for the client. However, the need for observation, engagement, support and accessibility must all be taken into consideration, especially if the client requests a time-out.
- Do not act before you have to or do more than is necessary to resolve the situation. Over-intervening is as bad as under-intervening.

system with all other professionals concerned with the care of the patient, to ensure continuity of care and, if possible, prevention of future relapse.

Support

The support required is twofold: firstly, for the person and, secondly, for the staff involved. Crisis intervention is high-stress, emotionally intensive and draining for those involved. Support for the person suffering the crisis is essentially a post-crisis stage where nursing staff can measure the effects of the interventions they have used, whilst enabling time for reflection and the use of social support strategies.

Staff support should be available post crisis by supervision, discussion with the patients' Community Mental Health Team members and other people involved in the crisis. Management of situations requires excellent communication and some of the important issues about two-way communication are outlined in Box 9.10. Jones and Bowles (2005) identify that:

Box 9.10 Communication between crisis teams, acute and community areas/teams

- **Communication**: essential between patient, carer, community mental health team, acute wards and crisis team
- **Liaison**: essential for follow up after crisis – identified team/ward members
- **Care plans**: must include plans for crisis and be available to crisis teams – patient should have copy
- **Copies of advance statements**: must be available for crisis teams and patient/carer encouraged to have copy to show crisis team if possible
- **Ability to access nursing notes**: essential to ensure continuity of care
- **Care plan/advance statement in medical records**: as these are the only records available out of hours
- **Electronic care plan**: ideal for out of hours team
- **Access to Mental Health Act status**: detentions under the Mental Health Act not available unless record accessed

Some essentials that crisis team should have knowledge of:

- CPN/acute ward staff let team know of crisis
- Give care plan
- Medication regime and when required medication
- Enhanced access list
- Early warning signs
- Crisis plan
- Carer details or support available to prevent hospital admission

> new systemic relationships have come 'on-line' between... acute wards and crisis/home treatment teams, changing the previously established arrangements between Community Mental Health Teams (CMHTs) and wards. Hence, practice development within one setting, especially 'a hub' service such as a ward, may require systemic implementation and will, at the least, seek to clarify and strengthen links within the system.

Jones and Bowles (2005, p. 642) also give an example of 'whole systems working' and proposed standards for both a 'well informed admission' and for 'connectedness and continuity'. These whole systems are relatively new but are already being aimed for at policy level, so the items given in Box 9.10 will assist in developing such systems.

Conclusion

Crisis intervention has come a long way in a short time. It is now an important part of overall care, but it has further to go to become a fully integrated part of continuous whole systems care. It also has to become fully geared towards supporting recovery from long-term problems. Carers are included in crisis care and in early intervention, but they are not yet wholly viewed and supported as partners in care. Their role remains undervalued and this must change if recovery models of care are to be fully implemented in the future.

There has been a distinct lack of research into the nursing role within teams. There are studies and randomised controlled trials about the effectiveness of the teams and the prevention of admission. Surprisingly there is little about the teams' relationship to acute wards or community teams, nursing management of care and the transition process. There is undoubtedly a need for more research in this area, especially with the advent of whole systems working.

References

Addis, J. and Gamble, C. (2004) Assertive outreach nurses' experience of engagement. *Journal of Psychiatric and Mental Health Nursing*, **11**, 452–60.

Adesanya, A. (2005) Impact of a crisis assessment treatment service on admissions into an acute psychiatric unit. *Australasian Psychiatry*, **13**(2), 135–9.

Aguilera, D. C. and Messick, J. M. (1982) *Crisis Intervention: Theory and Methodology*. C. V. Mosby, St Louis.

Birchwood, M., McGorry, P. and Jackson, H. (1997) Early intervention in Schizophrenia. *British Journal of Psychiatry*, **170**(1), 2–11.

Birchwood, M., Smith, J., MacMillan, F., Hogg, B., Prasad, R., Harvey, C. and Bering, S. (1989) Predicting relapse in schizophrenia: the development and implementation of an early signs monitoring system using patients and families as observers, a preliminary investigation. *Psychological Medicine*, **19**, 649–56.

Bowers, L. (2005) Reasons for admission and their implications for the nature of acute inpatient psychiatric nursing. *Journal of Psychiatric and Mental Health Nursing*, **12**, 231–6.

Brimblecombe, N., O'Sullivan, G. and Parkinson, B. (2003) Home treatment as an alternative to inpatient admission: characteristics of those treated and factors predicting hospitalisation. *Journal of Psychiatric and Mental Health Nursing*, **10**(6), 683–7.

Burns, T., Beadsmoore, A., Bhat, A. V., Oliver, A. and Mathers, C. (1993) A controlled trial of home-based acute psychiatric services. 1: Clinical and social outcome. *British Journal of Psychiatry*, **163**, 49–54.

Caplan, G. (1961) *An Approach to Community Mental Health*. Grune and Stratton, New York.

Caplan, G. (1964) *Principles of Preventive Psychiatry*. Basic Books, New York.

Caplan G. (1974) *Support Systems and Community Mental Health*. Behavioural Publications, New York.

Coffey, M. (1998) Provision of out-of-hours support to a forensic population: strategies and research potential. *Journal of Psychiatric and Mental Health Nursing*, **5**(5), 367–78.

Coffey, M. and Bishop, N. (2000) Crisis plans in forensic mental health nursing. *Mental Health Practice*, **4**(4), 22–5.

Crisis 211 (2006) http://211palmbeach.org/ab_about.shtml

Department of Health (2000) *The NHS Plan: a Plan for Investment: A Plan for Reform*. HMSO, London.

Duffy, D., Doyle, M. and Ryan, T. (2004) Risk assessment and management in acute mental health care. In: *Acute Mental Health Nursing; From Acute Concerns to the Capable Practitioner* (eds. M. Harrison, D. Howard and D. Mitchell), Chapter 7. Sage, London.

Gournay, K. and Carson, J. (2001) Staff stress, coping skills and job satisfaction. In: *Forensic Nursing and Multidisciplinary Care of the Mentally Disordered Offender* (eds. D. Robinson and A. Kettles), Chapter 12. Jessica Kingsley, London.

Hall, J. (2004) Integrated care pathways: the 'acute' context. In: *Acute Mental Health Nursing; From Acute Concerns to the Capable Practitioner* (eds. M. Harrison, D. Howard and D. Mitchell), Chapter 6. Sage, London.

Howard, D. (2004) An introduction to acute mental health care: from acute concerns to the capable practitioner. In: *Acute Mental Health Nursing; From Acute Concerns to the Capable Practitioner* (eds. M. Harrison, D. Howard and D. Mitchell), Chapter 1. Sage, London.

Johnson, S., Nolan, F., Pilling, S., Sandor, A., Hoult, J., McKenzie, N., White, I. R., Thompson, M. and Bebbington, P. (1995) Randomised controlled trial of acute mental health care by a crisis resolution team: the North Islington crisis study. *British Medical Journal*, **331**(7517), 586–7, 599.

Jones, A. and Bowles, N. (2005) Best practice from admission to discharge in acute inpatient care: considerations and standards from a whole system perspective. *Journal of Psychiatric and Mental Health Nursing*, **12**(6), 642–7.

Langsley, D. G., Machotka, P. and Flomenhaft, K. (1971) Avoiding mental hospital admission: a follow-up study. *American Journal of Psychiatry*, **127**, 127–30.

Marshall, M. and Lockwood, A. (1998) *Assertive Community Treatment for People with Severe Mental Disorders*. Cochrane Systematic Reviews, York.

Marino, T. W. (1995) Crisis counselling: helping normal people cope with abnormal situations. *Counseling Today*, **38**, 40–6.

Marks, I. M., Connolly, J., Muijen, M., Audini, B., McNamee, G. and Lawrence, R. E. (1994) Home-based versus hospital-based care for people with serious mental illness. *British Journal of Psychiatry*, **165**, 179–94.

McAdam, M. and Wright, N. (2005) A review of the literature considering the role of mental health nurses in assertive outreach. *Journal of Psychiatric and Mental Health Nursing*, **12**(6), 648–60.

McDermott, G. (1998) Relapse: helping clients to recognise early signs. *Mental Health Nursing*, **18**(6), 22–3.

McGrew, J., Wilson, R. and Bond, G. (1996) Client perspectives on helpful ingredients of assertive community treatment. *Psychiatric Rehabilitation Journal*, **19**, 13–21.

Merson, S., Tyrer, P., Carlen, D. and Johnson, T. (1996) The cost of treatment in psychiatric emergencies: a comparison of hospital and community services. *Psychological Medicine*, **26**, 727–34.

Mitchell, T. T. (2004) Characteristics of successful early intervention programs. *International Journal of Emergency Mental Health*, **6**(4), 175–84.

Moos, R. H. (1982) Coping with acute health crises. In: *Handbook of Clinical Health Psychology* (eds. T. Million, C. Green and R. Meagher). Plenum Press, New York.

Pullen, I. and Nisbet, E. (2001) A second survey of Scottish emergency psychiatry. *Health Bulletin*, **59**(4), 228–32.

Reading, B., Birchwood, M. (2005) Early intervention in psychosis. *Disease Management and Health Outcomes*, **13**(1), 53–63.

Reding, G. R. and Raphelson, M. (1995) Around-the-clock mobile psychiatric crisis intervention: another effective alternative to psychiatric hospitalisation. *Community Mental Health Journal*, **31**(2), 179–87.

Reynolds, I., Jones, J. E., Berry, D. W. and Hoult, J. E. (1990) A crisis team for the mentally ill: the effect on patients, relatives and admissions. *Medical Journal of Australia*, **152**(12), 646–52.

Roberts, A. R. (2000) *Crisis Intervention Handbook: Assessment, Treatment and Research*, 2nd edn. Oxford University Press, New York.

Roberts, A. R. (2002) Assessment, crisis intervention and trauma treatment: the integrative ACT intervention model. *Brief Treatment and Crisis Intervention*, **2**(1), 1–21.

Sutherby, K. and Szmukler, G. (1995) Community assessment of crisis. In: *Emergency Mental Health Services in the Community* (eds. M. Phelan, G. Strathdee and G. Thornicroft). Cambridge University Press, Cambridge.

Ward, M. F. (1995) *Nursing the Psychiatric Emergency*. Butterworth-Heinemann, Oxford.

CHAPTER 10

Forensic aspects of discharge planning from acute care: transition to community

Michael Coffey, Julie Morgan and Tina Gronow

Introduction

Movement between varying levels of secure care and eventual discharge to the community are significant transition points in the care and treatment of people with mental distress. When working with people with a history of criminal offending and mental distress, however, these events can be fraught with anxiety for staff and the person alike. These anxieties may lead to restrictions and limits being placed upon the options made available to the person as they seek to build recovery and reintegrate into the wider community. This chapter explores the issue of community return for people with acute mental health problems who may have, for want of a better description, a 'forensic' history. It does so by first outlining a concept of transition and linking this to the process of community return and reintegration. That we talk of reintegration at all says much about how successful mental health services have been in isolating people from their communities and their support networks. A central theme in discharge work is the idea that planning for discharge should begin immediately upon admission. This necessarily involves maintaining and sustaining the social networks which people have in place on admission and, in many instances, this should be a fundamental focus for mental health nurses. More than this, however, this chapter covers the breadth of practical considerations that mental health nurses and others must address in ensuring and smoothing the person's transition to community living.

Transition

The concept of transition is one that suggests movement. This movement is not necessarily a physical one, however, and we must resist this easy interpretation, especially when considering the person moving from higher levels of security through lower levels towards community living.

Transition is often about how people make movements in the ways in which they perceive themselves and others, and their place within the wider social context. It can be about shifting and rebuilding a sense of self and of identity. For people with enduring mental health problems, these shifts may be forced upon them as a paternal society reacts to mental distress by isolating and, in some cases, incarcerating individuals for treatment and management.

Transition is composed of at least three distinct phases: the separation phase, the transition or liminal phase and the reintegration or incorporation phase (VanGennep, 1960). *Separation* involves loss of identity. This can be abrupt, violent and lead to ruptures in links to the self, family and the community. It may involve alienation, punishment, and journey. It may be characterised by losing friends, termination of a previous self and changing name or appearance. For people with mental health problems and criminal offending, the index offence and the immediate aftermath might be characterised in this way. For example, it is physical in the sense that people are removed to prisons or hospitals and ritualistic in that there are procedures that are followed in this regard, e.g. assessment in hospital or a court case. There is, in effect, an enforced distancing and separation.

The *transition* or liminal phase is the in-between stage. Here the person has lost their identity but has yet to be fully reintegrated into the community or society at large with a new identity. This can be a period of confusion, testing, learning new ways of being and of indeterminate identity. It can be a period full of paradox and ambiguity, and there may be ritual dislocation of the self. It may also be a time of revelation where the person discovers some new skill, spiritual awareness or personal truth. It could be considered to be a turning point or where change is fixed in place. It is a time of increased scrutiny and examination of the self by the person themselves and by others. It is painful and uncomfortable and in many ways it appears to be viewed as an ordeal, both physical, in terms of the restrictions on liberty/effects of treatment, and mental, in terms of the degree of attention placed upon the person's thinking and motivation. The person is required to change or alter their thinking and their behaviour and the degree to which they are successful at doing this or, indeed, convincing others that they have done so is often crucial in creating the opportunity to move to the next phase.

Incorporation is the phase in which the person moves from isolation to return to contact with the wider community. They do so with a new identity forged, if you will, in the crucible of the liminal phase. The person may receive emblems of their new status in the form of new clothes, a new name and keys to their new home. For some, preparation for leaving hospital and return to live in the community may be a new beginning, and the help of services in the form of finding somewhere to live and purchasing furniture are important events. The emblem might be the outpatient appointment or, more practically, a new sofa or bed for their flat. The person then has to go about the work of cementing their new identity in place. This newly formed identity, created in the relative safety of a closed environment, is now tested. Their history of offending, mental illness and incarceration must be reconciled with the societal requirements of normative behaviour. The person is challenged, in their everyday contact with the wider community, to demonstrate their new identity and to sustain this in the face of other identities imposed upon them by society. These are crucial junctures in the support needs of individuals and ones which mental health nurses must address. Service users have to find ways of negotiating and overcoming the various hurdles that they encounter, and mental health nurses, as the largest part of the workforce, must offer practical assistance.

Policy developments

In recent years, there has been significant focus upon discharge arrangements for people with long-term and enduring mental health problems from policy makers. Much of this focus has, unfortunately, followed in the wake of problems with the provision of community mental health care. In the early 1990s, a lack of sustained follow-up and communication across professional and geographical boundaries was clearly evident in what were termed failures in community care (see for example Ritchie *et al.*, 1994). The requirements of the Care Programme Approach will, if adequately supported, reduce the possibilities of people slipping through the net. People detained in hospital, and who are planning to return to community living, should have a care plan (including contingency plans and risk management plans), a key worker and a review date when they know their care will be reviewed. The National Service Frameworks (NSF) for the different parts of the UK all address aspects of discharge planning. In Wales, for instance, the most recent revised NSF outlines a key action requirement of teams to 'consider practicalities, such as keeping up rent or utilities payments as part of the care plan' and to 'work with housing and advice agencies to ensure that people will not be homeless following their discharge' (Welsh Assembly Government, 2005, p. 16). Given the complexity of the health needs of people with long-term and enduring mental health problems, and who have a history of criminal offences, it makes sense that care is provided by multidisciplinary teams. The following discussion is offered with this in mind.

Getting specialist advice

Mental health nurses working with people who have criminal offending histories and mental health problems may, at times, find it necessary to seek advice from specialist forensic mental health nurses when planning discharge. Multidisciplinary teams often make referrals for formal forensic opinion to help them plan with the person the most appropriate package of care post-discharge. Mental health nurses in acute settings, however, should consider whether a specialist forensic nurse assessment might be an appropriate avenue to explore in order to get expert advice on the practicalities of providing follow-up care and treatment in the community. Forensic community mental health nurses are the largest group of specialist practitioners working with people with forensic histories living in the community. They have more regular contact with service users and have accumulated a degree of experience and skill that should be accessible to colleagues in other specialist fields such as acute inpatient nurses. A referral for an opinion from a forensic community mental health nurse should be considered where the person has a history of criminal offending behaviour and there are concerns about future criminal offending, risk of harm to others, repeated relapses and admissions, non-compliance with care packages or loss of contact with services.

Assessment

In England and Wales, Health and Social Services are obliged, under section 117 of the Mental Health Act 1983, to provide aftercare to patients who have been detained for treatment under sections 3, 37, 47 and 48 of the Mental Health Act 1983 and section 5 of the Criminal Procedures and Insanity Act 1991. Planning for discharge should, therefore, occur in tandem with section 117 arrangements.

The need for detailed information and accurate data, as a prerequisite for the starting point of any risk assessment, is widely recognised. Accumulating information is the basis of any assessment. In addition to a thorough medical, psychiatric, social and forensic history, there is a need to gain a clearer understanding of the individual and family's perception of the illness and its relationship to risk. We need to know how the mental health, psychosocial problems, and cultural and ethnic needs of the person relate to their risk behaviour. Additionally, the appropriateness of past treatment plans and the individual's adherence to these will help to identify and inform current and future care plans.

One of the more consistent findings in inquiries of failures in mental health care is the need to improve communication, both within and between agencies (Reith, 1998). Communication and liaison with the service user, family and friends, the multidisciplinary team, professionals in other services and agencies such as the police, probation, housing, education and employers are imperative. Not only will this help to inform risk assessment, but it is crucial in providing a consistent and holistic approach to care and risk management.

An example of formal approaches to improving communication in risk assessment, as an integral part of working with mentally disordered offenders whilst in hospital and on their return to the community, is Multi-Agency Public Protection Arrangements (MAPPA). This is a statutory framework for collaborative working in assessing and managing violent and sexual offenders in England and Wales. Police, probation and prisons work together, supported by other agencies such as Local Authority housing, Social Services, Health, and Youth Offending Teams, to manage the risk that dangerous offenders may pose to the public. Offenders can be managed at one of three levels. Level one involves a single agency, most commonly the Probation Service, without the need for other agencies to be involved in managing the individual's risk. Level two indicates that the risk management plan requires more than one agency. Some offenders posing the highest risks can be managed through referral at Level two, where the plan is not complex and does not require commitment of resource at a senior level. The 'critical few' who are deemed to pose the highest risk of causing serious harm, and require multi-agency cooperation at a senior level, are referred to a Multi-Agency Public Protection Panel (MAPPP).

Risk assessment can be an imprecise science. Hart (1998) stresses that the purpose of risk assessment in mental health services should be to prevent, rather than predict, violence. Doyle and Dolan (2002) recommend a structured approach, combining actuarial approaches and the use of clinical judgement.

The information gathered from the risk assessment process should be summarised in an understandable formulation of the risk factors, ahead of planning management interventions. This risk formulation needs to encompass the information from the assessment and include prevention and treatment issues and the circumstances under which any identified risk is likely to increase or decrease. However, an important factor to highlight is that risk should be thought of as dynamic in nature rather than static. It should also communicate clearly an individual's risk status, summarising known information whilst considering any gaps in information about past behaviour, which might influence current risk. It should identify any specific people at risk and the circumstances under which the risk will increase or decrease, such as deterioration in mental state, fear or paranoia. This should also include any warning signs or any other considerations, such as medication adherence and substance misuse. This should be broken down into clear categories, identifying management plans and interventions to be taken as the different stages of risk present themselves.

Ideally decisions on risk should be made by a multidisciplinary team involving all the professionals involved in the individual's care, management and treatment. However, mental health nurses (MHNs) play an essential role in this process. They can provide a major source of clinical information that feeds into the risk assessment process, having access to 24-hour observation of behaviour and ideal opportunities to develop therapeutic relationships with service users, their families and carers. In the community, MHNs have a more autonomous role in assessing and managing risk; however, they also have a pivotal and continuous role in this process. Risk formulation should also involve the person being assessed, so they are aware of the intervention strategies and what is likely to happen and at what stage.

There is a need for mental health nurses to recognise that the risk behaviours demonstrated by people with mental health problems are significantly weighted towards themselves. In this regard, service users need increased support at critical times post-discharge. One instance of this has been highlighted in relation to self-harm and completed suicide, where there is now growing evidence of increased risk post-discharge. There is a peak within the first two weeks post-discharge, and 23% of completed suicides occur within three months of discharge. Most completed suicides happen prior to the person's first outpatient appointment. It has also been noted that many suicide completers have not been fully compliant with treatment post-discharge.

Gradual transfer and relational security

Identifying appropriate move-on accommodation will be a part of the discharge strategy. Due to the complex needs of many forensic patients, supported accommodation, specialist services and intense community follow-up may be indicated. Early involvement of funders such as Local Health Boards or Social Services will facilitate proactive planning for resource allocation. Close liaison with accommodation providers, such as hostel staff and other carers, prior to discharge, is important. A comprehensive knowledge of the service user's history, risk formulation, care plan, relapse indicators and risk management strategy will allow a safer and successful transition to the community.

Forensic service users can sometimes be detained in hospital for lengthy periods. Coupled with complex backgrounds and needs, many will come to rely on the relational security they have developed during their stay. It is important that this sense of security is transferred to the newly involved workers prior to discharge. Individual care planning should include plans for gradual introduction of the person to new workers and increasing time spent at the new accommodation to help smooth transition.

Medication management is an important consideration in the discharge planning process. Around 50% of outpatients with schizophrenia are reported to be non-concordant with medication in the first year following discharge, thus having an average relapse risk 3.7 times greater than concordant patients (Zygmunt *et al.*, 2002). Others report levels of non-concordance ranging from 11% to 80% (Corrigan *et al.*, 1990). This can involve dosage deviations as well as cessation. The critical period for problems in this area appears to be the first six months following discharge. However, clinical interventions to try to address possible non-concordance are recommended for much longer (possibly at least 18 months) with regular assessments to highlight any emerging issues, using standardised instruments to assess mental state and any side-effects of medication (Kemp *et al.*, 1998).

Substance misuse should also be considered both when planning for, and following, discharge, as people with a dual diagnosis of a psychiatric disorder and a drug or alcohol problem are recognised to have a significantly higher rate of readmission and reports of criminal or hostile behaviour than those diagnosed with psychosis alone (Vaughan and Done, 2000). Substance misuse can also be a sign that a person is self-medicating for psychotic symptoms and, therefore, be an indication for the need for assessment and possible intervention. The need for more awareness of these issues in members of community mental health teams and strategies for dealing with problems presenting as a result of substance misuse is vital (Champney-Smith, 2003). Links with substance misuse services are recommended to assist community mental health teams in developing plans to address these issues (Welsh Assembly Government, 2005).

Crisis intervention and relapse planning

Some of the key features of discharge planning include the involvement of the patient and carers in the planning and review of care, a multidisciplinary approach, robust communication between all individuals involved in the patient's care and proactive comprehensive care planning for a swift and appropriate response to crisis.

Relapse of illness, in patients with schizophrenia, is always a possibility, even when the ideal combination of treatments is present. Prevention of relapse is important, as it is felt that each relapse can have a compounding effect on the long-term prognosis of the illness in terms of duration, susceptibility to treatment and the long-term social disability associated with recurrent relapses. Service users also express a fear of a relapse and usually want to gain insight into their illness, gain a perceived control over this and avert a relapse and the associated distress and disruption to their own and their carers' lives. The use of early intervention techniques, instigated by the monitoring of early signs of psychotic relapse, has been shown to be effective in reducing relapse and readmission rates of people with schizophrenia (Herz *et al.*, 2000). The Care Programme Approach recommends that signs and symptoms of relapse should be included in aftercare packages (Department of Health, 1990). This, therefore, opens up the possibility of close collaborative working between the MHN, the person and their carers, in order to avoid a relapse by utilising early intervention strategies based on the identification of relapse indicators. The identification of relapse can help in identifying risk if violence is clearly associated with acute episodes of mental illness (Sutherby and Szmukler, 1995). It is, therefore, necessary to develop crisis plans with service users, especially those who are considered to be a high risk if a relapse occurs.

There has been much written in the literature about the existence of a prodromal phase prior to relapse in schizophrenia. This is a period consisting of symptoms and behaviour preceding the onset or recurrence of psychotic symptoms which can last for any time from a few days up to four weeks before a relapse of illness develops (Barrowclough and Tarrier, 1995). It is generally felt that this prodromal phase can be identified, and that interventions can be introduced on the basis of this, early enough in the process to avert a relapse. These signs and symptoms, and possibly even the sequence and timing of these episodes, are not universal and vary between individuals. Birchwood *et al.* (1989) suggest that it may, therefore, be more appropriate to think of these symptoms as the person's own 'relapse signature' and that people should be compared against their own individual baseline observations for the presentation and timing of their individual relapse signatures. In a study by Hamera *et al.* (1992) participants identified primary indicators (a symptom they particularly noted prior to relapse). When followed up a year later, 42% of these participants identified the same indicator, 8.3% identified an indicator from the same category as their primary indicator and 33% identified that their primary indicators had changed. This suggests that indicators of relapse are not static and that the stability of these indicators would increase if more than one indicator is used. Regular evaluation of relapse indicators, particularly following any further relapses, should be carried out to ensure that they are still relevant in order to increase the effectiveness of the monitoring of these symptoms.

Since patients appear to have their own relapse signatures, it is important to identify a person's specific patterns of change and to prioritise the events or experiences as the individual perceives them, using the patient's own language to describe events accurately. The use of technical terms can lead to experiences being perceived or documented differently from the person's actual meaning of it. Therefore, it is important to be specific with descriptions about signs and symptoms: for example, note that the patient says 'conversations are about me', rather than just stating 'paranoid ideas', which may not be specific enough to identify particular symptoms (McDermott, 1998).

Precise information regarding individuals' relapse signatures can be obtained by the careful interviewing of service users and carers about changes in thinking and behaviour leading up to a previous relapse. Birchwood *et al.* (1989) also suggests the use of an interview schedule to assist in the identifying of specific relapse indicators. Retrospective information can be open to the possibility of hindsight bias and, also, a degree of false reporting due to a poor memory of the events. However, a documented and accurate description of relapse indicators may improve predication for any future prodromal episodes. It is, therefore, important that the MHN document clearly state the observed and reported symptoms of the person when admitted and during their time spent on the ward. This information can be further built upon over time following subsequent relapses, thus helping to increase the accuracy of prediction with each relapse.

Service users and carers recognise symptoms of relapse themselves and are, indeed, monitoring and seeking help to deal with them (McCandless-Glimcher *et al.*, 1986). Proactive measures would, therefore, be welcomed by relatives who sometimes see mental health services as only responding to a crisis, rather than trying to avoid one (Barrowclough and Tarrier, 1995). Relatives and informal care givers can play an important and crucial role in securing and maintaining community tenure (Coffey, 2003).

Some difficulties that may arise when trying to instigate crisis intervention techniques could be that some people will refuse treatment, some may be guarded about their symptoms, especially if becoming paranoid, and not all carers will agree to collaborate with the reporting of relapse indicators, possibly for fear of the person being admitted to hospital. It is often thought that some service users may have little insight and that this affects the retrospective reporting of symptoms when collating information. However, it is known that a high proportion of people retain insight throughout the prodromal stage, some up until the day of relapse (Henrichs *et al.*, 1985).

Crisis plans incorporating intervention strategies should be agreed with the person in advance and be integrated into aftercare packages. As well as early signs of relapse, these crisis plans should include agreed plans of action to be taken if the patient develops these symptoms, including clear pathways for readmission. They could also include events that are likely to increase stress levels, what strategies are helpful or unhelpful if relapsing (including stress management skills), the patient's current treatment regime and details of any social networks that can be utilised to provide extra support to the patient during this time (Coffey and Bishop, 2000). Other factors, such as housing and education, should also be considered and integrated into discharge plans.

All members of the care team should be aware of these plans and alerted to any signs and symptoms which may indicate a possible relapse (Ritchie *et al.*, 1994). The patient, carers and any relevant others, such as housing support and out-of-hours staff, should have copies of these discharge plans in an appropriate format and be aware of what circumstances might result in a return to hospital (Coffey, 1998; Welsh Assembly Government, 2005). Comprehensive packages of care, including relapse indicators, may also make it easier to discharge patients to the community if professionals feel more able to rapidly identify an impending relapse in this client group.

Promoting reintegration

Users of mental health services can face discrimination in spheres of life including housing, immigration, insurance, health care, employment and access to justice (Kelly, 2005). Recognising the importance of combating discrimination against individuals and groups with mental health problems and promoting their social inclusion is well documented (Link and Phelan, 2001; Repper and Perkins, 2003). People with mental disorder who are also offenders (and therefore have the additional stigma of criminality) arguably have more difficulty securing social inclusion than other service users.

In England and Wales, under section 37 of the Mental Health Act 1983, a court can order an offender to be detained in a psychiatric hospital for treatment. When considering the nature of the offence, the offender's antecedents, and the risk of serious harm to the public, a judge also has the power to impose a restriction order under section 41. The aim of a restriction order is to protect the public by placing constraints upon the transfer and discharge of that offender from hospital. Restriction orders are usually made for an indefinite period. In some cases, this type of order may well lead to an offender being detained for longer than if they had been sentenced to a term of imprisonment. On the other hand, some offenders may be discharged from hospital after what would be seen by some as a comparatively short period, in relation to the crime committed. This is often difficult for the victims and society to comprehend and, consequently, may affect the social inclusion of the offender when discharged into the community.

Because of the nature of the offence, and consideration for the victims, it is sometimes deemed advisable that service users do not return to the area of the index offence. This means that they have to settle in an area that is unfamiliar to them. While this may have the advantage of 'anonymity' for the person in that community, it has the disadvantage of increased social isolation. Social circumstances are an important consideration, not only because they are an indication of a person's progress following discharge from hospital, but also because of the effect that situational factors can have upon the degree of risk that a person poses to others (Monahan and Steadman, 1994).

Mental health nurses can support the person in the transition to the new community by helping them to develop social networks in the area prior to discharge. Assisting the individual to become familiar with the area and the facilities it offers will allow them to make an informed choice about the suitability of the area. Accessing and securing vocational, educational, employment or social opportunities before the person leaves hospital will facilitate community reintegration.

Clearly, unemployment in the mentally ill population has perpetuated the current negative stereotypes and social exclusion associated with mental health problems (Evans and Repper, 2000). Service users who wish to re-engage with employment report that tacit expectations are usually very low and often the message is that work is unrealistic (Read, 1997; Webster, 1998).

Mental health nurses should attach greater importance in their direct practice to how employment (or lack of it) affects service users. An appraisal of employment history and skills should be conducted early in the assessment process. Constructive links with external organisations will help to prepare service users to take up employment opportunities in the community (Foster, 1999). Mental health nurses assisting service users to gain and maintain employment should carefully consider the suitability of the work for the individual. Identifying potential stressors in the environment and working with service users to develop coping strategies will aid them in maintaining employment and may prevent relapse of illness (Evans and Repper, 2000).

The issue of disclosure when seeking employment is a central consideration for most forensic service users, anecdotal evidence suggesting that disclosing the offence overrides any concerns of disclosing mental health problems. Concerns that workmates and the local community will gain information on the individual's offence, and the possible consequences of victimisation and social exclusion, deter some service users from seeking employment. Decisions about disclosure of information (other than medical information) are taken by the social supervisor and clinical team, with the full knowledge and agreement of the person. Guidance from the Home Office/Department of Health (1997) does not stipulate that information is shared with every prospective employer; the decision is left to professional judgement. Information should only be given against the person's wishes when there are strong overriding reasons for doing so (Home Office/Department of Health 1997). Practitioners need to provide service users with information that will allow them to make informed choices and offer practical and emotional support, should they choose to disclose information to prospective employers.

Conclusion

Discharge from acute mental health services can be a time both for celebration and of increased worry for people with long-term and enduring mental health problems. Mental health nurses, however, play a pivotal and strategic role in forming therapeutic alliances with people to enable them to successfully reintegrate on their return to community living. Given the complexity of health and social care provision, this is clearly no easy task, and takes commitment and tenacity on the part of the nurse and the person themselves. There appear to be significant long-term benefits for people who are adequately supported and who make successful transitions. Mental health nurses must ensure through their intervention that people in their care get this opportunity.

References

Barrowclough, C. and Tarrier, N. (1995) *Families of Schizophrenic Patients: Cognitive Behavioural Intervention*. Chapman & Hall, London.

Birchwood, M., Smith, J., MacMillan, F., Hogg, B., Prasad, R., Harvey, C. and Bering, S. (1989) Predicting relapse in schizophrenia: the development and implementation of an early signs monitoring system using patients and families as observers, a preliminary investigation. *Psychological Medicine*, **19**, 649–56.

Champney-Smith, J. (2003) Working with people with coexisting mental health and substance misuse problems. In: *The Handbook of Community Mental Health Nursing* (eds. B. Hannigan and M. Coffey). Routledge, London.

Coffey, M. (1998) Provision of out-of-hours support to a forensic population: strategies and research potential. *Journal of Psychiatric and Mental Health Nursing*, **5**(5), 367–78.

Coffey, M. (2003) Working with mentally disordered offenders. In: *The Handbook of Community Mental Health Nursing* (eds. B. Hannigan and M. Coffey). Routledge, London.

Coffey, M. and Bishop, N. (2000) Crisis plans in forensic mental health nursing. *Mental Health Practice*, **4**(4), 22–5.

Corrigan, P. W., Liberman, R. P. and Engel, J. D. (1990) From noncompliance to collaboration in the treatment of schizophrenia. *Hospital and Community Psychiatry*, **41**, 1203–11.

Doyle, M. and Dolan, M. (2002) Violence risk assessment: combining actuarial and clinical information to structure clinical judgements for the formulation and management of risk. *Journal of Psychiatric and Mental Health Nursing*, **9**(6), 649–57.

Evans, J. and Repper, J. (2000) Employment, social inclusion and mental health. *Journal of Psychiatric and Mental Health Nursing*, **7**(1), 15–24.

Foster, T. (1999) When will they ever work? *Journal of Forensic Psychiatry*, **10**(2), 245–8.

Hamera, E. K., Perterson, K. A., Young, L. M. and Schaumloffel, M. M. (1992) Symptom monitoring in schizophrenia: potential for enhancing self-care. *Archives of Psychiatric Nursing*, **VI**(6), 324–30.

Hart, S. D. (1998) The role of psychopathy in assessing risk for violence: conceptual and methodological issues. *Legal and Criminological Psychology*, **3**, 121–37.

Henrichs, D. W., Cohen, B. P. and Carpenter, W. T. (1985) Early insight and the management of schizophrenic decompensation. *Journal of Nervous and Mental Disease*, **173**, 133–8.

Herz, M. I., Lamberti, J. S., Mintz, J., Scott, R., O'Dell, S., McCartan, L. and Nix, G. (2000) A program for relapse prevention in schizophrenia: a controlled study. *Archives of General Psychiatry*, **57**, 277–83.

Home Office/Department of Health (1997) *Supervision and After-care of Conditionally Discharged Restricted Patients. Notes for the Guidance of Social Supervisors*. Stationery Office, London.

Kelly, B. D. (2005) Structural violence and schizophrenia. *Social Science & Medicine*, **61**(3), 721–30.

Kemp, R., Kirov, G., Hayward, P. and David, A. (1998) Randomized controlled trial of compliance therapy – 18 month follow-up. *British Journal of Psychiatry*, **172**, 413–19.

Link, B. G. and Phelan, J. C. (2001) Conceptualizing stigma. *Annual Review of Sociology*, **27**, 363–85.

McCandless-Glimcher, L., McKnight, S., Hamera, E., Smith, B. L., Peterson, K. A. and Plumlee, A. A. (1986) Use of symptoms by schizophrenics to monitor and regulate their illness. *Hospital and Community Psychiatry*, **37**(9), 929–33.

McDermott, G. (1998) Relapse: helping clients to recognise early signs. *Mental Health Nursing*, **18**(6), 22–3.

Monahan, J. and Steadman, H. (1994) *Violence and Mental Disorder: Developments in Risk Assessment*. University of Chicago Press, Chicago.

Read, J. (1997) What is a good day project? *A Life in the Day*, **1**, 7–11.

Reith, M. (1998) *Community Care Tragedies. A Practical Guide to Mental Health Inquiries*. Ventre Press, Birmingham.

Repper, J. and Perkins, R. (2003) *Social Inclusion and Recovery: A Model for Mental Health Practice*. Baillière Tindall, London.

Ritchie J. H., Dick, D. and Lingham, R. (1994) *The Report of the Inquiry Into the Care and Treatment of Christopher Clunis*. HMSO, London.

Sutherby, K. and Smukler, G. (1995) Community assessment of crisis. In: *Emergency Mental Health Services in the Community* (M. Phelan, G. Strathdee and G. Thornicroft). Cambridge University Press, Cambridge.

VanGennep, A. (1960) *Rites of Passage*. Kegan Paul and Routledge, London.

Vaughan, G. and Done, D. J. (2000) Recent research relevant to discharge planning from medium secure psychiatric units: re-examining the literature. *Journal of Forensic Psychiatry*, **11**(2), 372–89.

Webster, A. (1998) An uncharted journey. *A Life in the Day*, **2**(2), 9–12.

Welsh Assembly Government (WAG) (2005) *Raising the Standard: The Revised Adult Mental Health National Service Framework and Action Plan for Wales*. Welsh Assembly Government, Cardiff.

Zygmunt, A., Olfson, M., Boyer, C. A. and Mechanic, D. (2002) Intervention to improve medication adherence in schizophrenia. *The American Journal of Psychiatry*, **159**, 1653–64.

CHAPTER 11

The Pharmacaust and its relevance to nursing forensic mental health clients

Linda Hart

Introduction

I have to declare a biased interest for this chapter. For the best part of 40 years, I was prescribed huge amounts of almost every psychiatric drug ever invented, mostly in acute mental health hospitals under a section of the Mental Health Act, or in the 'community'. Five years ago, I stopped taking them all. I had to endure a year of withdrawal symptoms, which were horrendous, but around that time, I was transferred to what was known then as the Rehabilitation Service, and my new Consultant Psychiatrist promised I would no longer be detained or drugged against my will.

It was wonderful to experience no longer being a member of the living dead; wonderful to be able to walk in the countryside and wonderful to be able to be outrageously creative once again.

On the downside, there was a slow but inexorable decline in my physical health. Soon after I transferred to my new psychiatrist, I had a brain scan which showed extensive abnormalities. He has tested me (medically) for everything likely and unlikely, but although I fit many of the criteria for neurological diseases, I don't fit exactly any one. So although we do not have a name for what I undoubtedly have, that doesn't mean I do not have it. It is outside most doctors' experience to have a patient who was given forensic doses of antipsychotics plus a range of other treatments and drugs for such a length of time and to have come off them, and been off them for five years. The drug industry certainly has no light to shed on my condition and I suspect that they have a vested interest in not doing so. But, I am convinced that the drugs I was compelled to take have played a major part in my present predicament.

As for my mental health difficulties, they have not been cured and have not gone away, but under the new regime, they do not last as long as they did before, probably because I can be myself at last. I can remember saying long ago that I would rather be mad than drugged.

When I was heavily sedated, I wasn't interested enough to read anything (how many patients do you see reading a book?) let alone anything about the adverse effects of medication, and when I 'came to', there wasn't a lot of reading matter that I could get hold of and understand, although

Box 11.1 Applying Linda Hart's chapter to nursing forensic mental health patients: medication, its alternatives and therapeutic environments

Linda's account can enable nurses who work with forensic mental health patients to reflect on the following points:

- There is evidence that in some acute admission wards, there has been an over-reliance on medication (Barker, 2005; Faulkner, 2004) and anti-therapeutic ward environments (Garcia *et al.*, 2005; Higgins *et al.*, 1999; Royal College of Psychiatrists Audit Team, 2005). Elsewhere, Linda describes these problems in relation to an acute admission ward which included forensic mental health patients (Hart, 1999).
- Nurses, psychiatrists and other professionals need to be aware of:
  - The wide range of experiences of forensic and other mental health service users, related to the efficacy and acceptability of antipsychotic and other medication (Keen, 2003; Lehmann, 2001; Romme and Escher, 2000).
  - The sometimes devastating consequences, for individuals, of the side-effects of antipsychotics: for example, those affecting sexual functioning, and tardive dyskinesia (Keen, 2003).
- There is research evidence that, for some individuals with schizophrenia, low expressed emotion environments, including those provided in crisis houses, are a viable alternative to antipychotics (Barker, 2005; Mental Health Foundation and Sainsbury Centre for Mental Health, 2002).
- This relates to Linda's comment that there is a 'lack of places for people to go to who wish to come off psychiatric drugs'.

instinctively I knew all along that there was a sickness in the health profession itself. Now, there is an ever-growing body of academics who are taking up the subject, so I don't feel as isolated, mad, or radical.

The first formal paper I wrote on the subject of psychiatric drugs was one that I presented to the Mental Health Trust in 2002 (Hart, 2002). Essentially, it compared the drug pushers on street corners to the psychiatric drug reps selling their equally toxic substances, together with their 'perks', which I would describe as bribes. And I asked why, when thousands of pounds are spent on alcohol and drug advice services, there was no advice or place for people to go to who wished to come off psychiatric drugs. It is perhaps ironic when you consider that the Victorian asylums invested much of their money in the East India Company, which was well known for its trade in tea and opiates. In addition, the old asylums spent a good deal of their resources on tobacco, snuff, ale, wine and spirits. In 1852, the accounts for Leicester City Asylum (later Towers Hospital) showed that by far the largest single purchase was ales and beers, followed by wine and spirits, leeches, and tobacco and snuff. Ah, the good old days!

Psychiatric patients and their medication are so conjoined in most psychiatrists' and nurses' minds (and the media's and public's too) that it is almost a heresy to suggest that they may be separated.

Harm from psychiatric medication

My argument is not whether you agree with psychiatric medication or not, but the questions that arise from psychiatric over-dependency on its use and the harm it does to the patient and, indirectly, to mental health practitioners. This raises yet more complex questions that include complicity, coercion, treatment resistance, liability and compliance – now known as 'concordance' (does that make me discordant?) – and informed consent, which is linked to The Mental Capacity Act 2005 (H. M. Government, 2005).

Also, nurses will be faced with issues like 'choice of treatment': the latest theme which gives credence to the idea that mental health patients have a right to decide what is best for them. I wonder if this will become a reality or just another sop to get us loonies off the backs of the Mental Health Trusts.

Another interesting article I read was about nurses being prescribers of medicines. On the one hand, I can recognise the benefits of this, in that nurses will no longer have to solely administer drugs, acting like a doctor's maid, or doing their dirty work for them, as if by proxy. Nevertheless, upon reading a booklet published by the Department of Health, I was saddened to be confronted on the first page by a paragraph extolling the virtues of psychotropic medication, and all the way through, no mention was made of patients not wishing to take drugs; instead, a cosy scene was set of 'concordance' (National Prescribing Centre, National Institute for Mental Health in England and Department of Health, 2005). It made no reference to the input that good social workers can make. It also did not take into account how the pharmaceutical industry fails the test of their testing methods, in that they have a history of taking no account of the long-term, serious, bad effects

Box 11.2 Applying Linda Hart's chapter to nursing forensic mental health patients: 'therapeutic time' and staff–patient communication

Linda's account indicates the importance of:

- Professionals being prepared to listen and respond to service users' experiences, feelings, perspectives and views about treatment and nursing/multidisciplinary interventions (Faulkner, 2004; Meehan *et al.*, 2004; Secker *et al.*, 2004).
- Staff having dedicated therapeutic time with patients, without the distractions of paperwork and administrative duties (Clarke and Flanagan, 2003; Faulkner, 2004; Higgins *et al.*, 1999; Kent, 2005).

of their drugs; that they test for a short time only on healthy young people, and not on people at each end of their lifespan; that they are too big and powerful and the drugs far too expensive; and that placebos (sugar pills) have been proved to be more or less as effective.

Added to this, they suggest that a nurse should fill in the standard 'diagnostic' forms, which, as far as I can see, are about as useful as a predictor/diagnostic tool as those of astrological signs.

And what if the nurse 'who knows you so well' is so busy filling out forms that she no longer gets the time to speak to you? Not that nurses get much time now.

As long as the Diagnostic and Statistical Manual (DSM) (American Psychiatric Association, 2000) is inventing illnesses at the rate they have been for the past six years, and marketing the drugs that 'cure' these illnesses, I guess that a nurse will become like Halley's Comet, seen maybe once if you're lucky, and not again until the next time you are admitted – that is, if they are not on sick leave.

I came across a gem. It is a leaflet extolling a new nasal spray for establishing trust (Kosfeld *et al.*, 2005; Oxytocin Organisation, 2006). The drug was issued by Swiss researchers and seems only to include men making investment deals. It takes no account of young women being the prey of predatory males, and suggests that, although the drug increases trust, it doesn't make the trustees any more trustworthy.

A piece was written in the *Guardian* (14 January 2006) that said that the drug industry exploited people's hopes and wishes for good health, whilst ignoring the body's own natural healing mechanisms (Law, 2006).

Compliance

This is a tricky one, in that the patient, psychiatrist and nurse, not to mention the whole of the nation's Mental Health Trusts, have something to lose if there were no complicity, but I feel that it is the patient who has the least to lose, and the most to gain, although they do not necessarily know it.

Formerly, psychiatry had little status compared to other branches of medicine. The early psychiatrists who worked in the asylums were known as Alienists, and their patients as Aliens – I wonder if it is some historic, collective unconscious that leads many of today's patients to believe that their minds have been taken over by aliens!

It is only recently, in some medical schools, that any attention at all has been given to 'listening' to the patient, and a psychiatrist's training is heavily focused on the 'scientific', on their diagnostic skills (I would call it labelling rather than diagnosis), and the subsequent physical treatments which, over the decades, have rescued psychiatrists from the ignominy of being considered less than medical doctors. But getting back to a psychiatrist's training, the Industrial Revolution meant that people migrated from the rural environment to the urban and lived together in vast numbers. The mad and the simple were more visible and therefore more problematic, and so too were those who could not conform to Victorian moral values (usually women who were unwaged, unwed and pregnant). So they had to be confined and covertly punished, and the places of confinement were the asylums. Although all manner of indignities and privations were meted out in these institutions, I think that, although the words have changed, the existence of moral judgements levelled at the mad is alive and well today. There is some debate still going on about the goodness versus the badness of the asylums, but whenever you crowd together a population of the kind found in these institutions and force them to obey someone else's arbitrary rules for years and years, then the inmates are bound to become institutionalised. I would question whether the mad have really been released from institutional care, even in the 'community'. Now, what I see instead of straitjackets is a group of people given a chemical straitjacket and set before a TV for most of the day.

A nurse I was speaking to said that in his country, Zimbabwe, he had a friend and it wasn't until he came to this country and did his training as a psychiatric nurse, that he realised that, in the UK, his friend would be diagnosed as having schizophrenia. This is reminiscent of the view of the writer Maureen Duffy of the destructiveness of segregating people; and of labelling, and treating them solely as objects who are expected to conform (Duffy, 2006).

It was not long before doctors began to specialise in the insane, but it was not practical to offer all the thousands of people psychotherapy, even though the NHS had come into being, offering free medical treatment for all, as this was time-consuming and required a massive work force. The works of Freud and Jung, although outstandingly important, advocated this approach, but they worked largely with a few wealthy patients. By the 1950s, the drug Chlorpromazine was noted to be effective in calming the inmates of the asylums and the psychiatrists at the time seized upon it as a wonder drug.

During the 1960s, I was given antipsychotics, not to mention many other drugs and 'treatments' such as amphetamines, barbiturates, semi-narcosis, insulin-induced coma and ECT – the barbaric electrocution of the brain – which still goes on today. As Jung wrote in 1919:

> Psychiatry is a stepchild of medicine. All other branches of medicine have one great advantage; the scientific method. In all other branches there are things that can be seen and touched, physical and chemical methods of investigation to be followed. The microscope reveals the dreaded bacillus, the surgeon's knife halts at no anatomical difficulty and gives us glimpses into the most vital and inaccessible organs. Psychiatry, the art of healing the soul, still stands at the door, seeking in vain to weigh and measure.... We have long known what we have to do with a definite organ, the brain; but only beyond the brain, beyond the anatomical substrate, do we reach what is important to us – the psyche, as indefinable as ever. (From Jung, 1992; first published in 1919)

I think that psychiatry should be more of an art and less of a science. It is an art to understand the many manifestations and workings of the mad mind. It is an art to be able to communicate to that person. It is an art to be able to engender trust and to be able to make a professional relationship with those who have lost their faith and trust in people.

Hippocrates, the founder of medicine and the oath to which all doctors today swear, writing two and a half thousand years ago, defined medicine as an art and a calling. Hippocrates viewed medicine as being based on rigorous inquiry, with respect for patients, reduction of suffering and avoidance of harm (Wingate with Wingate, 1996).

Most psychiatrists who are faced daily with patients who present their torment and despair can feel helpless, because their training does not encourage or befit them for anything else, and to reach for the prescription pad is a way of 'doing' something to relieve their feelings of helplessness. But doing something, even if it could be said to be 'in the patient's best interest', does not equate with doing the patient any good or doing them no harm.

Many psychiatrists that I have met are not interested in how you actually feel or what has led to these feelings, but all they seem to be interested in is ticking a box that will lead to this diagnosis or that. And it is not unusual for every new psychiatrist you have to give you another label even though you yourself haven't changed. In our position as snivelling, disturbed and tormented patients, the psychiatrist sets himself up as a god-like figure that has all the answers, and many are reluctant to relinquish this power and admit that they don't or can't relieve our suffering. Or could it be that they actually believe in their divine status? Sometimes it seems so.

This also feeds many patients' expectations. After all, if you are given a drug, that must confirm that you are ill, and as the relationship to general medicine is so ingrained, a pill is what you are led to expect. Since most psychiatric patients have histories of unsatisfactory relationships and their needs are similar to everyone else's needs, not to mention the need for human contact, I wonder whether a small, hard pill will ever meet the needs of the patient. After all, you cannot cuddle a pill; or talk to it and have it answer you; it won't accompany to you to a café for a cup of tea and it won't give you a present on your birthday. Instead, it stops you from doing most of these things, turning you into a slobbering, unmotivated, socially apathetic, inarticulate patient. A well programmed robot could be just as effective as a psychiatrist and would be much cheaper. A robot wouldn't cause the patient to be delusional – you would know that you were talking to a robot, and wouldn't mistake the psychiatrist for a human being to whom you had come for help and hope.

I know many patients who humour their psychiatrist by taking the prescription but not the pills, but I don't expect many psychiatrists would see the joke. When I was doing an artwork of a woman being crucified, I constructed it out of pills that many patients sent me from all around the country. I called it 'Crucified by the Drug Industry, with a little help from my non-compliant friends'. They know that if they confessed to not taking the medication, the psychiatrist would not see them. I think that if a person is not taking their drugs, their need for support and advice is even greater.

If we consider that psychiatrists' training requires no evidence of self-reflection, or of the intricate dynamics involved in any patient–nurse–doctor situation, it is surprising that they have more power than medical doctors. This is reflected in psychiatrists making judgements that can lead to the kidnapping, incarceration and drugging of a person against their will, which will no doubt affect that person in some way for the rest of their life. We must ask how have we, as a society, given psychiatrists the power of an autocratic despot? Prisoners have more rights than a psychiatric patient, who has committed no crime other than being in torment.

Coercion, collusion and treatment resistance

I always think it is amusing to compare the words used in the context of us mad people with the words commonly used to describe psychiatrists and nurses. *Disassociation* is commonly used to describe us, yet when a psychiatrist or nurse is disassociating, it is called objectivity: i.e. treating a sentient human being as an object. *Coercion* is another such word. It could equally be said to be manipulation, but then such negative words are only assigned to us. This term interweaves with other themes contained in this chapter.

I was often called *treatment-resistant*, and so were many others I used to meet on the ward. I once said to my psychiatrist that, if the drugs worked as well as it was claimed, why is it that I knew 95% of patients here, because I had met them here on previous admissions? She replied that many patients were treatment-resistant, implying that somehow it was our fault – not that the drugs didn't work. And the 'revolving door syndrome' was also something that we were to be blamed for.

I attended a lecture in 2004 which was called 'What doctors may not tell you about psychiatric drugs'. The spokeswoman was Grace E. Jackson, MD, and what she said in her highly entertaining way, amongst other things, was that a patient can get a tolerance to the drugs (Jackson, 2006):

> ... what could happen is that the person who is taking the medication experiences an increase in the flow of messages – the neurotransmitters could actually get revved up. Dopamine or serotonin could get really revved up, and guess what? The body reacts to that. And when the flow of transmissions gets revved up, the number of receptors usually goes down. This may be an explanation why some people go back to their doctor and say 'I'm not feeling good. I've been on this medicine for six weeks, and I felt pretty good at first but now, either they gave me a bad dose at the pharmacy, or it was a bad lot, but the medicine is just not [helping] any more.' So this idea of down-regulation – when receptors disappear or stop responding – this is something that can result in people saying that the medicine has worn off. It means basically, that tolerance develops to the effects of a drug. This is precisely what happens to some people who drink alcohol and they eventually find that they can drink more and more, because their receptors keep going down and down. (From Jackson, 2006)

Box 11.3 Applying Linda Hart's chapter to nursing forensic mental health patients: consent, trust and 'doing no harm'

- The vulnerable and relatively powerless position of forensic mental health patients needs to be borne in mind in relation to issues of informed consent and concordance concerning medication and other treatments (Department of Health and Welsh Office, 1999; Mason and Mercer, 1998; Nolan, 2005).
- Linda's points related to professionals 'engendering trust', especially in service users 'who have lost faith and trust in people' is particularly applicable to many forensic mental health patients, especially some individuals with 'personality disorders', who have experienced traumatic and abusive relationships (Aiyegbusi, 2006).
- Linda refers to 'Victorian moral values' and her view that 'moral judgements' continue to be applied to individuals with mental health problems. To what extent is forensic mental health nursing (e.g. in relation to decisions about patients' restrictions and freedom) influenced by moral judgements in wider society? (Kettles *et al.*, 2006).
- 'Above all, to do no harm'. Hippocrates' injunction, quoted by Linda, reminds us of the need to constantly evaluate acute and forensic mental health services, to ensure that harm is avoided, e.g. from institutionalisation or failure to value patients as individuals (Kilshaw, 1999; Nolan, 2005; Williams and Dale, 2001).

When I was on vast amounts of psychiatric drugs, which I knew were to break me, to make me submit to their institutional insanity, to make me conform and above all to keep me quiet and stop me from saying 'uncomfortable' things that were too close to the truth for their liking, it was horrible. It was like screaming, yet no sound would come out. In other words I was non-compliant because my life depended on it. (And I am rather bolshy, too!)

Informed consent

When I wrote the book *Phone at Nine Just to Say You're Alive* (Hart, 1995), I was on section 3 of the Mental Health Act and had no choice, nor did I have the necessary information on the drugs. I did not then have sufficient knowledge to make sense of the little information I did have. From what I know now, psychiatrists, even today, have such a rudimentary knowledge of the brain and the nervous system, that my current psychiatrist said that psychiatrists know nothing about the brain, yet they can do everything, whilst neurologists know all about the brain and can do nothing.

In my book, I describe how I used to go the nurses who were drawing up my weekly Depixol depot of 400 mg, and say that they were damaging my brain. They would reply 'Oh no, the doctors wouldn't do that to you, after all they're trained'. It was put down to my 'paranoia'. Paranoia, my foot! I now have brain scans to prove that it was not paranoia.

There is a well-known phrase in the patient information leaflet that refers to tardive dyskinesia. It may be a well-known phrase, but that doesn't mean its pathology is at all well known, because no one has yet been able to explain it. And few nurses can even recognise it, which is surprising, since many base their professionalism on their observational skills. I have it, along with reduced facial expression, and on a few occasions health workers have had the cheek to say I was sneering at them. I can assure you that if I felt in any way antagonistic to a nurse or anyone else, I would say so, because being articulate stops the need for covert sign language.

It is usual on any psychiatric ward to see patients walking up and down. You may believe that this is due to the lack of meaningful occupation, but often its cause is the medication which is supposed to sedate, rather than agitate. The trouble is that the nurses often say to these unfortunate patients: 'Oh do sit down for goodness sake, you're driving me mad with your pacing up and down'.

In the Asylum 1
Each of us,
barely visible
like the wraiths that haunt us, circle
from the smoke room,
to the lounge.

Or else we pace the face
off the carpet,
feet follow and lead.

And in our circling,
we play the game of life;
the need for exercise,
the claim to territory,
the unacknowledged pleasures of sex, smoking, eating,
the need to be needed.

And all this without a word,
because words have proved purposeless
and we have a purpose:
to pace and circle,
because without the drugs
that make us pace and circle,
we might play the game of life for real.

Linda Hart 25/10/03

Often too, I have heard women complaining that their breasts are secreting milk, yet I have never heard of a nurse who has said the cause was the drugs. Isn't this odd when you are in a psychiatric hospital because your thinking isn't 'right', yet these strange things are happening to you and no one seems to offer reassurance, or information? It must be remembered that many patients don't even complain about what's happening to them for fear of being considered even madder, and the effects of psychiatric drugs are so insidious, they creep up on you, and soon you forget what it was like not be on them.

Sexual dysfunction is another side-effect and unless you have a sexual deviation, it is rarely mentioned at all. Yet we know that food, occupation, comfort and safety are important, so why does sex rank so low? It is ranked so low that it doesn't exist at all. Is it that doctors and nurses are too embarrassed to mention it, or could it be that they also suffer from sexual dysfunction? Some men cannot get or sustain an erection, and if you know anything about men, this is indeed high on their list of anxiety factors. But I have known many men who have been too embarrassed to discuss this with anyone because they think their manhood could be called into question. As for women – you must be an insatiable sex maniac if you even want to talk about sex, and many women, because of the drugs, don't fancy sex at all, believing that they have become frigid. Until fairly recently, women's sexual dysfunction wasn't even written about in the Patient Information Leaflets, which is no surprise because, as we all know, men's is of greater importance. Even now they mention 'loss of libido', assuming that all women are familiar with medical lingo. I might suggest that men write many of these leaflets, or are behind them, and what do they know of women's sexuality? I know from my own experience that it had a great impact on my self-esteem. If you feel sexy, you look on yourself differently, and you look on the world differently, and there is even a tinge of 'love' or well-being in the way you interact with yourself and others. I know that sexuality is a very difficult area to deal with appropriately in a hospital setting, but to ignore it and the problems that patients face, is a tragic disservice.

Another poem, just in case you didn't get the point!

Real Help from Psychiatry for Men
I have had my genitalia removed
which makes me like
Barbie's boyfriend Ken.

They did it with the utmost care,
my con-genital feelings of inferiority
paramount in their minds,
and to save any unnecessary embarrassment
they preferred not to mention it at all.

They did not use brutality or force,
showing their empathy
in the shape of pills
which I swallowed
with a glass of water.

You see, it was in my best interests.
I was just another worthless, dysfunctional patient,
prone to experiences of deep despair
which they were eager to exchange
for a new, sanitised torture.

They kindly eradicated any residual moments of pleasure
which could have led to the risk of my
forming a real relationship
by inventing the safest sex of all,
a chemical castration,
to make me feel better about myself.

But Ken,
an international heart throb
became famous for his cockless physique,
whereas with me
my heart was lost
along with my knob
which wouldn't throb
with anyone,
not even me.

Linda Hart 3/11/03

It is pertinent to ask why there should be any question around the notion of 'informed consent'. If the psychiatrist or the nurse were to carry out the spirit of informed consent, without coercion or complicity befuddling the issue, it would be reasonably easy. But I have heard such professionals saying 'we don't want to upset them'. Why? If these medications were as efficacious as they purport to be, why is there such a degree of non-compliance? If people who suffer from cancer can undergo what would seem to be horrendous treatment willingly, what is it about mad people and their treatment that produces such a reaction?

It is a fallacy to believe that a person labelled as having bipolar disorder will necessarily have it forever. I have known lots of people who were labelled with this disorder 10 or 17 years ago, and they are still on lithium and haven't had a proper review. Yet whenever they try to come off their drugs, the symptoms return. But is it the symptoms or withdrawal effects that can mimic the symptoms? It is surprising that, in any Patient Information Leaflet (PIL), the withdrawal effects are not listed. Instead, you are advised to continue taking your medication and to speak to your doctor if you are thinking of stopping. They are also known to be particularly unhelpful in giving cautions and not explaining why; for example, you should not drink alcohol. And this is only one criticism I have of the PILs. It is government policy not to give PILs until discharge, by which time I think it might be too late. In my neck of the woods, it is also customary not to give out PILs when a patient goes on leave.

I should like to give you an example of a fairly simple drug, Clopidogrel, which is like an aspirin but does not give the stomach irritation that aspirin does:

> Each tablet contains hydrogenated castor oil, mannitol [E421], microcrystalline cellulose and polyethelene glycol 6000 as inactive ingredients. The pink coating contains ferric oxide, hypromelloose 2910 [E464], lactose monohydrate, titanium dioxide and triacetin [E1518]. The tablets are polished with Carnuba wax. (From: Prescription List. The International Drug Index, 2006. Information about E numbers is from Food Additives and Ingredients Association, 2006)

Well, I wish I knew if I were allergic or not, and I wish I knew what all those E numbers were, and I expect any doctor would wish he knew too before I came hammering on his door for an explanation. And what if any of those ingredients were not allowed for ethical or religious reasons? I think the drug industry relies on the fact that vegetarians either can't, or choose not to, read the ingredients, and many are unaware of what constitutes gelatine. How did they get away with gelatine during the BSE outbreak?

It would not make much of a dent in their profits to substitute a vegetable equivalent in place of gelatine.

To round off this diatribe, I think it should be a matter of choice whether you take a drug or not – an informed choice. This would be possible if a patient were to have real information, including how the drug manufacturers make, market and test their wares; the profits they make; and the politics involved. A recent news item says that the Government has accepted a massive amount of money from the drug industry to 'finance' universities doing research. That effectively cuts out any independent research. Instead of patients being told about drugs in clinical settings where the medical model reigns supreme, it would be ideal if, instead, they could choose whom to ask for information about drugs, and where they met to discuss this. If the patient really had some knowledge about drugs, they would know how the drugs would affect their present and future lives, and how they would 'feel' when on them.

Sally Hughes, who amongst other things, does legal work for Mind, wrote notes on a lecture (Hughes, undated) she gave about the new Mental Capacity Act (H. M. Government, 2005) which introduces a presumption of capacity – 'you are deemed to have mental capacity unless shown otherwise, and lack of capacity cannot be determined on the basis of age, appearance, a 'condition' or behaviour that gives rise to 'unjustified assumptions'' (Section 2(3)).

Capacity is now 'decision-based', so it will be incumbent on health professionals to do all in their power to determine capacity by applying the tests, and taking 'all practical steps to help him/her' to make a decision, and if a substitute decision is taken, choosing the least restrictive alternative.'

I haven't been able to do Sally justice, as I have gone over my word allowance, but it would be worth getting many of Mind's information leaflets (Mind, 2006).

Finally, I know that the medical model, within which nurses will be expected to practise, is a hierarchy, and any hierarchy is only as good as the person who sits at the top and has the power to remain at the top; and being at the top is inevitably corrupting. I worry that the emphasis on the medical model, with drugs being its Holy Grail, together with Government dictates, is making nurses bureaucratic and risk-obsessed, kow-towing to the health and safety police, and stuffed to the ears with policies instead of intelligence – and where I wonder is the patient in all this? Whatever happened to nurses caring for their patients?

I leave you one of my favourite sayings – 'Question everything' (Question Everything, 2006).

References

Aiyegbusi, A. (2006) The emotional impact of working with people who have personality disorders. In: *Forensic Mental Health Nursing: Interventions with People with 'Personality Disorder'* (ed. National Forensic Nurses' Research and Development Group), Chapter 6. Quay, London.

American Psychiatric Association (2000) *Diagnostic and Statistical Manual of Mental Disorders. DSM–IV–R*, 4th edn, text revision. American Psychiatric Association, Washington, DC.

Barker, P. (2005) Putting acute care in its place. *Mental Health Nursing*, **23**(1), 12–15.

Clarke, L. and Flanagan, T. (2003) *Institutional Breakdown: Exploring Mental Health Nursing Practice in Acute Inpatient Settings*. APS Publishing, Salisbury.

Department of Health and Welsh Office (1999) *Mental Health Act, 1983. Code of Practice*. Stationery Office, London.

Duffy, M. (2006). Quotations from work in: Quotations Book (2006). http://www.quotationsbook.com/authors/2153/Maureen_Duffy. Accessed 16 November 2006.

Faulkner, A. (2004) Strategies for surviving acute care. In: *Acute Mental Health Nursing: From Acute Concerns to the Capable Practitioner* (eds. M. Harrison, D. Howard and D. Mitchell), Chapter 4. Sage, London.

Food Additives and Ingredients Association (2006). http://www.faia.org.uk/enumbers.php. Accessed 16 November 2006.

Garcia, I., Qugaishi, M., Kennett, C. and Duncan, C. (2005) *Acute Care, 2004: A National Survey of Adult Psychiatric Wards in England*. Sainsbury Centre for Mental Health, London.

Hart, L. (1995) *Phone at Nine Just to Say You're Alive*. Douglas Elliot Press, London.

Hart, L. (1999) The reliable kettle. *Openmind*, **96**, 20–1.

Hart, L. (2002) Unpublished paper.

Hart, L. (2004) *In the Asylum 2004*. Available from Mind Publications, London.

Higgins, R., Hurst, K. and Wistow, G. (1999) *Psychiatric Nursing Revisited: the Care Provided for Acute Psychiatric Patients*. Whurr, London.

H. M. Government. (2005) *The Mental Capacity Act*. Stationery Office, London.

Hughes, S. (undated) Unpublished lecture notes.

Jackson, G. E. (2004) *What Doctors May Not Tell You About Psychiatric Drugs*. Lecture.

Jackson, G. (2006) *What Doctors May Not Tell You About Psychiatric Drugs*. Text of a public lecture given at the University of Central England, Birmingham, on 9 June 2004. University of Central England Centre for Community Mental Health. Newsletter, November–December, 2006. Accessed 16 November 2006 through University of Central England Centre for Community Mental Health website: http://www.ccmh.uce.ac.uk/news.htm.

Jung, C. G. (1992) On the problem of psychogenesis in mental disease. In: Jung, C. G. (1992) *The Collected Works: Volume 3. The Psychogenesis of Mental Disease* (transl. R. F. C. Hull). Routledge, London. First published in 1919.

Keen, T. (2003) The person with schizophrenia. In: *Psychiatric and Mental Health Nursing: The Craft of Caring* (ed. P. Barker), Chapter 32. Arnold, London.

Kent, M. (2005) My mental health. *Mental Health Practice*, **8**(8), 22.

Kettles, A. M., Woods, P. and Byrt, R. (2006) Conclusions: themes, action and research for the future. In: *Forensic Mental Health Nursing: Interventions with People with 'Personality Disorder'* (ed. National Forensic Nurses' Research and Development Group), Chapter 16. Quay, London.

Kilshaw, J. (1999) Can medium secure units avoid becoming total institutions? In: *Forensic Mental Health Nursing. Strategy and Implementation* (P. Tarbuck, B. Topping-Morris and P. Burnard). Whurr, London.

Kosfeld, M., Heinrichs, M., Zak, P. J., Fischbacher, U. and Fehr, F. (2005) Oxytocin increases trust in humans. *Nature*, 435(7042), 571–2.

Law, J. (2006) The fool's gold that heals. *The Guardian*, 14 January 2006. Accessed, 16 November 2006 through http://www.books.guardian.co.uk/extracts/storyo,,1686011,, 00.html.

Lehmann, P. (2001) Coming off neuroleptics. In: *This is Madness Too: Critical Perspectives on Mental Health Services* (ed. C. Newnes, Holmes, G. and Dunn, C.), Chapter 8. PCCS Books, Ross-on-Wye.

Mason, T. and Mercer, D. (eds.) (1998) *Critical Perspectives in Forensic Care: Inside Out*. Macmillan, Basingstoke.

Meehan, T., McIntosh, W. and Bergen, H. (2006) Aggressive behavior in high-secure settings: the perceptions of patients. *Journal of Psychiatric and Mental Health Nursing*, **13**(1), 19–25.

Mental Health Foundation and Sainsbury Centre for Mental Health (2002) *Being There in a Crisis: a Report of the Learning from Eight Mental Health Crisis Services*. Mental Health Foundation and Sainsbury Centre for Mental Health, London.

Mind (2006) Website: http://www.mind.org.uk/.

National Prescribing Centre, National Institute for Mental Health in England and Department of Health (2005) *Improving Mental Health Services by Extending the Role of Nurses in Prescribing and Supplying Medication: Good Practice Guide. March, 2005*. National Prescribing Centre, National Institute for Mental Health in England and Department of Health, London.

Nolan, P. (2005) The historical context. In: *Multidisciplinary Working in Forensic Mental Health Care* (eds. S. Wix and M. Humphreys), Chapter 1. Elsevier Churchill Livingstone, Edinburgh.

Oxytocin Organisation (2006) http://www.oxytocinorg/oxytoc/trust.html. Accessed 20 November 2006.

Prescription List. The International Drug Index (2006) *Cholesterol Management*. Accessed 16 November 2006 through http://www.rxlist.com/cgi/generic/clopidog.htm.

Question Everything (2006) http://www.questioneverythingplace.com. Accessed 20 November 2006.

Romme, M., Esher, S. (2000) *Making Sense of Voices: the Mental Health Professional's Guide to Work with Voice Hearers*. Mind, London.

Royal College of Psychiatrists Audit Team (2005) *The Health Care Commission National Audit of Violence, 2003–2005*. Royal College of Psychiatrists, London.

Secker, J., Benson, A., Balfe, E., Lipsedge, M., Robinson, S. and Walker, J. (2004) Understanding the social context of violent and aggressive incidents on an inpatient unit. *Journal of Psychiatric and Mental Health Nursing*, **11**(2), 172–8.

Williams, P. and Dale, C. (2001) The application of values in working with patients in forensic mental health settings. In: *Forensic Mental Health: Issues in Practice* (eds. C. Dale, T. Thompson and P. Woods), Chapter 13. Baillière Tindall/Royal College of Nursing, London.

Wingate, P. with Wingate, R. (1996) Hippocrates of Cos. In: *The Penguin Medical Encyclopaedia*, 4th edn (ed. P. Wingate with R. Wingate). Penguin, Harmondsworth.

CHAPTER 12

Forensic aspects of caring for people with personality disorder in acute settings

Jean Woodally and Michele McGunnigle

Introduction

This chapter considers how nurses can care for people with a personality disorder in the acute ward setting. Nurses sometimes hold negative expectations of their patients and may feel that individuals with personality disorder may not benefit from treatment (Byrt *et al.*, 2005; National Forensic Nurses' Research and Development Group, 2006; Peplau, 1952). This attitude may precipitate disengagement with a person who is most in need of help. Nurses may make assumptions that, because an individual is diagnosed as having a 'personality disorder', this means that they will always break rules and test boundaries (Schafer, 2002).

However, some moves forward have been made. Whilst a detailed review of the literature found few evidence-based nursing interventions (Woods and Richards, 2003), research findings suggest that certain approaches, particularly cognitive behavioural therapies (Doyle *et al.*, 2006) and therapeutic community principles (Byrt, 2006) are effective in relieving individuals' distress and enabling positive coping strategies. However, many nurses express feelings of disempowerment when involved with these individuals (Bowers, 2002). Within this chapter, we would like to empower our colleagues by discussing and outlining the current state of knowledge to enable a more professional, holistic, person-centred approach, reflecting service users' expressed needs in a recent research report to Greater Glasgow Health Board (Ferguson *et al.*, 2003).

Discussing how we nurse individuals who have been diagnosed with a personality disorder will enable us to improve our knowledge and skills, which will ultimately improve our clinical practice. Box 12.1 outlines the symptoms commonly found in those diagnosed with a personality disorder. Many mental health nursing interventions are concerned with these symptoms.

The Mental Health (Care and Treatment) (Scotland) Act 2003, includes personality disorder in such a way that individuals can be solely diagnosed as having a personality disorder, as opposed to the Mental Health Act (Scotland) 1984, when those diagnosed with personality disorder were

Box 12.1 Individuals with personality disorder: some features (quoted from Byrt and Woods, 2006, p. 3)

- Compared with most people in their cultural and social groups, individuals with personality disorders are described as having particularly **fixed, rigid and habitual** (i.e. frequent and repetitious) **patterns of behaviour, thinking and ways of responding to situations.**
- Personality disorder usually results in **(often considerable) distress** to individuals with this diagnosis, and sometimes, to other people. The personality disorder **adversely affects aspects of the individual's life**, such as his/her close relationships, ability to trust or relate to people, feelings of satisfaction with life and desired educational, work and other achievements.
- Individuals with personality disorders **generally lack coping strategies to respond to stress in creative ways** that do not cause harm to themselves and/or others. However, the extent that different personality traits and ways of coping are 'adaptive or nonadaptive' **depends on the individual's culture** (Paris, 2004, p. 139).
- In general, people with personality disorders do not have signs and symptoms of mental illness as part of the personality disorder. However, some individuals can have **both** a personality disorder **and** a mental illness and/or problems related to alcohol and/or other drugs...

required to have another mental disorder diagnosed as the primary illness. The current Mental Health Act 1983 for England and Wales is currently under review and may deal with the diagnosis of personality disorder in a similar way to the Mental Health (Care and Treatment) (Scotland) Act 2003.

The *Diagnostic and Statistical Manual of Mental Disorders* (DSM-IV-TR) (American Psychiatric Association, 2000, p. 685), defines personality disorder as an:

> Enduring pattern of inner experience and behaviour that deviates markedly from the expectation of the individual's culture, is pervasive and inflexible, has an onset in adolescence or early adulthood, is stable over time, and leads to distress or impairment.

The Diagnostic and Statistical Manual (DSM-IV; American Psychiatric Association, 1995) has been criticised for listing features of personality disorder that sound more like moral judgments than 'symptoms' (see the lists under 'symptomatology' in Boxes 12.2–12.4). This reflects evidence that the term 'personality disorder' has sometimes been used to negatively judge and label individuals seen as having 'personality disorder' (Byrt *et al.*, 2006; Byrt and Woods, 2006; Pilgrim, 2001). In addition, the DSM-IV definition of personality disorders gives the impression that these conditions are not treatable, and this is supported by a report of a former USA Surgeon General (Satcher, 1999) who stated: 'An armamentarium of the efficacious treatments is available to ameliorate symptoms'. The report goes on to say that most treatments fall into psychosocial and pharmacological groups; moreover, the combination of the two can sometimes be more effective than each group individually.

According to Labelle (2005), for individuals to heal, they must have the desire to change; they need to gain insight into and face their inner experiences and behaviour. This would involve changing their thinking about themselves, relationships and the world, and would also involve changing their behaviour. (Labelle, 2005). In contrast, some cognitive behavioural approaches focus mostly on the achievement of specific goals, the relief of particular symptoms and the development of positive coping strategies (Byrt *et al.*, 2005; Doyle *et al.*, 2006).

Vaknin (2005) states that individuals with personality disorders have many symptoms and other features in common. This author does not propose a unified theory of psychopathology, as he considers there is still much to learn about causative factors in personality disorder. Vaknin (2005) also considers that personality disorder shows its own unique manifestations through the individual's personal story or narrative, although there is limited evidence supporting a psychodynamic explanation that can be universally applied to all individuals with personality disorder.

It is also important to note that some people diagnosed with borderline antisocial, schizoid and obsessive-compulsive personality disorders may be suffering from an underlying biological disturbance. A strong genetic link (Siever, 1997) has been found in antisocial and borderline personality disorders. Causative factors are briefly reviewed in Byrt and Woods (2006).

To gain a better understanding, we will first look at the types of personality disorder and the classifications of these types according to DSM-IV.

Types of personality disorder

Besides 'Personality Disorder Not Otherwise Specified' (American Psychiatric Association, 2000, p. 685), according to the Diagnostic and Statistical Manual (American Psychiatric Association, 2000), there are 10 different types of personality disorder within three cluster classifications (see Boxes 12.2–12.4):

- '**Cluster A** includes the Paranoid, Schizoid and Schizotypal Personality Disorders. Individuals with these disorders often appear odd or eccentric.
- '**Cluster B** includes the Antisocial, Borderline, Histrionic and Narcissistic Personality Disorders. Individuals with these disorders often appear dramatic, emotional or erratic.
- '**Cluster C** includes the Avoidant, Dependent and Obsessive–Compulsive Personality Disorders. Individuals with these disorders often appear anxious or fearful'

(American Psychiatric Association, 2000, p. 685f)

Considering these classifications whilst assessing clients with personality disorder, will ensure that we are offering the best treatment that is available for them. Assessing and identifying the individual symptoms that they portray enables the appropriate nursing care planning and interventions with the patient (National Forensic Nurses' Research and Development Group, 2006). This will be addressed later in the chapter.

Box 12.2 Symptoms of Cluster A personality disorders with associated nursing interventions (symptoms are quoted from American Psychiatric Association, 2000)

	Symptomatology experienced by some individuals	Nursing interventions for some Cluster A symptoms
1	Distrust of others	Establish and maintain therapeutic relationship and communication
2	Others' motives are interpreted as malevolent	Timeline assessment of life experience and/or behaviour
3	Morbid jealousy	Relate past experience to present behaviour
4	Persistently bears grudges	Use of tools to control symptoms
5	Withdrawn	Specific therapeutic interventions: e.g. cognitive behavioural therapy (CBT), dialectical behavioural therapy (DBT), therapeutic community principles
6	Cognitive distortion	Social skills training
7	Acute discomfort in social relationships	Family/relationship discussion
8	Identity problems	Individual and group work
9	Intimacy problems	Medication
10	Substance misuse	Enable social inclusion and acceptance in society

Service users' expectations

In this section, consideration will be given to service users' views and experiences in relation to a diagnosis of personality disorder, with particular reference to what they would find helpful (see Box 12.5) (Ferguson *et al*., 2003). We will also try to explore the problems that service providers have faced whilst working with people who have a personality disorder.

Ferguson *et al*. (2003) found in their research that service users experienced the most difficulties in being able to build and maintain a relationship, loneliness, problems in managing situations (in particular those that can be seen as stressful), coping with daily tasks, low motivation; they also had problems in holding down a job and in dealing with past abuse. Individuals with personality disorder felt that the cause and contributory factors to their illness are childhood trauma, current life circumstances, managing emotions in childhood and coping with feelings of loss later on in life. Two factors in particular are worth pointing out: their difficulties in learning to trust and in identifying and managing emotions/feelings.

The views of service providers concerning what would help were as follows: building a trusting relationship, clear boundaries and lines of responsibilities between workers and service users and

Box 12.3 Symptoms of Cluster B personality disorders with associated nursing interventions (symptoms are quoted from American Psychiatric Association, 2000)

	Symptomatology experienced by some individuals	Nursing interventions for some Cluster B symptoms
1	Excessive emotionality and 'attention-seeking' behaviour	Establish and maintain therapeutic relationship and communication
2	Suggestible and easily influenced by others	Assess effects of personality disorder on self and others
3	Dissocial	Motivational interviewing
4	Impulsive	Well structured care plans, easy for patients and staff to understand
5	Lack of remorse	Effective multidisciplinary working and communication
6	Disregard and violation of others	Specific therapeutic interventions: e.g. CBT, DBT, therapeutic community principles
7	Financially draining	Consistent boundaries
8	Substance misuse	Enable behaviours which are constructive for self and others (within the individual's social and cultural context)
9	Deceitful	Staff and client feedback about behaviours in a non-threatening way
10	Inability to maintain close personal relationships, in particular, intimate ones	Peer group pressure
11	Need for admiration	Contracts related to boundaries and/or symptoms
12	Lack of empathy	Recognise triggers – impulse control – problem solving – break the loop
13	Grandiosity	Anger management
14	Arrogance	Zero tolerance of violence
15	Preoccupation with power, success, wealth or love	Staff persistence, in the face of patients' continued problems and stressful behaviours
16	Instability in interpersonal behaviours	Staff who can cope with enforcing boundaries
17	Unpredictable and impulsive	
18	Recurrent suicidal behaviour/self-mutilation	
19	Identity disturbance	
20	Suicidal tendencies (Paris, 2002)	

Box 12.4 Symptoms of Cluster C personality disorders with associated nursing interventions (symptoms are quoted from American Psychiatric Association, 2000)

	Symptomatology experienced by some individuals	Nursing interventions for some Cluster C symptoms
1	Preoccupation with orderliness	Establish and maintain therapeutic relationship and communication
2	Perfection and control	Assessment of the causes, nature and frequency of symptoms and problematic behaviours
3	Compulsivity	Assessment of patient's strengths, aptitudes and positive qualities
4	Rigidity and stubbornness	Motivational interviewing
5	Over-conscientious	Nursing/multidisciplinary responses to crisis
6	Submissive	Specific therapeutic interventions: e.g. CBT, DBT, therapeutic community principles
7	Behaviour relates to expressive need to be cared for	Counselling focused on specific behaviours
8	Difficulty in decision making	Assertiveness training
9	Insecure attachment	Establish and maintain clear, consistent boundaries
10	Social inhibition	Contracts, with limit-setting
11	Feelings of inadequacy	
12	Hyper-sensitivity to negative evaluations	
13	Social withdrawal but with a longing for a close relationship	
14	View of self as socially inept and inferior to others	
15	History of sexual dysfunction	

between different workers and agencies, a multidisciplinary approach, consistency, basic therapeutic skills, good engagement and relationship skills and empowerment (Ferguson *et al.*, 2003).

Ferguson *et al.* (2003) identified the risks in working with people with personality disorder as self-harm and/or suicide, risk to others in the form of aggressive and/or violent behaviour, and the associated loss of home, relationships and unemployment.

In the Ferguson *et al.* (2003) report service providers named self-harm and suicide as major risks to people with personality disorder. The National Institute for Mental Health in England (NIMHE) (2001) found that, amongst these individuals, there is a high rate of self-injury without suicidal intent, as well as a significant rate of suicide attempts and completed suicide in severe

Box 12.5 What people with personality disorder have found helpful or unhelpful while in care (after Ferguson *et al.*, 2003)

Helpful	Unhelpful
■ Having contact with services	■ Excessive use of medication
■ Helpfulness of service	■ Judgemental views
■ Help to reduce self-harm	■ Inflexible services
■ Information about illness	
■ Hospital respite care	
■ Trust based on empathy	
■ Challenge manipulative behaviour	
■ Understanding and acceptance	
■ Giving service users a voice	

cases. Patients often need extensive mental health services, and this accounts for around 20% of psychiatric hospitalisations.

Pidd *et al.* (2005) found that clinicians and practitioners are reluctant to venture into areas where they feel they have limited skills and capacity and that mental health services have little to offer. In practice, mainstream health services respond as best they can to the needs of a person with personality disorder.

When staff were asked their views, they stated that people with personality disorder were challenging to work with (Ferguson *et al.*, 2003). The report found a wide variation in staff confidence in working with individuals with personality disorder. The most confident workers possessed a more theoretical framework and knowledge, which allowed them to contextualise the individual behaviour.

Markham and Trower (2003) found that patients labelled with borderline personality disorder (BPD) attracted more negative responses from staff than did individuals with a label of schizophrenia or depression. Staff reported less sympathy and optimism towards patients with a BPD and rated their personal experiences of working with these individuals as more negative, compared with patients with a diagnosis of schizophrenia or depression.

Forensic issues related to acute settings

In the open acute ward, for some individuals with personality disorder, there are many dangers around the issue of security (Haglund and von Essen, 2005). Problems in relation to assessed risk in some patients include (Harrison *et al.*, 2004):

- Open door policies and access to an easy exit, mean that individuals can, and will, abscond from the ward (Bowers *et al.*, 2000). On their return they are often abusive and aggressive to nurses and other members of the team.
- Informal status in patients who, arguably, should be detained under a section of the relevant Mental Health Act.
- The lack of checking for illicit substances when visitors enter the ward. This can be a problem, especially as some individuals with personality disorder use these substances as a means to alleviate difficult and complex problems (Kettles, 2006).
- The extent that staff have the right to check patients' belongings to ensure that there are no weapons or tools for harming self or others.
- The relatively easy access to alcohol or drugs.
- The need for boundary setting to ensure safety

Often it is difficult for staff to know precisely who is in or out of the ward, which visitor is in the ward and which part of the public ward areas they are in. Many wards have multi-bedded bays as their structure and this provides many possible places where illicit substances can be exchanged or consumed by individuals with personality disorder, as well as other patients (Kettles, 2006). Often, because of their regard for patients' rights, staff may think it is not right to 'interfere' or are not confident to ask for the names of patients' visitors. Within a secure environment, this is accessed prior to coming on to the ward. Visits are observed and held in a designated area, which is small enough to ensure a minimal risk of passing items that are restricted to ensure the safety of patients and other people. Restricted items may include glass, knives, scissors, blades, chewing gum, tins, computers, mobile phones and illicit substances (Dale and Gardner, 2001). Windows that open on to hospital grounds, where there is public access means that restricted items can be exchanged.

Glass, knives, scissors and tins can be used by certain patients, including some with personality disorders, to harm themselves or others, while chewing gum can be used to block locks. Wires within mobile phones can be used in the making of weapons, as well as calling persons who have expressed no wish for contact. For a minority of people with personality disorder, unsupervised use of computers in hospital has issues around illegal use of the Internet such as cyber-stalking, pornography and other banned sites such as paedophile and weapons-making sites. This may also include easy access to spending money in ways later regretted by patients (e.g. through the use of credit cards when in a manic phase of bipolar mental illness).

With the high numbers of patients on acute admission wards, in comparison to low staffing, there are many areas where individuals can hide to harm themselves until they wish staff to know of their expression of need. The ward office is often a room with minimal windows onto patient areas (Bowers *et al.*, 2002).

In one study conducted in acute wards in our area, up to 10% of patients (both male and female) expressed a concern that they felt vulnerable to unwanted sexual advances and aggression from other male patients in particular (Kettles, 1997). This may reawaken trauma in individuals with personality disorder who have previously experienced sexual and physical abuse (Aiyegbusi and Byrt, 2006).

In the authors' experience, personal alarms for individual staff are rarely provided in acute wards, particularly ones that go off within a unit of several wards; consequently, the need to telephone a neighbouring ward to gain assistance is frequent. In secure environments, alarm systems are in place where immediate response will come to staff's aid from neighbouring wards.

There are also ethical and legal issues about other clients who do not need to be in an area where the door is locked. Because of the lack of beds in more secure environments, patients who need to stay for periods of time in an acute ward, when the secure areas are full, are kept locked in open door wards. Staff shortages and budget restrictions result in inadequate numbers of staff to ensure all individuals' safety or to prevent absconding if the doors were unlocked. An acute admission ward is not a secure environment. It should be an area where individuals are cared for in the least restrictive way possible, as described in the Mental Health (Care and Treatment) (Scotland) Act 2003.

In this era, when beds are at a premium and there are not enough low and medium secure beds within the forensic system, the courts are placing individuals who have been sent to hospital to have an assessment and this can take place in acute areas. Patients with a forensic history can be treated for personality disorder or a mental illness in the same area as an older woman who is depressed because of bereavement, or a young person with an onset of a major debilitating illness. While dealing with distressing mental health problems, non-forensic patients may also have to cope with individuals intimidating them, and perhaps with staff who are not equipped (e.g. through appropriate clinical supervision and education) to feel in control of the situation (Watson and Kettles, 2006). This does not give an appropriate environment for the therapeutic relationship to develop. In such circumstances, ensuring safety and security is essential not only to the well-being of all patients (whether informal or detained under a Mental Health Act), but as a prerequisite for effective therapeutic interventions (Dale and Gardner, 2001).

Aptitudes of staff working with people with a personality disorder

A wide range of knowledge, skills and experience is required on an acute area when nursing these clients. There is a need for strong leadership for the team to feel confident and motivated. The ward manager will have to support their team when some individuals with personality disorders attempt to split the team, isolate a member of staff or bully and intimidate either patients or staff (Schafer, 2002). However, not all individuals with personality disorders engage in such behaviours (Byrt *et al.*, 2006). To ensure that communication is effective, the team need to have debriefing time on a regular basis and specific time where clinical supervision can take place, with appropriate stress and emotion management. Very experienced staff who have several years of experience, who have worked in different areas of psychiatry, and who have seen and nursed many different people, can take on the role of group facilitator for debriefing sessions. Nurses who have confidence in their practice and who have a number of life experiences behind them, so that they can empathise more effectively, can help more junior staff by mentoring and providing assistance with stress management. Newly qualified staff can learn from more experienced staff, but can also bring new and evidence-based practices into the ward environment. They can also bring in motivation to the team when the team feel that it is all just a matter of routine (Shimmins and Storey, 2000; Watson and Kettles, 2006).

All nurses who work with people with personality disorder need to be resilient. Staff will often experience challenges from patients, verbal and physical abuse, manipulation and attempts to split the team, as well as encountering the results of self-harm and aggression.

Lifelong learning is an important factor, especially at the present time, with changes in the role of interventions with patients who have a personality disorder. New and innovative ways of treating and caring for the symptoms of personality disorder are being researched and practised (National Forensic Nurses' Research and Development Group, 2006). More research results will become available with time. We have to be open and welcome these changes. Box 12.6 outlines some of the skills, attitudes and aptitudes that nurses require in order to be able to work effectively with people with personality disorder.

The nurse who works with this group of individuals will have motivational skills to help to encourage individuals with personality disorder. However, often the nurse–patient relationship is going to be hard to establish and can be harder to keep going for lengthy periods of time (Prins, 2005), especially in acute wards where admissions are now of short durations. Often the client will fall at a hurdle and staff can feel that they have failed the patient. We have to accept that with this client group this will occur, and we have to keep going and not give up (Bowers, 2002).

All the team must be consistent in their care. Many individuals with personality disorder have never had consistency in their life (Prins, 2005). It is much easier for the patient to run when the going gets tough. We have to encourage them to maintain contact with services over time and to ensure that they know that identified staff will maintain a recovery-based approach to care (Coffey, 2006).

Ideally, every ward would have at least one specialist nurse who can teach, advise and support their peers. These specialist nurses would be trained in therapeutic processes, such as Cognitive Behavioural Therapy (CBT) or Dialectical Behaviour Therapy (DBT) and Counselling (National Forensic Nurses' Research and Development Group, 2006). These nurses would be able to carry out group and individual therapies, as well as providing clinical supervision for the other staff in the ward, for the benefit of both staff and patients

The management of risk behaviours must be organised, explicit and easy to follow for staff to use in a crisis situation, and in relation to other issues such as aggression and substance abuse. Strong, clear ward and hospital policies that staff can easily use are essential to help staff to know their boundaries in care (Kettles, 2006; Watson and Kettles, 2006). All staff working in these

Box 12.6 Some skills, attributes and aptitudes that nurses require to work with people with personality disorder

- Strong leadership
- A variety of levels of staff
- Lifelong learning
- Values of care
- Therapeutic alliance skills
- Motivational skills
- Resilience
- Empathy
- Consistency
- Honesty
- Non-judgementalism
- Perseverance
- Assertiveness
- Supervision

wards should have access to appropriate clinical supervision, on the ward or outwith the ward environment (Watson and Kettles, 2006).

The client must have an awareness of engaging in risky behaviours and their consequences. A contract which has been negotiated, explained and agreed with the patient is a very handy tool. Such a contract allows the patient to feel in control of their care and treatment but also to know where the boundaries are and what is, or is not, accepted as appropriate behaviour (Marlowe and Sugerman, 1998).

In the last 10 years, there has been a shift from psychologist-led to multidisciplinary teams, including nurses, carrying out the assessment and treatment of mentally disordered persons, using particular approaches and therapeutic models such as cognitive behavioural therapy. It is recognised that nurses trained as nurse therapists compare equally to psychologists and psychiatrists in the therapeutic outcomes of clients (Marks *et al.*, 1975, 1978; Marks, 1985). Their selection and management decisions match those of psychiatrists (Marks *et al.*, 1977). Box 12.7 summarises 20 principles of good nursing practice and Box 12.8 the therapeutic environment for people with a personality disorder.

Interventions found to be effective with people with personality disorder

It is difficult to do justice to this subject in a chapter such as this, and the reader is directed to the first book in this series for a much fuller discussion of the interventions listed here (National Forensic Nurses' Research and Development Group, 2006). Prior to using any intervention, a risk assessment should be carried out. From this, decisions can be taken on what intervention is most appropriate to alleviate the assessed risk, especially in less secure environments (i.e. acute adult mental health areas). Box 12.9 gives a few examples of risk assessment items to be aware of when assessing risk with people with personality disorder. Some interventions that have been found to be effective with some individuals with personality disorder are discussed below.

Cognitive Behavioural Therapy (CBT) is any mode of therapy that attempts to change clients' thinking, behaviours and affect through the use of the pragmatic implementation of sound evidence (Rogers and Gournay, 2002; Guy and Hume, 1998; Leichsenring and Leibing, 2003).

Dialectical Behavioural Therapy (DBT) is an eclectic form of psychotherapy that combines group therapy and individual therapy designed specifically to treat patients with borderline personality disorder (BPD). This approach uses behavioural techniques, contingency management, problem solving, contracting strategies and social skills training (Linehan, 1993; Jones, 2002; Wix and Humphreys, 2005).

Community mental health teams, outpatient services and day services are now part of the effective care of patients on discharge from acute hospital care (Coffey, 2006; Karterud and Pedersen, 2004).

Regular, planned case reviews ensure that all members of the team are involved in the care of the individual with personality disorder, and that he/she has a clear, concise plan of care in a specific time-scale, with identified team members (Anon, 2003)

Box 12.7 Twenty principles of good nursing practice (after Duff *et al.*, 2003)

1. Actively work towards a therapeutic relationship with the service user.
2. Maintain good clear records.
3. Ensure clear pathways of information sharing, both within the team caring for the service user and with outside agencies.
4. Be vigilant about access to corroboration of good quality, detailed information regarding the service user (from a wide variety of sources such as self-report and professional, family and social contacts), including both static and dynamic risk factors.
5. Complete a full chronology of the service user's past life and match those events to current behaviours/events.
6. Identify and record the type, severity, frequency and circumstances of the specific risks.
7. Be sensitive towards race, culture and gender differences.
8. Ensure the team acknowledges and manages its blind spots and personal anxieties.
9. Ensure the team discusses and analyses information in relation to the context of personal circumstances.
10. Have a clear mechanism for regularly updating the risk assessment information, taking into account not only information relating to the service user, but also factors relating to the carers, nursing staff, other parts of the organisation and environmental influences.
11. Link assessment information to management plans by documenting clearly made, collective decisions, which articulate reasonable actions to minimise the potential for future harm.
12. Spend time listening to the concerns of non-professional carers and give consideration to their needs.
13. Support the potential to maximise the gains from positively taking risks.
14. Include relapse-preventing elements.
15. Focus on clear, explicit warning signs and the practical subsequent actions that should be take if these warning signs become present (i.e. crisis management plan).
16. Have regard for the vulnerability of the service user and make sure the team does not return the service user to a situation in which risk behaviours can be re-enacted.
17. Make plans that are contributed to and agreed by all that are involved in the person's care, including the individual himself/herself and identified carers, wherever possible or appropriate.
18. Have discussions about when it is appropriate to tell others in the service user's environment about the risks to themselves, and about whom it is appropriate to tell.
19. Be seen to have considered the service user's ability to change his or her risk behaviours.
20. Ask the unaskable, think the unthinkable and imagine the unimaginable.

Box 12.8 The therapeutic environment for people with a personality disorder (see National Forensic Nurses' Research and Development Group, 2006)

Therapeutic environment should include:

- Set boundaries
- Support groups
- Structured day
- Regular ward reviews
- Consistency in treatment and team
- Incorporate patient suggestion
- Peer group pressure
- Discuss/challenge specific problems
- Structured OT groups

Box 12.9 Examples of risk assessment items (Anon 2003)

Items to be asked during risk assessment:

- Possible triggers
- Emotional antecedents
- Continual or temporary nature
- Use of drugs and/or alcohol
- Towards whom – general or specific
- Intensity, e.g. delusional or not
- Plans
- Reaction of interviewer/team, e.g. fear

In anger management (Marlowe and Sugerman, 1998), specific measures for intervention with individuals with personality disorder are applied, using techniques for managing anger in patients with aggressive behaviour. Anger management often involves the application of CBT principles, including nursing and other interventions, to identify the causes of the anger that are enacted through maladaptive aggressive behaviour (Rogers and Gournay, 2002). There is also evidence that prayer and meditation can be useful tools to use within anger management (Ingram, 2005). Assertiveness training (Marlowe and Sugerman, 1998) can help to increase the low self-esteem that people with personality disorder suffer from. Contracts (Marlowe and Sugerman, 1998) help staff to establish boundaries and give the person clear guidelines to work within.

Therapeutic community principles (outlined in Chapter 4 and in Byrt, 2006) enable some individuals with personality disorders to learn about themselves and their problems, safely express and explore difficult feelings, and try out new ways of behaving and relating to others. This is achieved, in part, through regular community meetings, where events in the life of the therapeutic community are examined, including specific issues, such as an individual returning intoxicated or absconding. Discussion allows for peer support and pressure, as well as staff input (Bree *et al.*, 2003; Byrt, 2006).

Art therapy and occupational therapy are also used in the treatment of some individuals with personality disorders (Campling and Haigh, 1999). One use of art therapy is the application of art media to enable emotional expression in a supportive environment, using a variety of materials. Nurses may work with qualified art therapists in the ward or in an art therapy department. Some mental health nurses are also qualified as art therapists (Murphy, 2001). Occupational therapy (OT) is the use of activity in a structured environment to intervene in an individual's problems with daily living, thus addressing the symptoms of the personality disorder to enhance the quality of the individual's life. Activities such as diversional therapy, specific behavioural programmes and social activities will aid the individual to a 'normal work day' life pattern, when they have lived in a disorganised life pattern for a period of time. Again, nurses, with occupational therapists, can utilise the acute ward environment to assist the patient, or the nurse can refer the patient to participate in an organised OT programme (Humphreys, 2005).

Appreciation of adverse childhood and later experiences can enable nurses to work with patients in understanding the reasons for present behaviours and to enable appropriate use of the recovery approach to care (Aiyegbusi, 2006).

The nurse in an acute ward has the responsibility to enable a patient to have a positive experience of the care they receive and to be able to develop trust with an individual who has seldom had anyone who has taken the time to accept them, without first judging them on their behaviour. The nurse needs to use effective communication skills to enable the individual to understand, and when he/she desires, to change behaviours that cause distress to self and/or others (Bateman and Fonagy, 2004).

Often individuals with personality disorder will find it initially difficult to change behaviours, but with consistency and a willingness to persevere they will be able to do so.

Ward environment

A ward that incorporates patient suggestions, where appropriate, through group participation in care and management, will help the client to feel that they are in control (Bree *et al.*, 2003). This is especially the case when a lot of their choices have been taken from them, such as decisions about leaving the ward, legal detention and limits to behaviour, treatment against their wishes, loss of family contact, unemployment, divorce and social isolation.

In the authors' experience, boundaries which are clear and consistent will allow the person with a personality disorder to know what is acceptable and what is not. By having these boundaries displayed around the ward at strategic points, such as at their bedside, and a booklet explaining these on admission, the patient can clearly see what is expected of them. Many people with personality disorder work more effectively in an environment which is organised and where the activities are structured on a daily basis. This allows the individual to know what is expected of them and enables the opportunity to respond (Schafer, 2002). Structured occupational therapy groups are an effective treatment to allow the person with a personality disorder to acquire a daily routine, save the person from boredom and reinforce a normal adult daily life pattern (Humphreys, 2005).

The most important issue in the ward environment is consistency in treatment and care within the team (Wix and Humphreys, 2005). Good and effective communication is essential to effective care. For many individuals with a personality disorder it may be the first time in their lives that they have had a period of consistency and anyone willing to persevere. Once a therapeutic relationship has developed, the nurse can develop positive coping strategies that the person with a personality disorder can use to express their feelings in ways that minimise distress to self and others (Byrt, 2006).

Management of wards with people with a personality disorder

The management of the ward where any person with a personality disorder is treated must have a leader who will ensure that clear, concise communication is practised on a continuous basis. Ensuring that national and (particularly) local policies and procedures are clear, concise and explicit so that staff and the person with a personality disorder are sure of the position will allow for less animosity and give greater structure to the environment (Lyons, 2005). This will allow the practitioner to be more confident when explaining why a boundary is set and the consequences of breaking that boundary (Schafer, 2002).

By ensuring that education is facilitated and that practitioners have adequate knowledge, a greater consistency in care will be achieved, to the benefit of the patient. Facilitating supervision on a regular basis, both in house and in more official clinical supervision, will allow staff to let go of emotional 'baggage', to enable appropriate stress management and allow them to continue to practice effectively (Watson and Kettles, 2006). The use of specialist trained nurses within the team, who have a sound and experienced knowledge in the treatment of these individuals, must be cost-effective in the long haul (Wing *et al.*, 1998). The supporting of staff is crucial, to make them feel valued, empowered and confident in their care delivery (NIMHE and Department of Health, 2003).

Ensuring staff–patient ratios and adequate staffing to practise safely is crucial to the care of patients with personality disorder (Shimmins and Storey, 2000). People with personality disorders are not the cheapest patients to care for, but effective treatment now may cost less in the long run because of early identification of the need for care and management for patients with complex, and sometimes enduring, problems.

Conclusion

This chapter has considered the nature and types of personality disorder, and service users' expectations in relation to nursing and multidisciplinary interventions. Various difficulties have been outlined, in relation to caring for individuals with personality disorder on acute admission wards.

Despite past pessimism and limited research findings, the authors' clinical experience and the literature suggest that some people within this diagnostic category benefit from certain nursing skills and aptitudes and from therapeutic interventions. Of crucial importance are high quality staff support, clinical supervision and relevant education.

References

Aiyegbusi, A. (2006) The emotional impact of working with people who have personality disorders. In: *Forensic Mental Health Nursing: Interventions with People with 'Personality Disorder'* (ed. National Forensic Nurses' Research and Development Group), Chapter 6. Quay, London.

Aiyegbusi, A. and Byrt, R. (2006) Gender and sexuality issues. In: *Forensic Mental Health Nursing: Interventions with People with 'Personality Disorder'* (ed. National Forensic Nurses' Research and Development Group), Chapter 8. Quay, London.

American Psychiatric Association (1995) *Diagnostic and Statistical Manual of Mental Disorders*, 4th edn (DSM-IV). American Psychiatric Association, Washington.

American Psychiatric Association (2000) *Diagnostic and Statistical Manual of Mental Disorders*. DSM-IV-TR, 4th edn, text revision. American Psychiatric Association, Washington, DC.

Anon (2003) *Effective Management of Personality Disorder: Principles of Management*. National Institute for Mental Health in England, London.

Bateman, A. and Fonagy, P. (2004) *Psychotherapy for Borderline Personality Disorder: Mentalization Based Treatment*. Oxford University Press, Oxford.

Bowers, L. (2002) *Dangerous and Severe Personality Disorder. Response and Role of the Psychiatric Team*. Routledge, London.

Bowers, L., Jarrett, M., Clark, N., Kiyimba, F. and McFarlane, L. (2000) Determinants of absconding by patients on acute psychiatric wards. *Journal of Advanced Nursing*, **32**(3), 644–9.

Bowers, L., Crowhurst, N., Alexander, J., Callaghan, P., Eales, S., Guy, S., McCann, E. and Ryan, C. (2002) Safety and security policies on psychiatric acute admission wards: results from a London-wide survey. *Journal of Psychiatric and Mental Health Nursing*, **9**, 427–33.

Bree, A., Campling, P. and Liderth, S. (2003) Empowerment in mental health: the therapeutic community model. In: *Empowerment and the Health Service User* (eds. J. Dooher and R. Byrt), Chapter 10. Quay, Salisbury.

Byrt, R. (2006) Nursing interventions in therapeutic communities. In: *Forensic Mental Health Nursing: Interventions with People with 'Personality Disorder'* (ed. National Forensic Nurses' Research and Development Group), Chapter 14. Quay, London.

Byrt, R. and Woods, P. (2006) Introduction. In: *Forensic Mental Health Nursing: Interventions with People with 'Personality Disorder'* (ed. National Forensic Nurses' Research and Development Group), Chapter 1. Quay, London.

Byrt, R., Wray, C. and 'Tom' (2005) Towards hope and inclusion: nursing interventions in a medium secure service for men with 'personality disorders'. *Mental Health Practice*, **8**(8), 38–43.

Byrt, R., Graley-Wetherell, R., 'R'., Studley, R., D'Silva, K., James, L. and Pocock, T. (2006) Service user experiences and professional attitudes. In: *Forensic Mental Health Nursing: Interventions with People with 'Personality Disorder'* (ed. National Forensic Nurses' Research and Development Group), Chapter 4. Quay, London.

Coffey, M. (2006) Community interventions. In: *Forensic Mental Health Nursing: Interventions with People with 'Personality Disorder'* (ed. National Forensic Nurses' Research and Development Group), Chapter 9. Quay, London.

Dale, C. and Gardner, J. (2001) Security in forensic environments: strategic and operational issues. In: *Forensic Mental Health: Issues in Practice* (eds. C. Dale, T. Thompson and P. Woods), Chapter 23. Baillière Tindall/Royal College of Nursing, Edinburgh.

Doyle, M., Aiyegbusi, A. and Burbery, P. (2006) Personality disorder: specialist psychological approaches. In: *Forensic Mental Health Nursing: Interventions with People with 'Personality Disorder'* (ed. National Forensic Nurses' Research and Development Group), Chapter 15. Quay, London.

Duff, A., Meredith, B. and Woodridge, K. (2003) *Making Positive Connections*. Pavilion, Brighton.

Ferguson, I., Barclay, A. and Stalker, K. (2003) *'It's a Difficult Life to Lead'. Supporting People with Personality Disorder: Service User and Provider Perspectives*. Department of Applied Social Science, University of Stirling.

Guy, S. and Hume, A. (1998) A CBT strategy for offenders with personality disorders: Part one. *Mental Health Practice*, **2**, 12–16.

Haglund, K. and von Essen, L. (2005) Locked entrance doors on psychiatric wards – advantages and disadvantages according to voluntarily admitted patients. *Nordic Journal of Psychiatry*, **59**(6), 511–15.

Humphreys, M. (2005) The multidisciplinary team and clinical team meetings. In: *Multidisciplinary Working in Forensic Mental Health Care* (eds. S. Wix and M. Humphreys). Elsevier Churchill Livingstone, Edinburgh.

Ingram, L. (2005) *Court Ordered Anger Management Course: Anger Management Training for Domestic Violence Offenders*. http://www.angermgmt.com/courtorder.html.

Jones, T. (2002) DBT and treating personality disorder. *Mental Health Nursing*, **22**(92), 6–9.

Karterid, S. and Pedersen, G. (2004) Short-term day hospital treatment for personality disorders: benefits of the therapeutic components. *The International Journal for Therapeutic & Supportive Organisations*, **25**(1), 43–54.

Kettles, A. M. (1997) A survey of patients' preferences for mixed-or single-sex wards. Research in brief. *Journal of Psychiatric and Mental Health Nursing*, **4**, 55–7.

Kettles, A. M. (2006) Dual diagnosis of personality disorder and substance misuse. In: *Forensic Mental Health Nursing: Interventions with People with 'Personality Disorder'* (ed. National Forensic Nurses' Research and Development Group), Chapter 13. Quay, London.

Labelle, L. (2005) *Personality Disorders*. http://www.focuas.com/personalitydisorders.html.

Leichsenring, F. and Leibing, E. (2003) The effectiveness of psychodynamic therapy and cognitive behaviour therapy in the treatment of personality disorders: a meta-analysis. *American Journal of Psychiatry*, **160**, 1223–32.

Linehan, M. M. (1993) *Cognitive-Behavioral Treatment of Borderline Personality Disorder*. Academic Press, New York.

Lyons, K. (2005) The role of the manager. In: *Multidisciplinary Working in Forensic Mental Health Care* (eds. S. Wix and M. Humphreys). Elsevier Churchill Livingstone, Edinburgh.

Markham, D. and Trower, P. (2003) The effects of the psychiatric label 'borderline personality disorder' on nursing staff's perceptions and causal attributions for challenging behaviours. *British Journal of Clinical Psychology*, **42**(3), 243–56.

Marks, I. M. (1985) *Psychiatric Nurse Therapists in Primary Care, RCN Research Series*. Royal College of Nursing, London.

Marks, I. M., Hallam, R. S. and Connelly, J. C. (1975) Nurse therapists in behavioural psychotherapy. *British Medical Journal*, **3**(5976), 144–8.

Marks, I. M., Hallam, R. S., Connolly, J. C. and Philpott, R. (1977) *Nursing in Behavioural Psychotherapy: an Advanced Clinical Role for Nurses*. Royal College of Nursing, London.

Marks, I. M., Bird, J. and Lindley, P. (1978) Behavioural nurse therapists – developments and implications. *Behavioural Psychotherapy*, **6**, 25–6.

Murphy, J. (2001) *Art Therapy with Young Survivors of Sexual Abuse*. Brunner-Routledge, Hove.

National Forensic Nurses' Research and Development Group (ed.) (2006) *Forensic Mental Health Nursing: Interventions with People with 'Personality Disorder'*. Quay, London.

NIMHE and Department of Health (2003) *Personality Disorder: No Longer a Diagnosis of Exclusion. Policy Implementation Guidelines for the Development of Services for People with Personality Disorder*. Department of Health, London.

Paris, J. (2002) Implications of long term outcome research for management of patients with borderline personality disorder. *Harvard Review of Psychiatry*, **10**(6), 315–23.

Peplau, H. E. (1952) *Interpersonal Relations in Nursing*. G. P. Putnam's Sons, New York.

Pidd, F., Benefiel, N. and Duggan. M. (2005) *Personality Disorder, Everybody's Business*. http://www.findarticles.com/p/articles/mi_qa4120/is_200509//ai_n15668230.

Pilgrim, D. (2001) Disordered personalities and disordered concepts. *Journal of Mental Health*, **10**, 253–65.

Prins, H. (2005) *Offenders, Deviants or Patients?*, 3rd edn. Routledge, Taylor & Francis, Hove.

Rogers, P. and Gournay, K. (2002) Nurse therapy in forensic mental health. In: *Therapeutic Interventions for Forensic Mental Health Nurses* (eds. A. M. Kettles, P. Woods and M. Collins), Chapter 10. Jessica Kingsley, London.

Satcher, D. (1999) *Mental Health: a Report of the Surgeon General*. US Department of Health and Human Services. Office of the Surgeon General SAMHSA. http://www.surgeongeneral.gov/library/mentalhealth/toc.html.

Schafer, P. (2002) Nursing interventions and future directions with patients who constantly break rules and test boundaries. In: *Therapeutic Interventions for Forensic Mental Health Nurses* (eds. A. M. Kettles, P. Woods and M. Collins), Chapter 4. Jessica Kingsley, London.

Shimmins, H. and Storey, L. (2000) Social therapy: a case study in developing a staffing model for dealing with personality disordered offenders. In: *Forensic Mental Health Care: A Case Study Approach* (eds. D. Mercer, T. Mason, M. McKeown and G. McCann). Churchill Livingstone, Edinburgh.

Siever, L. J. (1997) the biology of borderline personality disorder. *Journal of the California Alliance for the Mentally Ill*, **8**(1), 18–19.

Vaknin, S. (2005) *Malignant Self-love: Narcissism Revisited*. Narcissus Publications, Skopje.

Watson, C. and Kettles, A. M. (2006) Education training and support for staff working with clients with a diagnosis of personality disorder: some thoughts. In: *Forensic Mental Health Nursing: Interventions with People with 'Personality Disorder'* (ed. National Forensic Nurses' Research and Development Group), Chapter 7. Quay, London.

Wing, J., Marriott, S., Palmer, C. and Thomas, V. (1998) *Management of Imminent Violence: Clinical Practice Guidelines to Support Mental Health Services*. Royal College of Psychiatrists Research Unit, Oxford.

Wix, S. and Humphreys, M. (eds.) (2005) *Multidisciplinary Working in Forensic Mental Health Care*. Elsevier Churchill Livingstone, Edinburgh.

Woods, P. and Richards, D. (2003) Effectiveness of nursing interventions in people with personality disorders. *Journal of Advanced Nursing*, **44**(2), 154–72.

CHAPTER 13

Cultural and diversity issues

Richard Byrt, Anne Aiyegbusi, Tim Hardie and Mary Addo

Introduction

This chapter considers respect for patients' individuality and diversity related to forensic mental health nursing. Issues concerning ethnicity, culture, gender, sexual orientation and disability will be considered, with reference to recent literature, including Department of Health policy.

Diversity has been defined as 'social variety across and within groups of people' (Thompson, 2003, p. 10) The term 'cultural diversity' has been criticised for concentrating unduly on difference, and for comparing variations with an assumed superior, and generally white, 'norm' (Andrews and Boyle, 2003). However, Thompson (2003) comments that a 'managing diversity approach' (p. 9) has the advantage of positively valuing and affirming individuals' differences, as well as their common humanity. Such an approach, which respects each individual and his or her unique needs (Addo, 2006) is relevant to the care of all forensic mental health and other patients (O'Brien and Morrison-Ngatai, 2003, p. 532):

> The encounter between a nurse and a service user may involve an interaction between two people from very different backgrounds. For both the nurse and the service user, a wide range of beliefs, experiences, norms and values will influence perceptions of mental health, mental health care and treatment. Many of these have their origin in cultural identity. The therapeutic relationship is influenced by two sets of cultural beliefs and values – those of the nurse and those of the service user...
>
> ... Although the term 'culture' is most frequently used to refer to ethnic culture, it can usefully be applied to a range of differences, including those of gender, sexuality, physical ability, age and religion...

Culture has also been defined as the values and beliefs shared by a group of people, and as the sense of how individuals 'do and view things in their group' (Henley and Schott, 1999, quoted in Narayanasamy and White, 2005, p. 106). 'Ethnic culture' refers to the shared values, beliefs, customs and knowledge of the members of an ethnic group (Papadopoulos, 2001). The term *ethnicity* is used in the literature in a variety of ways, often to indicate both 'race' and 'culture', as well as 'the sense of being together' experienced by members of a particular group (Fernando, 2002, pp. 10 and 12).

Stigma, prejudice, negative discrimination and social exclusion

Some individuals, including many forensic mental health patients, are the recipients of negative attitudes and behaviours related to perceived 'differences', which are emphasised at the expense of their shared humanity. This results in stigma, prejudice, negative discrimination and social exclusion. Stigma has been defined as 'an attribute that makes [an individual] different from others.... He is thus reduced in our minds from a whole and usual person to a tainted, discounted one' (Goffman, 1963, p. 12). In general, individuals with mental health problems have been widely stigmatised in the UK since at least the Middle Ages (Porter, 2004), and this is said to deter many individuals, including those from minority ethnic groups, from seeking help from mental health services (Cochrane, 2001; Gary, 2005). Associated with stigma are prejudice and negative discrimination:

> Prejudice can be defined as a set of attitudes which cause, support and justify discrimination, i.e. an emotionally rigid attitude or predisposition in response to a group of people. [Negative] discrimination is the acting out of prejudicial beliefs, which can originate from the desire to maintain one's privileges or power in a particular situation... (Knowles, 2001, p. 231)

Discrimination often results in social exclusion, which involves both experience of discriminatory and stigmatising attitudes from others; and lack of opportunities, choices and life chances available to most people (Office of the Deputy Prime Minister, 2004, quoted in Dooher, 2006; Sayce, 2000; Repper and Perkins, 2004).

Stigma, prejudice, negative discrimination and social exclusion are reflected in generally negative media reporting on individuals with mental health problems (Crisp, 2004; Smith, 2004). The latter are frequently associated with images of violence, with little or no change in public attitudes over time, despite several extensive campaigns to lessen stigma and increase awareness. In addition, nurses working with forensic mental health patients tend to acquire a 'courtesy stigma', reflected in generally negative media reporting (Phillips, 2003). Campaigns to reduce stigma have included those by Mind, the Department of Health and the Royal College of Psychiatrists (Byrt with Dooher, 2006; Crisp, 2004; National Institute for Mental Health in England, 2004; Smith, 2004).

Why issues of diversity are important in forensic mental health nursing

Issues concerning diversity are important in relation to forensic mental health patients for the following reasons:

- Forensic mental health service users face double prejudice, negative discrimination and social exclusion from their dual roles of 'psychiatric patient' and 'offender' (Bartlett, 2004).
- Many of these individuals face possible further social exclusion in society because of one or more of the following: ethnic group, culture, religion, gender, sexual orientation, gender identity, age, disability (Andrews and Boyle, 2003; Cope, 2001; Crisp, 2004).
- Some individuals' discrimination in wider society is mirrored within forensic and other mental health services.
- Furthermore, it can be argued that diversity issues are important to all forensic mental health patients and staff, not just those who are in the most obviously stigmatised groups. This is because each individual, whilst sharing a common humanity, has his/her unique experiences and background (Addo, 2006). All of us may face discrimination at some time in our lives, e.g. as teenagers or older people (Bishop, 2002).
- Government legislation and policy requires recognition of individuals' diversity, and avoidance of discrimination in health and other public services.

Institutional and overt racism and other forms of discrimination

It is important to distinguish between:

- Institutional racism and other institutional discrimination: the lack of availability of appropriate health services to particular groups of clients and their carers, and insensitivity to their needs (Blofield, 2003; Prins *et al.*, 1993; Secker and Harding, 2004).

and

- Overt or intentional racism or other overt discrimination which is deliberate (Blom-Cooper, 1992; MacPherson, 1999; Secker and Harding, 2004).

The National Institute for Mental Health in England (2004, p. 37) states that institutional racism:

> ... is defined as a feature of institutions where there are pervasive racist attitudes and practices, assumptions based on racist differences, practices and procedures which are discriminatory in outcome, if not in intent, and a tolerance or acceptance of such differences.

There has been evidence of discrimination in some forensic and other mental health services in relation to individuals from black and minority ethnic groups (Blofield, 1999; Blom-Cooper, 1992; Prins *et al.*, 1993; Secker and Harding, 2002; see Box 13.1); women (Byrt *et al.*, 2001; Parry-Crook, 2000; Jeffcote and Watson, 2004); and individuals who are gay, lesbian, bisexual or transsexual (Aiyegbusi and Byrt, 2006; Blom-Cooper, 1992; King *et al.*, 2003).

Box 13.1 Evidence of racism in mental health services (Bhui *et al.*, 1998; Cope, 2001; National Institute for Mental Health in England, 2003; Pilgrim and Rogers, 2005; Secker and Harding, 2002)

Research has found that people of black African and African-Caribbean origin are significantly more likely to be:

- Diagnosed as having a mental illness
- Prescribed antipsychotic medication
- Admitted to mental health units, rather than be treated in the community
- Detained by police under section 136 of the Mental Health Act 1983
- Compulsorily admitted under the Mental Health Act 1983
- Admitted to locked and physically secure mental health services
- Subject to more stringent court sentences
- In the case of men in some forensic and other mental health services, viewed as especially 'dangerous', sometimes because of racist assumptions (Blofeld, 2003; Blom-Cooper, 1992; Prins *et al.*, 1993)

Many writers on discrimination have argued that, as members of oppressed groups recognise discrimination, they may become creatively angry: challenging oppression instead of internalising others' negative attitudes. This process is often experienced as an empowering 'raising of consciousness' by the oppressed individual (Byrt and Dooher, 2002; Barnes and Mercer, 2003). Forensic and other mental health nurses may recognise such anger as creative, justified and assertive – or deny or 'pathologise' it (Hopton, 1995). Sometimes, attitudes held by nurses and other professionals have reflected those in wider society, e.g. 'women clients should not be assertive', 'young black patients tend to be dangerous' (Prins *et al.*, 1993). In addition, certain forms of cultural expression or communication have been misinterpreted by professionals as 'aggressive' or 'rude', when this is not intended by the patient (Arnold, 2003). These findings should lead us to reflect on the attitudes of ourselves and our colleagues in relation to the care of forensic mental health patients.

Transcultural nursing

Transcultural nursing provides a framework to provide care that competently meets individuals' needs, including those related to culture and diversity (Andrews and Boyle, 2003; Narayanasamy, 2002; Narayanasamy and White, 2005):

> ... The goal of transcultural nursing is to develop a scientific and humanistic body of knowledge in order to provide culture-specific and culture-universal nursing care practices. Culture-specific refers to particular values, beliefs and patterns of behaviour that tend to be special or unique to a group and that do not tend to be shared with members of other cultures. Culture-universal refers to the commonly shared values, norms of behaviour and life patterns that are similarly held among cultures about human behaviour and lifestyles (Andrews 2003a, pp. 3ff, citing Leininger, 1978, 1991, 1995 and Leininger and McFarland, 2002).

Transcultural nursing is concerned with the cultures of all individuals, including people from groups constituting either an ethnic 'minority' or an ethnic 'majority' in a particular area (Andrews, 2003). Although much of the literature on transcultural nursing is on issues related to individuals' ethnic groups, it considers also aspects of nursing assessment and care relevant to individuals' spirituality, gender, sexuality, disability and other aspects of diversity (Andrews and Boyle, 2003).

Critical perspectives of transcultural nursing

Many proponents of transcultural nursing propose that nurses need to acquire knowledge of specific religious and other beliefs from a variety of cultures (Andrews and Boyle, 2003; Leighton, 2004; Narayanasamy and White, 2005). Criticisms of transcultural nursing include the observation that this is impracticable. Substantial training would be needed to acquire useful knowledge, in view of the enormous breadth of human experience. Further, some transcultural nursing texts and related resource packs have been criticised for assuming that all members of particular ethnic and cultural groups share similar characteristics, beliefs and values, rather than enabling nurses to be concerned with variations within supposed groups. It has been argued that of more importance is a preparedness to respond to each patient as a unique individual and to endeavour to gain understanding of, and learn from, his/her experiences (Andrews, 2003; Gustafson, 2005; Leighton, 2004). However, Narayanasamy (2002) has evolved a model of transcultural nursing that has been found to be applicable in the UK.

Other criticisms relate to a perceived tendency to ignore the social and political context and related power issues, and the ways that these influence nurses' perceptions; and some nurse theorists' implicit assumptions of the superiority of white Western perspectives, and (by implication) the 'difference' or inferiority of other perspectives (Gustafson, 2005; Leighton, 2004, 2005).

A theme in the literature on transcultural nursing (Andrews and Boyle, 2003; Burford, 2001; Kavanagh, 2003; Narayanasamy and White, 2005) concerns the need for nurses and other professionals to acquire what Papadopolous (2001) refers to as 'cultural awareness, cultural knowledge, cultural sensitivity and cultural competence' (Papadopolous *et al.*, 2001, cited in Addo, 2006, p. 71):

- The nurse's **cultural awareness** involves cognisance of her/his attitudes, cultural identity and ways of perceiving the world.

- **Cultural knowledge** includes an understanding of patients' cultures and of their beliefs and actions related to health.
- **Cultural sensitivity** involves attempts to empathetically understand the forensic mental health patient's own experiences and meanings, i.e. the understanding that he or she has of specific problems. It also involves building 'acceptance' and a trusting relationship, with (as part of cultural competence) non-verbal and verbal communication skills appropriate to the individual's culture (Addo, 2006).
- **Cultural competence** refers to the nurse's specific skills related to assessment and interventions that are appropriate to the individual and his/her culture, and to abilities to challenge stigmatisation, negative discrimination and social exclusion. Cultural competence reflects the rationale for nurses to have an awareness of power and racism, as a necessary skill in relation to cultural and diversity issues in forensic mental health nursing practice.

(Addo, 2006, citing Papadopolous *et al.*, 2001; Andrews and Boyle, 2003; Narayanasamy, 2002; Narayanasamy and White, 2005)

Cultural sensitivity

In the nursing of forensic mental health patients, cultural sensitivity involves an appreciation that the patient may not share the perspectives of professionals related to her/his specific 'mental health problems', 'offending' or the need for particular interventions (Mason and Chandley, 1990; Schafer, 2002). Differences in perspective concerning these issues may be related, in part, to variations in cultural background. What is seen as a 'psychiatric problem' in professional culture may be perceived as a 'spiritual problem', a 'moral problem' or 'no problem at all', in the context of the patient's culture (Fernando, 2002; Gary, 2005; Kavanagh, 2003). These authors refer to a wide range of people's understandings, across cultures, concerning what is seen as 'mental illness' in Western societies. In relation to this, cultural sensitivity includes incorporating patients' health beliefs and practices into the planning and implementation of care and treatment, and sometimes, the collaboration between people involved in care or healing across cultures (Bhui and Bhugra, 2001; Fernando, 2002; Kavanagh, 2003; Khalifa and Hardie, 2005). For this to be effective, it is necessary that there is reciprocal respect between the people involved, and the avoidance of unwarranted assumptions that one method is necessarily 'superior' to the other (Fernando, 2002). It is important to note that most people are content to use biomedical treatment methods whilst retaining traditional explanatory models for illness (Dein, 2002). Therefore, making use of culturally pertinent treatments, or working with religious and other authorities who might not share biomedical explanations, can be perfectly legitimate (Khalifa and Hardie, 2005).

Khalifa and Hardie (2005) describe the collaboration between Islamic faith healers and Western mental health professionals in working with individuals who are possessed by jinn (a type of spirit). In a collaborative approach, Western professionals respect the individual and his/her belief, and recognise that the belief in jinn is not usually delusional, but an aspect of Muslim faith. The individual's perspective is invited, and assessed, in order to enable his/her participation in treatment, which may involve biomedical methods, as well as those used by the faith healer:

> ... Clearly, in any case of alleged jinn possession... any underlying mental disorder should be treated by usual psychiatric methods, but *the clinician should respect the cultural issues*, and avoid directly contradicting statements from the patient or relatives about the reality of possession. *When medicine [or, it could be added, nursing] invites conflict with culture and religion, the therapeutic alliance suffers...* There may be a strong case for involving an Imam or religious leader... (Khalifa and Hardie, 2005, p. 352; emphasis added)

In addition, achieving cultural sensitivity depends on the exercise of power and implementation of policy, by government departments and health service managers and providers, to ensure provision of services that respects cultural and diversity issues affecting a variety of individuals and communities (Lester and Glasby, 2006).

Patients' and nurses' cultural beliefs in forensic mental health services

Mason and Chandley (1990) describe the difficulties of implementing nursing models in a high-security hospital because nurses perceived patients as 'sick', whilst the latter viewed themselves as offenders 'doing time', who did not desire nursing interventions, or necessarily see nurses as having a therapeutic role. These findings have considerable implications for forensic mental health nursing in relation to the need for negotiation and finding 'common ground' with individuals who are often reluctant patients. This often begins with attempts to appreciate the individual's specific perspectives and ways of seeing the world related to his/her cultural background. The nurse's attempts in these areas may enable the establishment of trust and a therapeutic alliance, with eventual shared agreement: e.g. related to care planned goals (Byrt *et al.*, 2006; Kirby and Cross, 2002; Schafer, 2002).

Related to this, Department of Health policy documents emphasise the importance of listening to, and appreciation of, the perspectives and experiences of people who are deaf (National Institute for Mental Health in England and Department of Health, 2005), women (Department of Health, 2003, 2006) and individuals from black and minority ethnic groups (Department of Health, 2005a,b). The investigation into the death of David Bennett at a medium secure unit concluded that there was insufficient appreciation of Mr Bennett's cultural needs and a lack of practical action in response to his complaints about the racism of another patient (Blofeld, 2003). Diversity issues are being increasingly emphasised in much of the professional forensic mental health literature, including reference to validation of the individual's experience in relation to gender (Jeffcote and Watson, 2004), ethnicity (Addo, 2006; Khalifa and Hardie, 2005), sexual orientation and gender identity (Aiyegbusi and Byrt, 2006). For example, several authors outline the importance of understanding women's self-harming and offending behaviours in relation to their experiences of oppression in society, and within family and other relationships, in particular (Busfield, 2003; Doy, 2003; Jeffcote and Watson, 2004).

Faulkner (2004, p. 81) states, based on her experience as a service user and a researcher, that:

> One of the more serious implications of the medical model is the invalidation of the individual and her views. This can often lead to treatment and care delivery that does not fully include or involve the patient or service user, on apparently valid grounds. Yet, people continue to be whole human beings throughout periods of distress, and can be consulted about their views and involved in their treatment

Cultural sensitivity, disability and deafness

People may be discriminated against on the basis of a disability, but sometimes a 'disability' is not perceived as such by a 'disabled' person but as an attribute which signifies belonging to a cultural group (Barnes and Mercer, 2003). Deafness is a good example of this, with particular relevance to forensic mental health nursing, but similar considerations can apply to other disabilities. Sociologists of disability have distinguished between medical and social models of disability. The former are concerned with diagnosis, treatment and rehabilitation and the physiological and psychological effects of disability. Social models of disability study the political and social consequences of disability for the individual in relation, for example, to stigmatisation and social exclusion (Barnes and Mercer, 2003).

About one in 1000 people are born with a degree of deafness (Fortnum *et al.*, 2001). Deafness before language has been acquired (i.e. before about 2–3 years) can significantly affect the ability of that person to acquire speech through hearing, and should, therefore, be distinguished from deafness after speech has been acquired. For over a century, many people born deaf were prevented from using sign language as result of a stringently applied educational philosophy (Sacks, 1989). As a consequence, many of these individuals failed to acquire full use of any language, sign or speech. Language impairment leads to impaired communication which causes impeded psychological and social development, and educational achievement (Gregory *et al.*, 1995).

This set the scene for a strongly argued educational debate, but also for the evolution of the deaf community, who see themselves as a distinct cultural group (as opposed to a group of disabled people) with its own language, history and social etiquette. Deafness is, therefore, not something that requires a 'cure', for example in the form of a cochlear implant, and such a view would be condemned as the 'medicalisation' of deafness (Lupton and Seymour, 2004). Individuals who are deaf view themselves as having been systematically discriminated against by a society that has deprived potential new members of sign language, and failed to recognise its existence in any official capacity. The situation has changed in recent years because 'Deaf awareness' is increasing, specialist services are developing and sign language has been recently officially recognised (Lupton and Seymour, 2004).

For professionals working in forensic psychiatry, an understanding of the issues related to 'deafness' and 'Deaf' culture has particular relevance. Deaf people influenced the early development of the law related to fitness to plead and insanity (Jackson, 1997). Further, they require special consideration when they present to the criminal justice system because of communication problems and the need to ensure fairness (Hindley *et al.*, 2000). In addition, the offending behaviour may be rendered understandable in the light of Deaf awareness. Importantly, mental health problems are more common amongst deaf individuals (du Feu and Fergusson, 2003), and therefore, an understanding of the cultural issues related to deafness is essential for healthcare professionals in general, and forensic mental health professionals, in particular.

Deaf people, in this sense, have acquired a particular cultural identity, but similar considerations apply to other 'communities' of people who have been considered 'disabled', including blind people, physically disabled people and those with specific illnesses or mental health problems (Barnes and Mercer, 2003; Lupton and Seymour, 2004). The 'communities', as such, may be more informal or goal-directed and not consider themselves to have a culture specific to them. Nonetheless, in every case it is important to apply the principles of cultural sensitivity in order to ensure good nursing care.

A psychodynamic perspective on diversity and difference

Discrimination can also be understood from a psychodynamic perspective (Fernando, 2003). In order to achieve change at a social level, it is crucial to understand why people should be emotionally and behaviourally challenged by the interpersonal task of relating to others who are seen as different. Indeed, it has been argued that a psychological dimension is required to gain a full understanding of discrimination on the basis of difference, whether this manifests in sexism, racism, homophobia or other forms of exclusion and persecution (Bird and Clarke, 1999; Dalal, 2002; Frosh, 2005). A psychodynamic perspective on diversity and difference may be helpful in terms of providing a psychological framework that addresses the susceptibility of human beings to behave in a negative, sometimes attacking, manner when faced with what they perceive to be difference in other people.

The paranoid–schizoid position

The psychoanalyst Melanie Klein (1975) introduced the concept of the paranoid–schizoid position to describe a structure of early intrapsychic defences against anxiety. According to Klein (1975), the paranoid–schizoid position involves the self becoming deeply split into good and bad parts. Good parts represent the life instinct and are reflected in the pull towards life, love, nurturing and caring. Bad parts are associated with the death instinct and are reflected in a pull towards death, hatred, danger and damage. In the paranoid–schizoid position, difference, as represented by good and bad parts of the self, cannot be held together within the mind because of overwhelming anxiety. In the paranoid–schizoid position, good parts are retained and experienced as a part of the self; while bad parts are felt to be unacceptable and so have to be evacuated. Evacuation takes the form of unconscious projection onto a suitable object: invariably, but not necessarily, another person. The other person who functions as a receptacle for unwanted projections is then experienced as embodying unpalatable characteristics. This enables the projector to witness their unwanted qualities from a distance, within another who can then be interacted with disdainfully (Klein, 1975). An example would be of a young man, uncertain of his parental and racial heritage, who racially abuses a young black man and supports the idea that all 'aliens' should be repatriated 'back to where they came from'.

Projective identification

Psychodynamic theory can not only inform us of why people have a tendency to project their anxieties onto other people when feeling threatened, but also explains why some people may be prone to becoming receptacles for other people's unwanted psychic detritus. Horowitz (1983) explains how we can more fully appreciate the intricacy of group relating, when we take account of the way that people 'may transfer mental contents from one another and back and forth' through interpersonal relating. Not only do people project unwanted parts of themselves onto, and into, others, but the recipients can act in accordance with such projections, often experiencing them as a part of the self. This has important implications for the relationship between nurses and service users in mental health services. The risk is that the service user may be required to contain the

Case example

Joseph arrived in the UK in 1964, having emigrated from overseas. Joseph is a large black man, and when he arrived in the UK he found the indigenous population to be very wary of him. He found employment difficult to secure and was often called racially abusive names, such as 'monkey' and 'gorilla', as he walked in his local town. On a couple of occasions, Joseph was stopped by police officers who questioned him about his motives for looking in shop windows. When a bar room brawl occurred in a local pub where Joseph was having a quiet drink of soda, he was accused by the attending police officers of instigating violence. Wherever Joseph went, accusations of his presenting a physical threat to local white people seemed to follow.

After Joseph had been in the UK for two years, he became depressed. He was admitted to a psychiatric hospital. Because of his body size, mental health professionals decided to take no chances and he was frequently placed in seclusion and given large doses of tranquillisers, lest he be violent to others. Therapeutic relationships were not offered to Joseph in the psychiatric hospital and he was frequently surrounded by large numbers of nurses who appeared to be standing guard when he was not locked in a room. One day, Joseph became extremely violent and assaulted six nurses, causing significant injury to two of them.

Joseph had no history of violence towards other people prior to his emigration to the UK, where he was subject to massive and repeated hostile projections from other people. His large body size and his difference made him a convenient receptacle for projections about violence and menace. Other people's reactions were experienced by Joseph as unrelenting interpersonal pressure until he eventually broke down. Rather than leading to an opportunity for Joseph to recover from what he had experienced in a hostile society, admission to a psychiatric hospital resulted in an increase in interpersonal hostility until Joseph eventually acted on what was being so forcefully projected into him. The process by which Joseph transformed from a 'gentle giant' to a violent, depressed risk to others may be understood as projective identification (Perlin, 2005).

projected, disturbed aspects of mental health nurses and other workers (O'Brien and Morrison-Ngatai, 2003).

The importance of psychodynamic explanations

It is argued that social explanations for discrimination, on the grounds of difference, may offer an incomplete account for practice. A psychological dimension may also need to be included in any attempts to understand the human proclivity to discriminate on the grounds of difference. There is also the need to consider both the social and psychological dimensions, in order to fully understand the issue of discrimination based on differences among people.

The tendency of human beings to locate unwanted aspects of the self into those who are regarded to be 'other' may offer an explanation as to how this pattern of human relating persists over time and in so many contexts (Fernando, 2003). The intention to provide equal opportunities across the boundaries of human diversity may be continually undermined because of a failure to take account of unconscious processes operating at the level of the individual, the team or the organisation in mental health services. One way to address this is to increase the self-awareness of group members. In mental health services, this may take the form of supervision and reflective practice groups where the unconscious dynamics of teams are explored and thought about. This process will aim to reduce the extent to which members of the group project alien parts of themselves into others (Halton, 2004).

Conclusion

This chapter has considered the meaning of diversity and related concepts, and the stigma, negative discrimination and social exclusion faced by many forensic mental health patients. This relates to their experience of both mental health problems and offending; and, in many instances, to other factors, including their ethnic group, gender, disability, sexuality and gender identity. Discrimination in wider society is sometimes mirrored in forensic and other health services.

Despite criticisms which have been made of some of its assumptions, transcultural nursing provides a framework which can usefully inform nurses' cultural sensitivity and cultural competence. Differences in cultural perspectives between forensic mental health patients and nurses are considered, in relation to individuals' ethnic groups and deafness. The chapter concludes with the consideration of a psychodynamic perspective of diversity and difference.

References

Cited Acts of Parliament are listed in Appendix 14.1 at the end of Chapter 14.

Addo, M. (2006) Culture, spirituality and ethical issues in caring for clients with personality disorder. In: *Forensic Mental Health Nursing: Interventions with People with 'Personality Disorder'* (ed. National Forensic Nurses' Research and Development Group), Chapter 5. Quay, Salisbury.

Aiyegbusi, A. and Byrt, R. (2006) Gender and sexuality. In: *Forensic Mental Health Nursing: Interventions with People with 'Personality Disorder'* (ed. National Forensic Nurses' Research and Development Group), Chapter 8. Quay, Salisbury.

Andrews, M. M. (2003) Theoretical foundations of transcultural nursing. In: *Transcultural Concepts in Nursing Care* (eds. M. M. Andrews and J. S. Boyle), Chapter 1. Lippincott, Williams and Wilkins, Philadelphia.

Andrews, M. M. and Boyle, J. S. (eds.) (2003) *Transcultural Concepts in Nursing Care*. Lippincott, Williams and Wilkins, Philadelphia.

Arnold, E. (2003) Intercultural communication. In: *Interpersonal Relationships*, 4th edn (eds. E. Arnold and K. U. Boggs), Chapter 11. Saunders, St Louis.

Barnes, C. and Mercer, G. (2003) *Disability*. Polity Press, Cambridge.

Bartlett, A. (2004) Fashions in psychiatric care: implications for sense of self. In: *Every Family in the Land: Understanding Prejudice and Discrimination Against People with Mental Illness* (ed. A. H. Crisp), Chapter 49. Royal Society of Medicine Press, London.

Bhui, K. and Bhugra, D. (2001) Training and supervision in cross-cultural mental health services. In: *Psychiatry in Multicultural Britain* (eds. D. Bhugra and R. Cochrane), Chapter 14. Gaskell/Royal College of Psychiatrists, London.

Bhui, K., Brown, P. Hardie, T. Watson, J. P. and Parrott, J. (1998) African-Caribbean men remanded to Brixton Prison: psychiatric and forensic characteristics and outcome of final court appearance. *British Journal of Psychiatry*, **172**, 337–44.

Bird, J. and Clarke, S. (1999) Racism, hatred and discrimination through the lens of projective identification. *Journal of Psychoanalysis of Culture and Society*, **4**, 158–61.

Bishop, A. (2002) *Breaking the Cycle of Oppression in People*, 2nd edn. Fernwood Publishing, Halifax.

Blofeld, J. (2003) *Independent Inquiry into the Death of David Bennett. An Independent Inquiry Set Up Under HSG (94) 27*. Department of Health, London.

Blom-Cooper, L. (1992) *Report of the Committee of Inquiry into Complaints at Ashworth Hospital*. HMSO, London.

Burford, B. (2001) The cultural competence model. In: *Managing Diversity and Inequality in Health Care* (ed. Baxter, C.), Chapter 9. Baillière Tindall/Royal College of Nursing, Edinburgh.

Busfield, J. (2003) Disordered minds. In: *Women's Minds, Women's Bodies: An Interdisciplinary Approach* (eds. G. Boswell and F. Poland), Chapter 2. Palgrave Macmillan, Basingstoke.

Byrt, R. and Dooher, J. (2002) Empowerment and participation: definitions, meanings and models. In: *Empowerment and Participation: Power, Influence and Control in Contemporary Healthcare* (eds. J. Dooher and R. Byrt), Chapter 2). Quay, Salisbury.

Byrt, R. with Dooher, J. (2006) The social consequences of a 'personality disorder' diagnosis. In: *Forensic Mental Health Nursing: Interventions with People with 'Personality Disorder'* (ed. National Forensic Nurses' Research and Development Group), Chapter 3. Quay, Salisbury.

Byrt, R., Lomas, C., Gardiner, J. and Lewis, D. (2001) Working with women in secure environments. *Journal of Psychosocial Nursing and Mental Health Services*, **39**(9), 42–50.

Byrt, R., Graley-Wetherell, R., 'R', Studley, R., D'Silva, K., James, L. and Pocock, T. (2006) Service user experiences and professional attitudes. In: *Forensic Mental Health Nursing: Interventions with People with 'Personality Disorder'* (ed. National Forensic Nurses' Research and Development Group), Chapter 4. Quay, Salisbury.

Cochrane, R. (2001) Race, prejudice and ethnic identity. In: *Psychiatry in Multicultural Britain* (eds. D. Bhugra and R. Cochrane), Chapter 4. Gaskell/Royal College of Psychiatrists, London.

Cope, R. (2001) Forensic psychiatry. In: *Psychiatry in Multicultural Britain* (eds. D. Bhugra and R. Cochrane), Chapter 13. Gaskell/Royal College of Psychiatrists, London.

Crisp, A. H. (ed.) (2004) *Every Family in the Land: Understanding Prejudice and Discrimination Against People with Mental Illness*, rev. edn. Royal Society of Medicine Press, London.

Dalal, F. (2002) *Race, Colour and the Process of Racialization: New Perspectives from Group Analysis and Sociology*. Brunner-Routledge, London.

Dein, S. (2002) Transcultural Psychiatry. *British Journal of Psychiatry*, **181**, 535–6.

Department of Health (2003) *Mainstreaming Gender and Women's Mental Health. Implementation Guidance*. Department of Health, London.

Department of Health (2005a) *Delivering Race Equality in Mental Health Care. An Action Plan for Reform. Inside and Outside Services and The Government's Response to the Independent Inquiry Into the Death of David Bennett*. Department of Health, London.

Department of Health (2005b) *New Blueprint to Tackle and Eradicate Discrimination in Mental Health Services Over the Next Five Years*. Contains summary of action plan of 'Delivering Race Equality in Mental Health Care'. Department of Health, London.

Department of Health (2006) *Supporting Women into the Mainstream. Commissioning Women Only Community Day Services*. Department of Health, London.

Dooher, J. (2006) Social exclusion. Box 3.3, p27 in Byrt, R. with Dooher, J.: The social consequences of a 'personality disorder' diagnosis. In: *Forensic Mental Health Nursing: Interventions with People with 'Personality Disorder'* (ed. National Forensic Nurses' Research and Development Group), Chapter 3. Quay, Salisbury.

Doy, J. (2003) Women and deliberate self-harm. In: *Women's Minds, Women's Bodies: an Interdisciplinary Approach* (eds. G. Boswell and F. Poland), Chapter 3. Palgrave Macmillan, Basingstoke.

du Feu, M. and Fergusson, K. (2003) Sensory impairment and mental health. *Advances in Psychiatric Treatment*, **9**, 95–103.

Faulkner, A. (2004) Strategies for surviving acute care. In: *Acute Mental Health Nursing: From Acute Concerns to the Capable Practitioner* (eds. M. Harrison, D. Howard and D. Mitchell), Chapter 4. Sage, London.

Fernando, S. (2002) *Mental Health, Race and Culture*, 2nd edn. Palgrave, Basingstoke.

Fernando, S. (2003) *Cultural Diversity, Mental Health and Psychiatry: The Struggle Against Racism*. Brunner-Routledge, Hove.

Fortnum, H. M., Summerfield, A. Q., Marshall, D. H., Davis A. C. and Bamford, J. M. (2001) Prevalence of permanent childhood hearing impairment in the United Kingdom and implications for universal neonatal hearing screening: questionnaire based ascertainment study. *British Medical Journal*, **323**(7312), 536–40.

Frosh, S. (2005) *Hate and the 'Jewish Science': Anti-Semitism, Nazism and Psychoanalysis*. Palgrave, Basingstoke.

Gary, F. A. (2005) Stigma: barrier to mental health care among ethnic minorities. *Issues in Mental Health Nursing*, **26**, 979–99.

Goffman, E. (1963) *Stigma: Notes on the Management of Spoiled Identity*. Penguin, Harmondsworth.

Gregory, S., Bishop, J. and Sheldon L. (1995) *Deaf Young People and Their Families*. Cambridge University Press, Cambridge.

Gustafson, D. L. (2005) Transcultural nursing theory from a critical perspective. *Advances in Nursing Science*, **28**(1), 2–16.

Halton, W. (2004) Some unconscious aspects of organisational life: contributions from psychoanalysis. In: *Communication, Relationships and Care. A Reader* (eds. M. Robb, S. Barrett, C. Komaromy and A. Rogers), Chapter 22. Routledge, Taylor & Francis Group/The Open University, London.

Hindley, P., Kitson, N. and Leach V. (2000) Forensic psychiatry and deaf people. In: *Mental Health and Deafness* (eds. P. Hindley and N. Kitson), Chapter 9. Whurr, London.

Hopton, J. (1995) The application of ideas of Frantz Fanon to the practice of mental health nursing. *Journal of Advanced Nursing*, **21**(4), 723–8.

Horowitz, L. (1983) Projective identification in dyads and groups. *International Journal of Group Psychotherapy*. **33**(3), 259–79.

Jackson, P. (1997) *Deaf Crime Casebook*. Cox and Jackson, Ipswich.

Jeffcote, N. and Watson, T. (eds.) (2004) W*orking Therapeutically with Women in Secure Mental Health Settings*. Jessica Kingsley, London.

Kavanagh, K. H. (2003) Transcultural perspectives in mental health nursing. In: *Transcultural Concepts in Nursing Care* (eds. M. M. Andrews and J. S. Boyle), Chapter 10. Lippincott, Williams and Wilkins, Philadelphia.

Khalifa, N. and Hardie, T. (2005) Possession and jinn. *Journal of the Royal Society of Medicine*, **98**, 351–3.

King, M. and Mckeown, E. with Warner, J., Ramsay, A., Johnson, K., Cort, C., Davidson, O. and Wright, L. (2003) *Mental Health and Quality of Life of Gay Men and Lesbians in England and Wales*. Mind/University College, London, London.

Kirby, S. D. and Cross, D. (2002) Socially constructed narrative interventions: a foundation for therapeutic alliances. In: *Therapeutic Interventions for Forensic Mental Health Nurses* (eds. A. M. Kettles, P. Woods and M. Collins), Chapter 12. Jessica Kingsley, London.

Klein, M. (1975) Notes on some schizoid mechanisms. In: *Envy and Gratitude and Other Works, 1946–1963*. Hogarth Press and Institute of Psychoanalysis, London.

Knowles, J. (2001) Developing individuals. In: *Managing Diversity and Inequality in Health Care* (ed. C. Baxter), Chapter 10. Baillière Tindall/Royal College of Nursing, Edinburgh.

Leighton, K. (2004) Anglo-American nursing theory, individualism and mental health care: a social conflict perspective. *International Journal of Nursing Studies*, **41**, 21–8.

Leighton, K. (2005) Transcultural nursing: the relationship between individualist ideology and individualised nursing care. *Journal of Psychiatric and Mental Health Nursing*, **12**(1), 85–94.

Lester, H. and Glasby, J. (2006) Mental health: policy and practice. Palgrave Macmillan, Basingstoke.

Lupton, D. and Seymour, W. (2004) Technology, selfhood and physical disability. In: *Communication, Relationships and Care. A Reader* (eds. M. Robb, S. Barrett, C. Komaromy and A. Rogers), Chapter 18. Routledge, Taylor and Francis Group/The Open University, London.

MacPherson, Sir W. (1999) *The Stephen Lawrence Inquiry*. Cm. 4262-1. Stationery Office, London.

Mason, T. and Chandley, M. (1990) Nursing models in a special hospital: a critical analysis of efficacy. *Journal of Advanced Nursing*, **15**, 667–73.

Narayanasamy, A. (2002) The ACCESS model: a transcultural nursing practice framework. *British Journal of Nursing*, **11**(9), 643–50.

Narayanasamy, A. and White, E. (2005) A review of transcultural nursing. *Nurse Education Today*, **15**, 102–11.

National Institute for Mental Health in England (NIMHE) (2004) *Developing Positive Practice to Support the Safe and Therapeutic Management of Aggression and Violence in Mental Health In-patient Settings*. NIMHE, London.

National Institute for Mental Health in England (NIMHE) and Department of Health (2005) *Mental Health and Deafness. Towards Equality and Access*. Department of Health, London.

O'Brien, A. J. and Morrison-Ngati, E. (2003) Providing culturally safe care. In: *Psychiatric and Mental Health Nursing: The Craft of Caring* (ed. P. Barker), Chapter 63. Arnold, London.

Papadopolous, I. (2001) Antiracism, multiculturalism and the third way. In: *Managing Diversity and Inequality in Health Care* (ed. E. Baxter). Baillière Tindall/Royal College of Nursing, Edinburgh.

Papadopolous, I. *et al.* (2001) Culturally appropriate care should be at the heart of mental health services. *Openmind*, **110**, July–August. Cited in: Addo, M. (2006) Culture, spirituality and ethical issues in caring for clients with personality disorder. In: *Forensic Mental Health Nursing: Interventions with*

People with 'Personality Disorder' (ed. National Forensic Nurses' Research and Development Group), Chapter 5. Quay, Salisbury.

Parry-Crooke, G. (2000) *Good Girls: Surviving the Secure System: a Consultation with Women in High and Medium Secure Psychiatric Settings.* WISH/University of North London, London.

Perlin, C. K. (2005) Social responses and personality disorders. In: *Principles and Practice of Psychiatric Nursing*, 8th edn. (ed. G. W. Stuart and M. Laraia), Chapter 22. Elsevier/Mosby, St Louis.

Phillips, R. (2003) The good, the bad and the ugly: the role of local radio as a medium for overcoming prejudice. In: *Empowerment and the Health Service User* (eds. J. Dooher and R. Byrt). Quay, Salisbury.

Pilgrim, D. and Rogers, A. (2005) *A Sociology of Mental Health and Illness*, 3rd edn. Open University Press, Maidenhead.

Porter, R. (2004) Is mental illness inevitably stigmatising? In: *Every Family in the Land: Understanding Prejudice and Discrimination Against People with Mental Illness*, rev. edn. (ed. A. H. Crisp), Chapter 1. Royal Society of Medicine Press, London.

Prins, H., Backer-Holst, T., Francis, E. and Keitch, I. (1993) *Report of the Committee of Inquiry into the Death in Broadmoor Hospital of Orville Blackwood and a Review of the Deaths of Two Other Afro-Caribbean Patients: 'Big, Black and Dangerous'?* Department of Health, London.

Repper, J. and Perkins, R. (2004) Social inclusion and acute care. In: *Acute Mental Health Nursing: From Acute Concerns to the Capable Practitioner* (eds. M. Harrison, D. Howard and D. Mitchell). Sage, London.

Sacks, O. (1989) *Seeing Voices.* Picador, London.

Sayce, L. (2000) *From Psychiatric Patient to Citizen: Overcoming Discrimination and Social Exclusion.* Macmillan Press, Basingstoke.

Schafer, P. E. (2002) Nursing interventions and future directions with patients who constantly break rules and test boundaries. In: *Therapeutic Interventions for Forensic Mental Health Nurses* (eds. A. M. Kettles, P. Woods and M. Collins), Chapter 4. Jessica Kingsley, London.

Secker, J. and Harding, C. (2002) African and African Caribbean users' perceptions of inpatient services. *Journal of Psychiatric and Mental Health Nursing*, **9**, 161–7.

Smith, M. (2004) What do surveys of public attitudes to mental health problems really mean (and do we mean what we say)? *Journal of Mental Health Promotion*, **3**(4), 40–7.

Thompson, N. (2003) *Promoting Equality: Challenging Discrimination and Oppression*, 2nd edn. Palgrave, Basingstoke.

CHAPTER 14

Cultural competence and patients' rights

Richard Byrt and Tim Hardie

This chapter considers specific aspects of cultural sensitivity and cultural competence in the nursing of individuals who are forensic mental health patients. Issues of social exclusion, patient advocacy, and related legislation and policy will also be considered.

Kavanagh (2003) emphasises the need for mental health nurses and other professionals to have cultural competencies in particular areas. In liaison with patients, their informal carers and non-statutory organisations concerned with patients' rights and needs, this includes the competencies listed below. Some of the latter are also related to cultural awareness, cultural sensitivity and cultural knowledge (Addo, 2006; Andrews, 2003b; Kavanagh, 2003; Narayanasamy, 2002; Narayanasamy and White, 2005; for definitions of cultural sensitivity and cultural competence see Chapter 13).

Cultural competencies

It is suggested that the following cutural competencies are crucial aspects of the nursing and multidisciplinary care and treatment of forensic patients in acute and other services.

Communication, information, the nurse–patient relationship and access to interpreting and translating services

- Effective non-verbal and verbal communication, including, for example, appreciating the individual's needs related to 'silence... eye contact... touch... space and distance' (Andrews, 2003b, pp. 27ff).
- Communicating with individuals whose first language is not spoken English, including individuals who are deaf (Andrews, 2003b; Arnold, 2003; Kenny, 2005).
- Enabling swift access, where necessary, to interpreters and translators, so that communication and information are readily available (Bavington, 2000; Kenny, 2005).

- Spoken and written information which is sensitive to, and reflects, individuals' varied diversity. Written information which is readily accessible to all patients, attractively produced by a variety of organisations, including those that are voluntary and community-based (Bavington, 2000; Rai-Atkins *et al.*, 2002).
- Endeavouring to develop and convey empathetic understanding of the patient and his/her unique perspectives and experiences.

Empathy, validation of the individual's experience and affirmative counselling

- As part of an empathetic relationship, taking steps to appreciate the individual's specific experiences of discrimination and social exclusion, and affirmation of his/her culture and lifestyle (Addo, 2006; Williams *et al.*, 2004).
- The use of specific affirmative counselling techniques to achieve this, related to culture (Kareem and Littlewood, 2000; see the account of Nafsiyat in Box 14.1); varying intellectual, sensory and physical abilities (Corker, 1994); gender (Jeffcote and Watson, 2004); sexual orientation (Davies and Neal, 1996) and gender identity (Aiyegbusi and Byrt, 2006).

Holistic assessments, cultural and other aspects of safety and risk

- Holistic assessments which are sensitive to the individual's needs related to her/his ethnic group, culture, spirituality, including religion, gender, sexual orientation, gender identity and specific disabilities and problems (Addo, 2006; Aiyegbusi and Byrt, 2006; Kavanagh, 2003; O'Brien and Morrison-Ngatai, 2003).
- Risk assessments, based on reliable and valid measures from piloting on a variety of ethnic and other groups. Avoidance of assumptions of risk that are based on racist, sexist or other biases (Morgan and Wetherell, 2004).
- 'Enabling clients to derive a sense of cultural safety' (Narayanasamy, 2002, p. 645). This involves respect for the individual and his/her 'cultural identity' (Narayanasamy, 2002, p. 646), rights and needs, with awareness of factors that may make it difficult to achieve this with forensic mental health patients (Dale and Gardner, 2001).
- The balancing of needs for 'cultural safety' with prevention of harm to others and to self, through the provision of physical and relational security (Dale and Gardner, 2001).

The individual's spiritual needs

- Within the parameters of safety, enabling the individual to practice his/her spiritual and other beliefs. Provision of space and time for prayer, quiet, reflection and meditation, as desired by the individual. Provision of a multi-faith room (Addo, 2006).

The individual's physical needs

- Provision of diet, access to exercise, rest and sleep and the meeting of the individual's other physical needs, related to his/her ethnic group, culture and other diversity needs (Addo, 2006; Kavanagh, 2003)

Gender-related needs

- Development or provision of separate services for women. Choice of gender of primary nurse, keyworker and other staff. Within mixed gender services, women only space, toilet, bathing and sleeping facilities. Availability of women only activities, but with avoidance of assumptions that certain activities are 'only for women' or 'only for men' (Byrt *et al.*, 2001; NHS Executive, 1999; Department of Health, 2005a).

Needs related to disability

- Ensuring that services are accessible to, and meet the needs of, individuals with physical and sensory disabilities, in accordance with the Disability Discrimination Act (H. M. Government, 2005; Department of Health and Disability Rights Commission, 2004).

Psychosexual and relationship needs, including those related to sexual orientation

- Recognition of the individual's psychosexual needs (Aiyegbusi and Byrt, 2006) and of people important in the individual's life. (The importance of this is indicated, for example, from research findings that lesbian and gay partners have not always been recognised as the individuals closest to patients, and chosen by the latter to be given important information; Aiyegbusi and Byrt, 2006; UNISON and Royal College of Nursing, 2004).
- Avoidance of assumptions, in assessment and nursing interventions, that all patients have a fixed gender identity or are heterosexual, as may be reflected, for example, by questions about 'marital status' (Aiyegbusi and Byrt, 2006; Godfrey, 2003).
- Provision of a culturally appropriate environment (Ludwig-Beymer, 2003; see the example of a local community mental health centre in Box 14.1).
- Enabling the individual to access independent voluntary and legal advocates of his/her choice, with the provision of unbiased information about these (Garman *et al.*, 2003; Kenny, 2005; Rai-Atkins *et al.*, 2002; see the section on advocacy in this chapter).
- Other measures to reduce patients' social exclusion.

- Involvement in the planning and running of services for patients and their informal carers from diverse backgrounds, and of community and religious groups and voluntary organisations representing their interests (CVS Consultants and Migrant and Refugees Communities Forum, 1999; Rai-Atkins *et al*., 2002).
- Policies and procedures to address and eliminate racism, sexism, homophobia, disabilism, ageism and other forms of discrimination, including harassment (Ludwig-Beymer, 2003; Warner *et al*., 2000). (Disabilism is discrimination related to individuals' perceived disabilities: Barnes and Mercer, 2003).
- Recruitment procedures that are non-discriminatory and ensure that staff are from a range of genders, ethnic groups, varying intellectual, physical and sensory abilities, sexual orientations and gender identities (Ludwig-Beymer, 2003).
- Provision of appropriate educational and clinical supervision for all staff (Bhui and Bhugra, 2001; Ludwig-Beymer, 2003).

Other measures to reduce patients' social exclusion

Repper and Perkins (2004) point out that social exclusion may increase as a result of admission to acute (and, it might be added, to secure forensic) services. Social exclusion may be associated with the stigma of being admitted, and loss of freedom, as well as loss of contact with partner, family (including, for some patients, children) and friends. In addition, unwelcome and drab sur-

Box 14.1 Services reflecting individuals' cultures

Elms (a pseudonym) is a community mental health centre, administered by an NHS Trust, in an inner city area. Information about a range of services is available in several languages that are spoken locally. The Centre is welcoming, with a garden in which some clients work. Pictures in the Centre reflect the cultural backgrounds of local people, including drawings of the Caribbean and of famous women from Southern Asia. (Based on the experience of one of the authors.)

Nafsiyat Intercultural Therapy Centre in London provides psychotherapy which endeavours to be sensitive to the cultures, including ways of experiencing the world, of individuals from a wide range of ethnic groups. There is a recognition that people's distress may be influenced by wider social factors, including their experiences of discrimination and social exclusion. Attempts are made to minimise power imbalances between client and psychotherapist and to enable individuals to involve advocates in sessions, if they wish (Kareem, 2000).

roundings, losses in freedom, family, work and other important roles, and lack of fresh air may also contribute to social exclusion. The latter may be worsened by negative staff attitudes and inaccessibility, unnecessarily restricted visiting, visiting areas that are unwelcoming and isolation from the local community (Faulkner, 2004; Hart, 1999; Repper and Perkins, 2004).

The following measures may help to increase patients' social inclusion:

- Making visitors welcome, with attractive visiting areas and facilities for visitors of a high standard (Garcia *et al.*, 2005; McMillan and Allen, 2005).
- Involving members of local communities, including participants in community, religious and voluntary organisations (Department of Health, 2003, 2005b; Ludwig-Beymer, 2003; Rai-Atkins *et al.*, 2002)
- In particular, NHS Trusts are now required to involve members of community and religious organisations concerned with members of black and minority ethnic groups (Department of Health, 2005c).
- Members of other organisations could also be involved, including those concerned with women, individuals with disabilities and people who are lesbian, gay, bisexual or transsexual. For example, WISH ('Women in Secure Hospitals') provides advocacy and befriending for women in secure services (Namdarkhan, 2004).
- Besides the involvement of NHS Trust Patient Advice and Liaison Services (PALs), the participation of independent advocates, welfare workers and legal rights workers (Garman *et al.*, 2003; Kenny, 2005).

Advocacy and the involvement of service users, local communities and voluntary organisations

Empathy on the part of nurses and other forensic mental health professionals involves, in part, appreciation of the multiple crises and problems with which patients are faced, especially at the time of their admission. Some authors have emphasised the 'action component' of empathy: i.e. translation of the nurse's appreciation of the patient's concerns into practical action (Kunyck and Olson, 2001, citing Hudson, 1993, and Sutherland, 1993). This can include action taken by forensic mental health nurses, with patients' agreement, for example, referring pressing problems, such as lack of money, to other professionals in the clinical team and enabling patients to contact an independent patients' advocate (Garman *et al.*, 2003) and a solicitor to discuss concerns about court hearings (Kenny, 2005). However, empathy also involves honest acknowledgement that there is no ready answer to many patients' concerns (such as the unknown outcome of a court hearing).

Access to independent advocates and solicitors is particularly important for forensic mental health patients because of their relatively limited power as detained patients under Mental Health Acts, and in relation to the views of many that they do not need treatment (Mason and Chandley, 1990). The forensic mental health nurse's role in ensuring patients' rights, and enabling access to legal and voluntary organisation advocates, is thus particularly important (Garman *et al.*, 2003). Some aspects of forensic mental health nursing involve assessment and interventions with which patients may not agree. This includes aspects of clinical risk assessment and clinical risk management, with, for example, a patient disagreeing with staff about the extent that he/she is likely to be at risk of harming others. Because of this potential for differing patient and staff perspectives, it is vital for patients to access independent legal and other advocates, including those employed by a voluntary organisation, such as Together (formerly the Mental Aftercare Association). Several secure services have such advocates (Garman *et al.*, 2003).

The need for independent advocates has been stressed in forensic (Garman *et al.*, 2003) and acute settings (Faulkner, 2004). Advocacy is particularly needed for individuals who face discrimination in wider society, and sadly, in some services. This includes patients from black and minority ethnic groups, women, individuals with physical or sensory disabilities and people who are lesbian, gay, bisexual or transsexual (Addo, 2006; Aiyegbusi and Byrt, 2006; Jeffcote and Watson, 2004). The need for independent advocacy in relation to women's services is emphasised in Department of Health (2002) and (2003). The Executive Summary of 'Delivering Race Equality' states that, in mental health services, 'black and minority ethnic voluntary and community organisations... can advise... and in some cases, act as partners in delivering services' (Department of Health, 2005c).

The European Convention on Human Rights

The Human Rights Act 1998 strengthened the European Convention on Human Rights for British citizens and made the Convention a matter on which British courts could make decisions and potentially trigger changes in the law (H. M. Government, 1998). It is possible that issues related to diversity could apply to most of the articles of the Convention, but exactly how much remains to be determined by the actions of the courts and other bodies.

Article 3 ('Prohibition of Torture') includes the statement: 'No one shall be subjected to torture or inhuman or degrading treatment or punishment'. In relation to forensic mental health patients, this might include failure to respect the client as an individual with unique needs and rights, including the unethical use of seclusion and control and restraint.

Part of Article 9 ('Freedom of Thought, Conscience and Religion') states:

> ... Freedom to manifest one's religion or beliefs shall be subject only to such limitations as are prescribed by law and are necessary in a democratic society in the interests of public safety, for the protection of public order, health or morals, or for the protection of the rights and freedoms of others

This article indicates the importance, as a right in law, for forensic mental health patients to be able to have access to the means to practice their beliefs, including access to visitors who are leaders or members of their belief systems. The only justifiable reason for a Registered Nurse to deny such access would be the prevention of serious harm, e.g. the likelihood of a client's directing violence at a leader of his/her religion.

Article 14 ('Prohibition of Discrimination') states:

> The enjoyment of the rights and freedoms set out in this Convention shall be secured without discrimination on any ground such as sex, race, colour, language, religion, political or other opinion, national or social origin, association with a national minority, property, birth or other status.

This has particular relevance to the specific needs related to individuals' culture, ethnic group, religion, gender, sexual orientation and identity, age, particular illness or disability.

Box 14.2 Points for consideration/discussion

1. Consider the applicability of the above Articles of the Human Rights Act 1998 to the group of forensic mental health patients with whom you work.
2. Are there situations where there is a danger that any of these Articles could be considered to be infringed?

Legislation and Department of Health policy relevant to forensic mental health and diversity

This chapter concludes by considering, in relation to mental health nursing, legislation and Department of Health policy to 'ensure that people accessing health care are not unfairly discriminated against on the grounds of culture, ethnic group, religion, sexual orientation or idenity, age or disability' (Department of Health, 2004, p. 18). The wide range of relevant documents (listed in Appendix 14.1) at the end of this chapter) include the following:

- Policy and other documents specifically concerning forensic mental health patients/clients and their care and treatment. The inquiry into the death of David Bennett is considered in Chapter 13.
- Policy, other documents and legislation relevant to a wide range of health services, including those concerned with forensic mental health.
- Legislation on diversity issues applicable to a wide range of public and other organisations, including forensic and other health services.

There is specific Department of Health policy concerning mental health services for women (Department of Health, 2002, 2003, 2006); individuals from black and minority ethnic communities (Department of Health, 2005b,c; National Institute for Mental Health in England, 2003); and people with learning disabilities (Department of Health, 2001) and who are deaf (National Institute for Mental Health in England and Department of Health, 2005). The Department of Health has not, at the time of writing, produced specific policy related to mental health and individuals with physical and visual disabilities, or who are lesbian, gay, bisexual or transsexual.

Acts of Parliament relevant to forensic mental health services

Various Acts of Parliament apply to all public services, including those for forensic mental health patients. For example, the Disability Discrimination Act (H.M. Government, 2005) is relevant to ensuring, for example, that a forensic service provides appropriate interpreting services, where needed, for individuals whose first language is not spoken English, including some people who are deaf. Department of Health and Disability Rights Commission (2004) considers progress and future work on implementing the Disability Discrimination Act in health services. Parts of the Equality Act 2006 are applicable to ensuring avoidance of discrimination, within forensic mental health and other services, on the basis of gender, ethnicity, religion, sexual orientation and gender identity (H. M. Government, 2006). The Civil Partnership Act (H. M. Government, 2004a) and Gender Recognition Act (H. M. Government, 2004b) include requirements, relevant to forensic services, related to gay/lesbian and transsexual individuals, respectively. Application of the Human Rights Act 1998 is considered earlier in this chapter.

Conclusion

In this chapter specific areas of cultural sensitivity and cultural competence are outlined with reference to communication, information and the development of empathetic relationships; ensuring patients' 'cultural safety' and the safety of others; the ward environment; and the individual's particular needs related to his/her ethnic group, gender, sexual orientation and disability. Organisational aspects of cultural competence are briefly considered. The chapter concludes with a consideration of measures to reduce social exclusion and provide advocacy, and the application of the Human Rights Act 1998 and other relevant legislation and policy.

References

Addo, M. (2006) Culture, spirituality and ethical issues in caring for clients with personality disorder. In: *Forensic Nursing: Interventions with People with 'Personality Disorders'* (ed. National Forensic Nurses' Research and Development Group), Chapter 5. Quay, Salisbury.

Aiyegbusi, A. and Byrt, R. (2006) Gender and sexuality. In: *Forensic Nursing: Interventions with People with 'Personality Disorders'* (ed. National Forensic Nurses' Research and Development Group), Chapter 8. Quay, Salisbury.

Andrews, M. M. (2003a) Theoretical foundations of transcultural nursing. In: *Transcultural Concepts in Nursing Care* (eds. M. M. Andrews and J. S. Boyle), Chapter 1. Lippincott, Williams and Wilkins, Philadelphia.

Andrews, M. M. (2003b) Culturally competent nursing care. In: *Transcultural Concepts in Nursing Care* (eds. M. M. Andrews and J. S. Boyle), Chapter 2. Lippincott, Williams and Wilkins, Philadelphia.

Arnold, E. (2003) Intercultural communication. In: *Interpersonal Relationships*, 4th edn (eds. E. Arnold and K. U. Boggs), Chapter 11. Saunders, St Louis.

Barnes, C. and Mercer, G. (2003) *Disability*. Polity Press, Cambridge.

Bavington, J. (2000) The Bradford experience. In: *Intercultural Therapy*, 2nd edn (eds. J. Kareem and R. Littlewood), Chapter 7. Blackwell Science, Oxford.

Bhui, K. and Bhugra, D. (2001) Training and supervision in cross-cultural mental health services. In: *Psychiatry in Multicultural Britain* (eds. D. Bhugra and R. Cochrane), Chapter 14. Gaskell/Royal College of Psychiatrists, London.

Byrt, R., Lomas, C., Gardiner, J. and Lewis, D. (2001) Working with Women in Secure Environments. *Journal of Psychosocial Nursing and Mental Health Services*, **39**(9), 42–50.

Corker, M. (1994) *Counselling. The Deaf Challenge*. Jessica Kingsley, London.

CVS Consultants and Migrant and Refugees Forum (1999) *A Shattered World: The Mental Health of Refugees and Newly Arrived Communities*. CVS Consultants and Migrant and Refugees Forum, London.

Dale, C. and Gardner, J. (2001) Security in forensic environments: strategic and operational issues. In: *Forensic Mental Health: Issues in Practice* (eds. C. Dale, T. Thompson and P. Woods), Chapter 23. Baillière Tindall/Royal College of Nursing, Edinburgh.

Davies, D. and Neal, C. (eds.) (1996) *Pink Therapy: a Guide for Counsellors and Therapists Working with Lesbian, Gay and Bisexual Clients*. Open University Press, Buckingham.

Department of Health (2001) *Valuing People. A New Strategy for Learning Disability for the Twenty First Century*. A White Paper. Department of Health, London.

Department of Health (2002) *Women's Mental Health: Into the Mainstream*. Department of Health, London.

Department of Health (2003) *Mainstreaming Gender and Women's Mental Health. Implementation Guidance*. Department of Health, London.

Department of Health (2004) *Standards for Better Health. Health Care Standards for Services Under the NHS*. Department of Health, London.

Department of Health (2005a) *Elimination of Mixed Sex Hospital Accommodation*. Department of Health, London.

Department of Health (2005b) *Delivering Race Equality in Mental Health Care. An Action Plan for Reform. Inside and Outside Services and The Government's Response to the Independent Inquiry Into the Death of David Bennett*. Department of Health, London.

Department of Health (2005c) *New Blueprint to Tackle and Eradicate Discrimination in Mental Health Services Over the Next Five Years*. Department of Health, London.

Department of Health (2006) *A Practical Guide to Ethnic Monitoring in the NHS and Social Care*. Department of Health, London.

Department of Health and Disability Rights Commission (2004) *Department of Health and Disability Rights Commission Framework for Partnership Action on Disability 2005/7*. Department of Health, London.

Faulkner, A. (2004) Strategies for surviving acute care. In: *Acute Mental Health Nursing: From Acute Concerns to the Capable Practitioner* (eds. M. Harrison, D. Howard and D. Mitchell), Chapter 4. Sage, London.

Garcia, I., Qugaishi, M., Kennett, C. and Duncan, C. (2005) *Acute Care, 2004: a National Survey of Adult Psychiatric Wards in England*. Sainsbury Centre for Mental Health, London.

Garman, G., Kelly, R. and Waldron, S. (2003) Setting up a successful patients' council. *Mental Health Practice*, **6**(7), 20–2.

Godfrey, J. (2003) The lesbian, gay man and transgendered experience as users of healthcare services. In: *Empowerment: and the Health Service User* (eds. J. Dooher and R. Byrt), Chapter 6. Quay, Salisbury.

Hart, L. (1999) The reliable kettle. *OpenMind*, **96**, 20–1.

H. M. Government (1998) *Human Rights Act 1998*. Stationery Office, London.

H. M. Government (2004a) *Civil Partnership Act 2004*. Stationery Office, London.

H. M. Government (2004b) *Gender Recognition Act 2004*. Stationery Office, London.

H. M. Government (2005) *Disability Discrimination Act 2005*. Stationery Office, London.

H. M. Government (2006) *Equality Act 2006*. Stationery Office, London.

Jeffcote, N. and Watson, T. (eds.) (2004) *Working Therapeutically with Women in Secure Mental Health Settings*. Jessica Kingsley, London.

Kareem, J. (2000) The Nafsiyat Intercultural Therapy Centre: ideas and experience in intercultural therapy. In: *Intercultural Therapy*, 2nd edn (eds. J. Kareem and R. Littlewood), Chapter 2. Blackwell Science, Oxford.

Kareem, J. and Littlewood, R. (eds.) (2000) *Intercultural Therapy*, 2nd edn. Blackwell Science, Oxford.

Kavanagh, K. H. (2003) Transcultural perspectives in mental health nursing. In: *Transcultural Concepts in Nursing Care* (eds. M. M. Andrews and J. S. Boyle), Chapter 10. Lippincott, Williams and Wilkins, Philadelphia.

Kenny, P. J. (2005) The place of a legal representative or advocate working for the client. In: *Multidisciplinary Working in Forensic Mental Health Care* (eds. S. Wix and M. Humphreys), Chapter 4B. Elsevier Churchill Livingstone, Edinburgh.

Kunyck, D. and Olson, J. K. (2001) Clarification of conceptualisations of empathy. *Journal of Advanced Nursing*, **35**(3), 317–25.

Ludwig-Beymer, P. (2003) Creating culturally competent organizations. In: *Transcultural Concepts in Nursing Care* (eds. M. M. Andrews and J. S. Boyle), Chapter 9. Lippincott, Williams and Wilkins, Philadelphia.

Mason, T. and Chandley, M. (1990) Nursing models in a special hospital: a critical analysis of efficacy. *Journal of Advanced Nursing*, **15**, 667–73.

McMillan, I. and Allen, D. (2005) National guidelines needed for ward staffing levels. *Mental Health Practice*, **8**(9), 4.

Morgan, S. and Wetherell, A. (2004) Assessing and managing risk. In: *The Art and Science of Mental Health Nursing: a Textbook of Principles and Practice* (eds. I. Norman and I. Ryrie), Chapter 8. Open University Press, Maidenhead.

Namdarkhan, L. (2004) A gender-specific advocacy model, or 'I found my voice and I love it! In: *Working Therapeutically with Women in Secure Mental Health Settings* (eds. N. Jeffcote and T. Watson), Chapter 15. Jessica Kingsley, London.

Narayanasamy, A. (2002) The ACCESS model: a transcultural nursing practice framework. *British Journal of Nursing*, **11**(9), 643–50.

Narayanasamy, A. and White, E. (2005) A review of transcultural nursing. *Nurse Education Today*, **15**, 102–11.

National Institute for Mental Health in England (NIMHE) (2003) *Inside Outside. Improving Mental Health Services for Black and Minority Ethnic Communities in England*. NIMHE, London.

National Institute for Mental Health in England (NIMHE) and Department of Health (2005) *Mental Health and Deafness. Towards Equality and Access*. Department of Health, London.

NHS Executive (1999) *Safety, Privacy and Dignity in Mental Health Units. Guidance on Mixed Sex Accommodation for Mental Health Services*. Department of Health, London.

O'Brien, A. J. and Morrison-Ngati, E. (2003) Providing culturally safe care. In: *Psychiatric and Mental Health Nursing: The Craft of Caring* (ed. P. Barker), Chapter 63. Arnold, London.

Rai-Atkins, A., Jama, A. A., Wright, N., Scott, V., Perring, C., Craig, G. and Katbamna, S. (2002) *Best Practice in Mental Health: Advocacy for African, Caribbean and South Asian Communities*. Policy Press, Bristol.

Repper, J. and Perkins, R. (2004) Social inclusion and acute care. In: *Acute Mental Health Nursing: From Acute Concerns to the Capable Practitioner* (eds. M. Harrison, D. Howard and D. Mitchell). Sage, London.

UNISON and Royal College of Nursing (2004) *Not Just a Friend: Best Practice Guidance on Health Care for Lesbian, Gay and Bisexual Service Users and Their Families*. UNISON, London.

Warner, L., Nicholas, S., Patel, K., Harris, J. and Ford, R. (2000) *National Visit Two. A Visit by the Mental Health Act Commission to 104 Mental Health and Learning Disability Units in England and Wales: Improving Care for Detained Patients from Black and Minority Ethnic Communities*. Sainsbury Centre for Mental Health, London.

Williams, J., Scott, S. and Bressington, C. (2004) Dangerous journeys: women's pathways into and through secure mental services. In: *Working Therapeutically with Women in Secure Mental Health Settings* (eds. N. Jeffcote and T. Watson), Chapter 2. Jessica Kingsley, London.

Appendix 14.1 Department of Health and other documents relevant to forensic mental health services (includes relevant documents up to June 2006. See http://www.dh.gov.uk/ for more recent policy and legislation)

Most of the documents listed in this Appendix are available via http://www.dh.gov.uk/.

The list is not comprehensive, but mentions many relevant documents. The most recent are listed first.

Policy specifically concerning forensic mental health patients/clients

Department of Health (2005) *Delivering Race Equality in Mental Health Care. An Action Plan for Reform. Inside and Outside Services and The Government's Response to the Independent Inquiry Into the Death of David Bennett*. Department of Health, London.

Blofield, J. (2003) *Independent Inquiry into the Death of David Bennet. An Independent Inquiry Set Up Under HSG (94) 27*. Department of Health, London.

Prins, H., Backer-Holst, T., Francis, E. and Keitch, I. (1993) *Report of the Committee of Inquiry into the Death in Broadmoor Hospital of Orville Blackwood and a Review of the Deaths of Two Other Afro-Caribbean Patients: 'Big, Black and Dangerous'?* Department of Health, London.

Blom-Cooper, L. (1992) *Report of the Committee of Inquiry into Complaints at Ashworth Hospital*. HMSO, London.

Policy and legislation relevant to a wide range of health services, including those concerned with forensic mental health

Several aspects of diversity mentioned

Department of Health (2004) *The National Service Framework for Mental Health. Five Years On*. Department of Health, London.

Department of Health (2004) *The NHS Improvement Plan. Executive Summary*. Department of Health, London.

Department of Health (2004c) *Standards for Better Health. Health Care Standards for Services Under the NHS*. Department of Health, London.

National Institute for Mental Health in England (2004) *From Here to Equality. A Strategic Plan to Tackle Stigma and Discrimination on Mental Health Grounds, 2004–2009*. Department of Health, London.

Office of the Deputy Prime Minister – Social Exclusion Unit (2004) *Taking Stock and Looking to the Future. Emerging Findings*. Office of the Deputy Prime Minister, London. http://www.socialexclusion.gov.uk/page.asp?id=213

Disability

National Institute for Mental Health in England (NIMHE) and Department of Health (2005) *Mental Health and Deafness. Towards Equality and Access*. Department of Health, London.

Department of Health and Disability Rights Commission (2004) *Department of Health and Disability Rights Commission Framework for Partnership Action on Disability 2005/7*. Department of Health, London.

Department of Health (2001) *Valuing People. A New Strategy for Learning Disability for the Twenty First Century. A White Paper*. Department of Health, London.

Ethnicity and race equality

Department of Health (2006) *A Practical Guide to Ethnic Monitoring in the NHS and Social Care*. Department of Health, London.

Department of Health (2005) *Delivering Race Equality in Mental Health Care. An Action Plan for Reform. Inside and Outside Services and The Government's Response to the Independent Inquiry Into the Death of David Bennett*. Department of Health, London.

Department of Health (2005) *New Blueprint to Tackle and Eradicate Discrimination in Mental Health Services Over the Next Five Years*. Contains summary of action plan of 'Delivering Race Equality in Mental Health Care'. Department of Health, London.

National Institute for Mental Health in England (NIMHE) (2003) *Inside Outside. Improving Mental Health Services for Black and Minority Ethnic Communities in England*. NIMHE, London.

Gender

Department of Health (2006) *Supporting Women into the Mainstream. Commissioning Women Only Community Day Services*. Department of Health, London.

Department of Health (2005) *Elimination of Mixed Sex Hospital Accommodation*. Department of Health, London.

Department of Health (2003) *Mainstreaming Gender and Women's Mental Health. Implementation Guidance*. Department of Health, London.

Department of Health (2002) *Women's Mental Health: Into the Mainstream*. Department of Health, London.

NHS Executive (1999) *Safety, Privacy and Dignity in Mental Health Units. Guidance on Mixed Sex Accommodation for Mental Health Services*. Department of Health, London.

Sexual orientation and gender identity

Department of Health (2006) *Information on Sexual Orientation and Gender Identity Group*. Department of Health, London.

Legislation applicable to diversity issues in a wide range of public and other organisations, including forensic and other health services

H. M. Government (2006) *Equality Act 2006*. Stationery Office, London.
H. M. Government (2005) *Disability Discrimination Act 2005*. Stationery Office, London.
H. M. Government (2004) *Civil Partnership Act 2004*. Stationery Office, London.
H. M. Government (2004) *Gender Recognition Act 2004*. Stationery Office, London.
H. M. Government (2000) *Race Relations (Amendment) Act 2000*. Stationery Office, London.
H. M. Government (1998) *Human Rights Act 1998*. Stationery Office, London.

CHAPTER 15

Observation with engagement in acute areas

Alyson McGregor Kettles and Richard Byrt

Introduction

The practice of observation as both a nursing duty (Porter *et al.*, 1998; Neilson and Brennan, 2001) and a skill (Dodds and Bowles, 2001; Dodds *et al.*, 2002; Clinical Resource and Audit Group, 2002; Cutcliffe and Barker, 2002; Jones and Jackson, 2004; Kettles *et al.*, 2004) has come under considerable scrutiny in recent years. All of the work that has gone into this priority area of nursing has taken place in acute areas, with some minor comparison with forensic areas. What has not happened is the turning of the spotlight onto the differing patient groups who may require some specific attention within this wider area of 'observation'.

Although much is now being made about professional decision-making (Paterson *et al.*, 2005), and this is an important area when related to risk assessment, there are still some groups of patients who, when observed on an individual basis, will require some specialist knowledge, and this is what this chapter aims to address.

The purpose of observation

> The key purpose of observation is to provide a period of safety for people during temporary periods of distress when they are at risk of harm to themselves and/or others (Clinical Resource and Audit Group, 2002, p. 10)

Jones and Jackson (2004) go further and state that the main purpose is to keep people safe when they are acutely mentally ill and disturbed, particularly those who are assessed as being at risk of harming themselves or others, or who are at risk of being harmed or exploited by others. This applies to those forensic patients who find themselves in acute wards, as well as to patients without a forensic history.

Jones and Jackson (2004) give an account of a patient who committed suicide in an acute ward where she should have been safe. It is the responsibility of all staff to be aware and accountable for care of the patient on all levels of observation, regardless of staff shortages or ward design or any other reason. However, forensic patients or patients who enter acute wards without a 'forensic' history, but who exhibit behaviour that could be classed as forensic in nature, may require specific care and may need to be observed at higher levels than general observation.

The nature of observations in forensic and acute areas

Observation is a fundamental skill of nursing. Acute mental health areas probably have the most difficult job in terms of observation. Not only do they tend to have greater numbers of patients requiring all levels of observation in the lowest secure areas but they also tend to have lower staffing ratios than forensic areas. Not only this, but acute areas tend to have a wider range of patient

Box 15.1 Clinical Resource and Audit Group (2002) definitions of observation levels

General Observation (Level 1)
The staff on duty should have knowledge of the patients' general whereabouts at all times, whether in or out of the ward. Patients on general observation are considered not to pose any serious risk of harm to self or others.

Close or Constant Observation (Level 2)
An allocated member of staff should be constantly aware at all times of the precise whereabouts of the patient through visual observation or hearing. The method and purpose of maintaining observation must be clearly determined. Respect for privacy should be an important consideration, but a balance should be struck on the side of safety in all matters, such as escorting to the toilet, bathroom or public telephone.

Special Observation (Level 3)
The patient should be in sight and within arm's reach of a member of staff at all times and in all circumstances. Considerations of privacy would be subordinated to those of safety. In some situations, more than one member of staff may be required. As this form of observation is potentially very intrusive, it should only be used when judged strictly necessary by the clinical team, and this level of observation should be subject to frequent review (at least every 24 hours).

problems (Kettles *et al.*, 2004) to deal with than forensic areas, and the patients being observed are in great distress or in a state of potential danger. All of this makes observation difficult enough, but when individuals with histories of offending are admitted to acute areas, as they can be either for acute problems or when coming out of forensic or intensive psychiatric care unit (IPCU) areas prior to discharge, they may require an observation level other than general (Clinical Resource and Audit Group, 2002). In Scotland there are currently three accepted levels of observation (Clinical Resource and Audit Group, 2002) in all areas of mental health, and these are illustrated in Box 15.1. However, other countries have different levels, and some include the fourth level (Jones and Jackson, 2004, p. 171) of 'Intermittent observation' which means the patient's whereabouts are checked at specific intervals, such as every 15, 20 or 30 minutes. Not all patients need to be kept in sight, and this level can be useful, especially when taking patients off the higher levels.

Forensic areas are substantially different from acute areas. They have higher staffing levels and better staffing ratios to the number and type of patient, as well as secure ward areas with substantial backup and well-defined policies and procedures for managing incidents. The delineation associated with the security of the ward means that patients' whereabouts are known at all times and everyone knows the status of each patient in the clinical area, in terms of index offence, risk assessment, formal legal status and observation status. This enables the staff to work as a team and to work with the primary nurse to the best care of the patient. Staff also tend to know the patients very well because the patients are in the forensic unit for substantial periods of time, whereas in acute units the throughput of patients is high, stays can be as short as a few days and the optimum length of stay is about three weeks.

The observation–engagement debate

The observation versus engagement argument (Dodds and Bowles, 2001; Dodds *et al.*, 2002; Cutcliffe and Barker, 2002) is no longer relevant here, as what has become evident from the debate in the last few years is that all patients requiring higher levels of observation also require adjusted levels of engagement. It is not a case of either observation or engagement. Rather, it is the case that staff should be using their judgement and clinical decision-making skills to decide what is in the patients' best interests. What matters is how nursing staff assess, plan for, implement and evaluate the appropriate 'observation with engagement' level. It also matters how staff engage with other staff and communicate the current state of risk assessment, observation level and engagement (therapeutic and conversational) with the patient on an increased level of observation (constant or close and special).

It is interesting to note that while observation has three accepted levels (Clinical Resource and Audit Group, 2004) engagement has no accepted levels other than that given by Butterworth (1994) of basic relational communication skills. Maybe this is the point at which this needs addressing, not necessarily for 'levels' as such, but certainly to enable nursing staff to respond, using therapeutic and counselling skills appropriate to the work of therapeutic observation. The two respective current Mental Health Nursing Reviews, in both Scotland (2006) and England (2006), have identified that nursing staff need more than just the 'basic skills' for what they are being expected to undertake with patients with complex needs.

The need for engagement is well supported by research on service users' views. When observation is carried out by staff who fail to interact with patients, the latter often perceived this as being custodial, invasive and untherapeutic (Cleary *et al*., 1999). Conversely, personal accounts by former patients and research findings suggest that patients experience observations as more beneficial and less restrictive if observing nurses establish therapeutic communication and relationships (Jones *et al*., 2000; Rose, 2000). Cardell and Pitula (1999) found that there were 'therapeutic gains when observers had a positive attitude and engaged the [patients] in supportive interactions' (Cardell and Pitula, 1999, p. 12). Jones *et al*. (2000) reported that the experience of observation was more positive if patients knew the nurse and the latter indicated her/his availability for communication.

Role and responsibility

The role of the psychiatric nurse (in any area) is to provide care on a 24-hour basis to patients and to carry responsibility for the observation of patients (Clinical Resource and Audit Group, 2002; Butterworth, 1994). However, there are circumstances in which other professionals may take over the responsibility for defined periods of time, as outlined in Section 6 of the Clinical Resource and Audit Group document (Clinical Resource and Audit Group, 2002, p. 22). When other staff or carers and relatives are involved in such observation issues, there are specific points that need to be addressed, and these are outlined in Box 15.2.

Box 15.2 Essentials for other staff/carers/relatives involved in observation

- Appropriate education and training of the nature and responsibilities involved in observation for all staff and especially for staff new to the role, followed by updates as per the local policy
- Boundaries and limit setting must be understood by all involved
- Liaison with the Primary nurse, or if triumvirate nursing is being implemented for patients with personality disorders, then liaison with the triumvirate (Melia *et al*., 1999) – essential, but simple, communication of changes in the level of observation
- Foolproof system of knowing *who* is responsible for observation at all times
- All staff must accept responsibility for carrying out observation duty to the local standards
- Confidentiality of patient information must be balanced with the need to know when the patient or anyone else may be at risk by others involved in observation not knowing specific information

General principles of observation

Observation is a high-level skill, not just a 'task' to be performed in a routine or rote manner. It requires not just skill but also effort on the part of the observing nurse. It is demanding, tiring and directly opposed to most other nursing interventions. Whereas most nursing interventions are designed to help and enable patients to achieve their own goals, observation is 'deliberately designed to frustrate patients' aims' (Department of Health, 1999). General principles for the process of observation are given in Box 15.3.

Box 15.3 Principles of observation (after Clinical Resource and Audit Group, 2002; Jones and Jackson, 2004)

At Trust, Board or Hospital level:

- A written policy for the supportive observation of patients formulated from wide consultation
- Local policies and procedures for the supportive and safe observation of patients which are included as part of the risk assessment and care planning process
- Regular review of the policies and regular audit of risk assessment, care planning and observation in clinical practice
- Adequate training and supervision for staff involved in observation duty and support mechanisms and skills to enable them to conduct the procedure
- Adequate written information for patients, carers and families about the observation process

At clinical practice level:

- Competent staff are required with a broad range of clinical skills and operational competencies
- The observation environment must be considered
- Privacy, respect and intrusion must be considered in the planning process
- Clinical supervision process must be in place
- The culture must value the role of observation
- Knowledge of the forensic nature of the patient with associated legal, ethical and practical issues being addressed
- Knowledge of the policies and procedures in place
- Appropriate planning, staff rotation and provision for staff breaks
- Access to advocacy, staff concerned with patient leave decisions and social work care
- An appropriate system of Critical Incident Review
- An audit trail on the use of observation procedures

Skills required for observation duty

Skills required for observation of forensic patients in acute areas include those listed in Box 15.4. Observation for forensic patients requires knowledge of the index offence. For example, if the index offence is arson, then close observation may be required to ensure that the patient does not deliberately or inadvertently set fires. In one case, a forensic patient with a history of arson was being rehabilitated through the auspices of the acute unit in an attached but separate house, under general observation. When staff went to check on him making his tea, they found him cooking chips with the chip pan full to the brim and splashing over the side, despite the occupational therapists having taught him cooking skills. Knowledge of the patient's history is important to ensure that any specific issues can continue to be dealt with appropriately and that care plans begun in forensic areas are carried out.

Complex pathologies are the norm in forensic care, with patients suffering from problems such as substance misuse difficulties compounded by personality disorders, immature emotional functioning, psychological trauma from past abuse and even psychosis. However, in acute care, although there are patients suffering from complex pathologies, the tendency is to work with the primary diagnosis. There are well-documented examples of how, even with dual diagnosis of substance misuse and an axis I disorder, for example, the patient is either not treated adequately or at all. Although this situation is now changing for the better, with

Box 15.4 Skills required for observation of forensic patients in acute areas

- Knowledge of forensic patients' histories
- Knowledge of the index offence
- Knowledge and understanding of complex pathologies
- Trained observational skills for the minutiae of change and the ability to 'notice'
- Awareness of research evidence about the nature of observation and engagement
- 'Basic' communication skills and some degree of advanced communication or counselling skills
- Assessment skills
- Care planning skills
- Management skills
- Caring practice
- Understanding of why the patient has been placed on a higher observation level
- Understanding of what is expected of the 'observer' in terms of noticing, engagement with the patient, reporting (verbal and written), ability to take appropriate action and evaluation skills
- Security and safety skills, such as overseeing the use of matches
- Operational skills and competencies, such as use of the bleep system

protocols for dual diagnosis treatment, the tendency still remains in acute clinical areas for staff to work with the primary diagnosis. Forensic patients and patients not yet charged by the police, but exhibiting escalating forensic behaviours, need more than just the primary diagnosis treated and the changing nature of patient populations in acute care means that this now needs to be recognised.

The 'Dos' of 'observation with engagement' duty

There is no one right approach to observation duty. However, there are some principles that can be applied to care of the person being observed.

- Do consider the patient as a person and think about how you would like to be observed if you were in their place.
- Do treat the person with respect and dignity, no matter how intrusive the observation level.
- Do introduce yourself.
- Do try to convey a sense of caring about the person.
- Do consider very carefully every word that you say to the patient. Do communicate with the patient therapeutically, as well as conversationally. Think about what you are going to say *before* saying it.
- Do follow guidelines as guidelines, not as rules. Remember that rigid practices can lead to negative attitudes.
- Do sign observation sheets and complete any recording accurately, as it may be required for legal purposes at a later date.
- Do consider the safety and security of your patient, yourself and the other patients and staff in the clinical area.
- Do complete handovers as accurately as possible.
- Do consider the ethical, confidentiality and privacy issues that arise for *every* patient in this uncomfortable situation.
- Do consider the prevention of harm to your patient and carrying out observation duty as a professional privilege.
- Do take action when action is required.
- Do ensure that the level of contact is tolerable for the patient.
- Do *always* know the bleep and emergency procedures that are in place to help you.
- Do protect yourself. Always have an appropriate support system in place and enable the patient to have a support system too, such as access to friends and family or other patients.
- Do know the legal situation *at all times*.
- Do help patients with legal issues such as appeals to Mental Health Tribunals.
- Do be familiar with policies/expectations of observing nurse.

The 'Don'ts' of 'observation with engagement' duty

- Don't ask the same questions repeatedly (i.e. 'How are you?') every time you take up the observation duty.
- Don't sit reading magazines and looking uninterested or as if the work is boring. If you are reading a magazine, then make sure it is for the right reason, i.e. that a magazine is light reading, not absorbing and can be left at a moment's notice to enable appropriate intervention.
- Don't say things that could be taken the wrong way.
- Don't leave the patient unattended for *any* reason.
- Do not expect the patient to be able to respond to anything you say or ask them to do. Remember: the patient may be unable to appreciate what you are saying because of their mental, emotional or physical state. Do not be surprised if they appear not to hear you, as they may have impaired cognitive reasoning. Modify what you are saying or asking so that you can be more fully understood.
- Do not assume that male and female patients need the same things or that they can be treated in the same way.
- Don't assume that self-disclosure is appropriate.
- Don't forget that you are striving to help the person to more than a sanitised or symptom-free existence; you are there to help the person towards health and all that health entails.
- Don't assume that your presence prevents the patient experiencing distortions of time, unresolved fears, past memories, feelings of helplessness, regression experiences, hallucinations, despair or any other problem that patients are in hospital and under observation for. You have to help and to be proactive. You have to be approachable, especially if you are sitting within reach.
- Don't assume that patients know what is going on at any time. Keep your patient informed and give blow-by-blow accounts of what investigations or meetings are about. Keep information at a level the patient can cope with. Where possible keep it factual. Liaise with the key worker or primary nurse.

These are merely some of the issues that every member of staff who undertakes 'observation with engagement' duty must begin to address. Observation should not be so routine that patients are effectively ignored in the process.

Risk assessment and observation

The initial risk assessment, on entering the clinical area, does relate to the observation level the patient is placed on at the time of admission (Kettles *et al.*, 2004; Shugar and Rehaluck, 1990). The primary indications of a higher observation level than general observation are:

1. Self-harm
2. Symptoms related to self-harm (actual self-harm and potential self-harm)

3. Safety (potential violence to others and actual violence to others)
4. Unpredictability
5. The patient is unknown to staff
6. Other reasons, such as for further assessment or to decrease stimulation

There is also a correlation between the level of observation and how well known the patient is to staff. For example, the better a patient is known to staff (or conversely, if the patient is unknown to staff), then the lower or higher level the level is likely to be.

Violence and self-harm are issues that forensic staff take very seriously and deal with on a daily basis. There are clear guidelines, protocols and staff education, supervision and support related to these issues. Staff also work very much as a team in managing and reducing risk. However, in acute areas, these issues are not just quite as straightforward as they might be for several reasons. These reasons include the many (and constantly changing) staff who work in acute areas; the lower staff-to-patient ratios; the low security level of the area; the moving of staff around much more freely than staff in forensic services, to cover other clinical areas; and the tendency to concentrate on the primary diagnosis. All these factors contribute to a less well-managed environment from a risk management point of view. This is not something staff can easily change; rather, it is the way acute wards function that is responsible. However, the quality of the risk assessment and its applicability to forensic patients can make a difference to the level of observation with engagement and the overall level of care.

Ongoing assessment and observation

Observation duty presents staff with an opportunity to get to know the patient better, which then allows for ongoing assessment of the patient's mental state. Just because a patient has come from a forensic area and has a history of being a 'mentally disordered offender' does not mean that the patient should be given minimum or less care or that observation levels should be carried out at a 'relational distance'. The procedures may be carried out to the letter, but the engagement part can be conducted with less enthusiasm because staff are frightened by the intensity of the violence and hostility that the patient may display, or the procedures take precedence because the staff are scared by the thought of Fatal Accident Inquiries (FAIs) and police involvement. The focus of care should be the relationship with the patient, rather than the quality of the report writing, the written care plans and the completion of observation charts. This improved relationship will enable self-harm thoughts to be voiced, the number and intensity of violent incidents to reduce and the real or imagined risk of being harmed by others to be explored fully (Davidson, 2006).

Therapeutic alliance and observation

The knowledge and skills required to participate effectively in observation procedures, as well as the attitudes and values that need to be explored, provide the basic competence for practice.

However, Watson (2002) states that additional knowledge and skill are needed to enhance this competence within the particular restraints of a therapeutic alliance in a secure setting. Acute areas are not secure settings. However, higher levels of observation act 'as if' they were secure settings, as the patient is under similar restraints as those in a secure setting. The therapeutic alliance (Kirby and Cross, 2002, p. 189) is the necessary relationship that must exist between a nurse and a patient for positive therapeutic change to take place; essentially, it is the ability to work together in a realistic relationship, based on mutual respect, liking, trust and commitment to the work of treatment. Forensic patients are often part of a therapeutic alliance and are used to working in this way; therefore, it would be beneficial to all parties if acute staff understood the principles of therapeutic alliance working.

Observation of individuals from specific patient groups

Patients with personality disorder

Individuals with personality disorders have traditionally been perceived to be the most difficult patients to work with in any area of mental health. However, in acute areas, they can be particularly difficult to manage, not only for the staffing and geographical reasons given previously, but also because of the nature of the acting out that patients with personality disorder present to staff. Kettles and Woodally (2006) explore this aspect of observation in depth and suggest that there are several issues that are relevant to high-level observation of the personality disordered patient. For example, Norton and Dolan (1995) and Kettles and Woodally (2006) suggest that such observation does not therapeutically meet the needs of the patient; rather it is thought to provoke responses from the patient and the staff which are detrimental to the person with a personality disorder. Therefore, where possible, people with personality disorders should not be placed on higher level observation. Norton and Dolan (1995) suggest that the psychiatric system provides for the acting out patient an early, if not immediate, response. Kettles *et al.* (2004) show that it tends to be the relatively junior and inexperienced staff who conduct risk assessments in acute areas and subsequently make decisions about observation level. In some areas, there are also policies about both risk assessments and observation. However, it does require more senior staff to make some of these decisions, especially in the light of the acting-out patient.

Norton and Dolan (1995) discuss the need for the patient to consciously experience dominant unconscious emotional conflicts rather than to enact them. For the patient to mature, the institution must not simply respond by placing the patient on high level-observation which suppresses or denies the patient's conflicting emotional aspects. This response colludes with one or other side of the patient's internal conflict and creates an interpersonal enactment between staff and patient. This is the situation in which engagement is more important than observation. The institution should be enabling staff to provide or to facilitate a wider range of responses, including honest emotional feedback indicative of both sides of the patient's conflict. Patients are then more able to experience themselves fully (as victims and as perpetrators).

Box 15.5 Forensic nursing principles that need to be maintained during observation of patients with dual diagnosis

1. There is a need to engage in a therapeutic nurse–patient relationship (alliance) with trust as the foundation and with clarity in the goals, purpose and direction of the relationship
2. Appropriate limit setting is essential
3. There is a need to recognise and avoid/deal with power struggles and/or withdrawal
4. The observer needs to recognise and obtain help with distorted forms of caring and to avoid splitting
5. An appropriate treatment programme needs to be implemented and to be delivered in an integrated manner that includes both aspects of personality disorder and substance misuse treatment
6. Maintain the relationship as it moves fully through the phases of the treatment programme and throughout the length of the observation period(s)

Dual diagnosis patients

The unpredictable nature of patients with a dual diagnosis makes observation for some periods of time essential, especially in the first 48 hours after admission. Not only are they unpredictable, but they also present with a very complex clinical picture with multiple intertwined problems that are difficult to disentangle. In terms of observation, there are some very specific difficulties, such as those presented by patients with antisocial personality disorder (APD). For example, patients with APD do not tolerate boredom well and feel victimised easily. They are impulsive and rebellious, with a history of chronic antisocial behaviour. As a result, when this is combined with polydrug use, as is often the case, they are particularly difficult to observe, as they will rebel against such an intervention. Boredom needs to be relieved and diversion instituted. Box 15.5 outlines the forensic nursing principles used in nursing the dual diagnosis patient.

Violent and hostile patients

Chandley (2002, p. 109) gives an excellent description of the issues involved in observing hostile, violent and severely assaultive patients in secure environments. Box 15.6 illustrates the key points that are important to include as part of observation for patients with these particular problems. There may be a need at some point in care to section off an area of the ward as an 'intensive care area' or the patient may need to be moved to the Intensive Psychiatric Care Unit (IPCU/PICU). Geographical restrictions may also be necessary.

Box 15.6 Other variables in the assessment of the circumstances of observation for hostile or assaultive patients

- Manipulation of the stimulation the patient experiences
- Use of the characteristics and qualities of the environment
- Structure to the time on increased levels of observation, including assessment and diversions
- Maintenance of space between the hostile patient and those at specific risk as well as other patients
- Monitoring of specific stressors the patient may experience and acting accordingly
- Staff selection
- Awareness of dangers that may increase due to the aggressor having access to significant others

Self-harming and suicidal patients

Duffy (1995) identified particular problems with special observation, such as the paternalism of staff towards the patient. In particular Duffy (1995, p. 949) points out that there should be:

> ... revision of official policies on special observation to recognise firstly, individual patient needs and nurses as responsible professionals should be officially acknowledged as capable of formulating tailor-made 'policies' for each patient they care for. This would help to enhance the status of special observation duty and promote a more consistent approach by requiring written care plans that were both individualised and 'official'.

Clinical Resource and Audit Group (2002, p. 18) supports Duffy's view by recommending that 'there must also be a specific plan for each patient, which outlines the agreed changes in behaviour that would facilitate a reduction in observation level and the exact procedure for this decision to be actioned'.

All of the 'Dos' and 'Don'ts' of observation apply to the patient at risk of self-harm or suicidal behaviour.

Gender, culture and ethnicity

Jones and Jackson (2004, p. 176) report that issues relating to gender, culture and ethnicity remain effectively invisible in research and reports dealing with observation. They also point out that the National Visit 2 (Sainsbury Centre for Mental Health, 2000) reports that patients from black and minority groups are not receiving care that is sensitive to their cultural backgrounds. In her study of patient preference for mixed- or single-sex ward areas, Kettles (1997) makes the point that female patients often feel at risk from exploitation by male patients. This makes it even more imperative that such issues are taken into consideration on an individual basis when dealing with patients on higher levels of observation.

What observation means to patients

Nurses' attitudes towards, and experiences of, observation have come under scrutiny for some time (Phillips *et al.*, 1977; Aidroos, 1986; Yonge and Stewin, 1992; Reid and Long, 1993; McKie, 1994a,b; Duffy, 1995; Cleary *et al.*, 1999; Bowers and Park, 2001; McKay *et al.*, 2005). However, patients' experiences of observation have not been adequately explored. The few studies (Pitula and Cardell, 1996; Moorhead *et al.*, 1996; Cardell and Pitula, 1999; Conway, 1999; Jones *et al.*, 2000) that have been conducted into patients' experiences report positive and negative experiences. However, more negative than positive experiences have been reported, including the discomfort of being observed, the lack of information and the lack of supportive interaction.

Conclusion

Observation duty requires experienced, qualified nursing staff to undertake such an important, skilled, therapeutic intervention. Forensic patients in acute wards requiring higher levels of observation also require some level of more specialist knowledge. Patients with personality disorder may not require higher levels of observation; rather, they may require more intensive therapeutic engagement and staff need to be trained to accomplish this.

This chapter has highlighted some of the very real issues and problems faced by nurses in acute areas dealing with and observing forensic patients. Patients' experiences of being observed need to be taken into consideration and the negative aspects of their experiences dealt with as appropriately as possible.

There is a lack of evaluation of the guidance that does exist for the practice of observation duty and there is a lack of research, but what does exist is beginning to build up into an evidence base. However, despite these problems, observation is a real issue that needs to be conducted in a professional manner to the best of the nurse's ability and with due consideration of the patient, regardless of the his/her history or index offence.

References

Aidroos, N. (1986) Nurses response to doctors' orders for close observation. *Canadian Journal of Psychiatry*, **31**, 831–3.

Bowers, L. and Park, A. (2001) Special observation in the care of psychiatric inpatients: a literature review. *Issues in Mental Health Nursing*, **22**, 769–86.

Butterworth, A. (1994) *Working in Partnership: a Collaborative Approach to Care. Report of the Mental Health Nursing Review Team.* HMSO, London.

Cardell, R. and Pitula, C. R. (1999) Suicidal in-patients' perceptions of therapeutic and nontherapeutic aspects of constant observation. *Psychiatric Services*, **50**, 1066–70.

Chandley, M. (2002) Nursing interventions and future directions with severely assaultive patients. In: *Therapeutic Interventions for Forensic Mental Health Nurses* (eds. A. M. Kettles, P. Woods and M. Collins), Chapter 7. Jessica Kingsley, London.

Cleary, M., Jordan, R., Horsfall, J., Mazoudier, O. and Delaney, J. (1999) Suicidal patients and special observation. *Journal of Psychiatric and Mental Health Nursing*, **6**, 461–7.

Clinical Resource and Audit Group (2002) *Engaging People: Observation of People with Acute Mental Health Problems: a Good Practice Statement*. Stationery Office, Edinburgh.

Conway, E. A. (1999) *A Multi-dimensional Study of the Process of Observation in Acute Mental Health Wards, Involving Policy Documentation, Staff and User Views*. Report to Newcastle City Health Trust, Newcastle.

Cutcliffe, J. and Barker, P. (2002) Considering the care of the suicidal client and the case for 'engagement and inspiring hope' or 'observations'. *Journal of Psychiatric and Mental Health Nursing*, **9**, 611–21.

Davidson, R. (2006) *The Implementation and Use of the Tidal Model in Acute Wards in Glasgow*. Workshop session given at the National Review of Mental Health Nursing Conference, Inchyra Grange Hotel, Polmont, 18 January (pers. comm.).

Department of Health (1999) *Practice Guidance: Safe and Supportive Observation of Patients at Risk: Mental Health Nursing: Addressing Acute Concerns*. Stationery Office, London.

Dodds, P. and Bowles, N. (2001) Dismantling formal observation and refocusing nursing activity in acute inpatient psychiatry: a case study. *The Journal of Psychiatric and Mental Health Nursing*, **8**(2), 183–8.

Dodds, P., Bowles, N., Hackney, D., Sunderland, C. and Thomas, P. (2002) Formal observations and engagement: a discussion paper. *Journal of Psychiatric and Mental Health Nursing*, **9**(3), 255–60.

Duffy, D. (1995) Out of the shadows: a study of special observation of suicidal in-patients. *Journal of Psychiatric and Mental Health Nursing*, **21**, 944–50.

Jones, J. and Jackson, A. (2004) Observation. In: *Acute Mental Health Nursing* (eds. M. Harrison, D. Howard and D. Mitchell), Chapter 8. Sage, London.

Jones, J., Lowe, T. and Ward, M. (2000) Inpatients' experiences of nursing observation on an acute psychiatric unit: a pilot study. *Mental Health Care*, **4**(4), 125–9.

Kettles, A. (1997) A survey of patients' preferences for mixed- or single-sex wards. Research in brief. *Journal of Psychiatric and Mental Health Nursing*, **4**, 55–7.

Kettles, A., Moir, E., Woods, P., Porter, S. and Sutherland, E. (2004) Is there a relationship between risk assessment and observation level? *Journal of Psychiatric and Mental Health Nursing*, **11**, 156–64.

Kettles, A. M. and Woodally, J. (2006) Observation and engagement with people with personality disorder. In: *Forensic Mental Health Nursing: Interventions with People with a 'Personality Disorder'* (ed. National Forensic Nurses' Research and Development Group), Chapter 12. Quay, London.

Kirby, S. and Cross, D. (2002) Socially constructed narrative interventions. In: *Therapeutic Interventions for Forensic Mental Health Nurses* (eds. A. M. Kettles, P. Woods and M. Collins), Chapter 12. Jessica Kingsley, London.

McKay, I., Paterson, B. and Cassells, C. (2005) Constant or special observations of inpatients presenting a risk of aggression or violence: nurses' perceptions of the rules of engagement. *Journal of Psychiatric and Mental Health Nursing*, **12**(4), 464–71.

McKie, A. (1994a) Do we need a new approach? Caring for suicidal patients in acute hospital settings. *Psychiatric Care*, September/October, 133–7.

McKie, A. (1994b) Negative attitudes that lead to poor assessment: a survey of attitudes towards caring for suicidal patients. *Psychiatric Care*, November/December, 186–9.

Melia, P., Moran, T. and Mason, T. (1999) Triumvirate nursing for personality disordered patients: crossing the boundaries. *Journal of Psychiatric and Mental Health Nursing*, **6**, 15–20.

Moorhead, S. M. L., Kennedy, J., Hodgson, C. M., Ruiz, P. and Junaid, O. (1996) Observations of the observed: a study of inpatients' perception of being observed. *Irish Journal of Psychological Medicine*, **13**(2), 59–61.

Neilson, P. and Brennan, W. (2001) The use of special observations: an audit within a psychiatric unit. *Journal of Psychiatric and Mental Health Nursing*, **8**, 147–53.

Norton, K. and Dolan, B. (1995) Acting out and the Institutional Response. *Journal of Forensic Psychiatry*, **6**(2), 317–32.

Paterson, B., Dowding, D., McComish, S., Morrison, R. and Aitken, I. (2005) Observation and acutely ill psychiatric in-patients: a social judgement analysis. *NMAHP Research Unit Newsletter*. Nursing, Midwifery and Allied Health Professions Research Unit, Glasgow. http://www.nmahpru.gcal.ac.uk/.

Phillips, M., Peacock, E. J., Hermanstyne, L., Rosales, A., Rowe, M., Smith, P., Steele, C. and Weaver, R. (1977) Continuous observation – Part 1. *Canadian Psychiatric Association*, **22**, 25–8.

Pitula, C. R. and Cardell, R. (1996) Suicidal inpatients' experience of constant observation. *Psychiatric Services*, **47**(6), 649–71.

Porter, S., McCann, I. and Kettles, A. M. (1998) Auditing suicide observation procedures. *Psychiatric Care*, **5**, 17–21.

Reid, W. and Long, A. (1993) The role of the nurse providing therapeutic care for the suicidal patient. *Journal of Advanced Nursing*, **18**, 1369–76.

Sainsbury Centre for Mental Health (2000) *The National Visit 2: Improving Care for Detained Patients from Black and Minority Ethnic Communities*. Sainsbury Centre for Mental Health, London.

Shugar, G. and Rehaluck, R. (1990) Continuous observation for psychiatric in-patients: a critical evaluation. *Comprehensive Psychiatry*, **30**, 48–55.

Yonge, O. and Stewin, L. L. (1992) What psychiatric nurses say about constant care. *Clinical Nursing Research*, **1**(1), 80–90.

Further reading

Chaloner, C. and Coffey, M. (eds.) (2000) *Forensic Mental Health Nursing: Current Approaches*. Blackwell Science, Oxford.

Dale, C., Thompson, T. and Woods, P. (2001) *Forensic Mental Health: Issues in Practice*. Baillière Tindall, London.

Kettles, A. M., Woods, P. and Collins, M. (2002) *Therapeutic Interventions for Forensic Mental Health Nurses*. Jessica Kingsley, London.

National Forensic Nurses' Research and Development Group (2006) *Aspects of Forensic Nursing: Interventions with the Person with a 'Personality Disorder'*. Quay, London.

Ward, M. (1995) *Nursing the Psychiatric Emergency*. Butterworth-Heinemann, Oxford.

CHAPTER 16

Issues in multi-professional working

Helen Walker

Introduction

The benefits of multi-professional working need little explanation when we consider the complexity of caring for forensic patients in any setting. It would be virtually impossible for one individual to acquire all of the knowledge and skills required to deal with the diverse range of issues presented. Some of the key advantages of joint working have been evident for years, namely, to cut down on duplication and overlap, prevent gaps in service delivery and help clarify roles and responsibilities (Leathard, 1994; Ovretveit *et al.*, 1997). The need to share expertise, pool knowledge and cross traditional boundaries has been portrayed, not as a choice, but as an essential ingredient of delivering high-quality health and social care (Owens *et al.*, 1995; Department of Health, 2001. Yet the emergence of a range of professionals working towards a common goal (improved health and quality of care), with a common focus (the patient) has not been without its problems. The issues that arise from multi-professional working might, arguably, feel unique to the particular care setting; however, past experience of working with teams in the community, primary, secondary and tertiary care settings indicates that they often share similar grievances.

Problems identified in multi-professional work

The problems of multi-professional working in health and social care are fairly well understood. Norman and Edward (1999) identified four key reasons why mental health professionals working within teams are reluctant to comply with operational directives. These are: loss of faith by mental health care professionals in the system within which they work; their strong adherence to uni-professional cultures; absence of a strong and shared philosophy of community mental health services; and a mistrust of managerial solutions to the problems of inter-professional working. He also identifies a range of other problems: over-ambitious and under-focused aims, confusion about accountability, and ambiguous roles and responsibility of health and social care staff working in mental health services. The problems highlighted here are not unique to the community setting, but are evident from time to time in both acute admissions and forensic settings. Staff working in inpatient settings have precisely the same issues to deal with and often find themselves torn between allegiance with their own profession and the desire to work more collaboratively with other professions.

A report issued from the King's Fund London Commission (1997) also highlighted 'systemic' problems with inter-agency and multi-professional working. The commission pointed to disagreements between mental health care professionals about what constituted mental health and illness and saw debates about effective approaches to treatment as a particularly diverse issue which causes tension in joint working at agency and team level. Communication difficulty, and conflict about leadership, effective team management and role identification, were seen to be issues that stunted the development of community mental health teams.

Our awareness of the difficulties inherent in multi-professional working draws us to the conclusion that there must be some effort made to address this. Each discipline has a professional responsibility to focus their energy on providing the best possible care to meet the needs of the patient, instead of getting caught up in professional rivalry.

Multi-professional working

There is reference made to features of good team-working listed in textbooks, some nursing curriculum documents and nursing research (Miller *et al.*, 1999; Norman *et al.*, 1998; Wix and Humphreys, 2005). 'Effective communication', 'shared values' and 'respect for other professionals' are but a few examples on offer.

Effective communication – both verbal and written – has historically been a bone of contention amongst team workers. Clinicians are well aware of the importance of good communication and know how vital this is, especially in dealing with people who have complex needs. Information is often gathered from many different sources and used for several different purposes during treatment, and it is crucial that key people have adequate access to resources, as and when they need them. Practitioners working in inpatient settings are perhaps at an advantage over those in rural communities, because the patients' notes are multidisciplinary and more readily accessible. The former practice of each discipline holding separate notes for the same patient was resource intensive and duplication was rife. The use of multidisciplinary case notes has gone a long way to improve the situation, but missing, poorly recorded or inaccurate information continues to be a source of complaint for both clinicians and patients alike. It is hoped that the development of electronic patient records will improve the opportunity to share information more readily and further reduce the duplication of work.

Since the early 1990s, patients have had access to their case notes, and this, in itself, has brought about change in clinical practice; for example, clinicians are more sensitive in the manner in which they document patient progress. The adherence to care plans and use of regular multi-professional team meetings have also helped improve the lines of communication and subsequent compliance with treatment plans.

Two very important features that emerge throughout the literature and contribute to successful multi-professional working are 'cooperation' and 'collaboration' (Falk and Allebeck, 2002).

These two elements help engender shared values and respect for fellow clinicians. Specialised psychiatric care, primary care, primary health care, social services and other organisations have to cooperate in order to meet the patients' multiple needs. The main difference between collaboration and cooperation is illustrated using the following quotations: 'it is important that you can trust the people you collaborate with' and 'personal acquaintance is important so you can trust the information you get from the persons you cooperate with' (Falk and Allebeck, 2002). An evaluation of the Swedish psychiatric care reform showed that collaboration and cooperation among different health care providers still needed to be improved on the individual and organisational level (National Board of Health and Welfare, 1997, 1999). In many instances, in accordance with anecdotal information, this could also apply to many of the services in the UK. So the question remains, how do we strengthen multi-professional collaboration?

Role definition

Quinn (1988) highlights the complexities inherent in becoming an effective team member, especially when allegiances to the shared values of the team may be contradictory to specific professional identities. The issue of role definition is something that crops up time after time, and, in many instances, the role adopted by various clinicians is dictated by the personalities within the team, as opposed to being defined by the professional competencies. Some clinicians stick very rigidly to their professional remit and others adopt a more flexible attitude and 'do what has to be done for the patient at the time', as opposed to waiting for it to be done by someone else. What people have to be aware of is 'professional boundaries' and what is acceptable to do 'as a favour' for another professional, contrary to 'overstepping the mark'.

Payne (2000) notes that good practice is evident when there are good working relations between all the caring professionals. He also points out that professional boundaries and culture can inhibit such relationships. Some feel threatened by it. Some are even afraid to question others because of the differing power relationships that exist, for example, between doctors and nursing staff. One of the solutions to this dilemma is proposed by Bradbury (1996), who suggests a number of ways to break down the barriers. She maintains that flexibility is fundamental to successful multi-professional working. Regardless of the setting within which we are placed, it is essential for any individual to be clear about the roles and responsibilities associated with our work in order to perform with any degree of competence.

Traditionally in forensic psychiatry, wide ranges of professional disciplines contributed to the multidisciplinary process of treatment planning, with a core group of professionals adopting a more proactive role. It is widely recognised that the provision of nursing care within secure environments requires staff with considerable expertise (Reed, 1994). Nurses are fast becoming more protective of their professional identity and steadily developing and broadening their skills. The introduction of psychosocial interventions fairly recently has seen nurses display an ability to work even more closely with their psychology peers in delivering cognitive behavioural therapy for individuals with psychosis. It is in instances such as this that we see a blurring of roles – but in a healthy way.

Leadership and management

Within forensic psychiatry inpatient and community settings, the consultant psychiatrist commonly remains the head of the multi-professional team, having the overall responsibility for the patient's welfare. This is also the case in many acute inpatient settings. Wix and Humphreys (2005) do, however, argue that the traditional medical dominance is no longer the case and, for a variety of reasons, the medical profession is coming under scrutiny: for instance, in the UK, in relation to performance-related audit, formal appraisal for all grades of doctor and consultant revalidation takes place. Historically, each profession has been line managed and supervised within its own discipline. These uni-disciplinary management structures remain steadfast and each discipline accepts responsibility for its own governance. More recently, there has been a suggestion that perhaps this will not always be the case and clinicians have been asked to consider the possibility of a multi-professional approach to management, for example, where the team could be managed by an occupational therapist or a psychologist. This move would require a sensitive approach, since it is a somewhat contentious issue, and cultural change, such as this, is not as simple as it might seem.

Leadership and management of the team are important to the smooth-running day-to-day activity. This is particularly important to the forensic patient, who very quickly realises the value of efficient workers. The system within which they are contained is very complex, often due to legal implications, and their demands on the team are considerable. Thus, the importance of coordination and guidance from competent, knowledgeable workers cannot be underestimated.

In many multi-professional teams there are multiple leaders, who have additional individual networks with whom they liaise in order to provide or gather information on behalf of the patient. This style of working is described as open team work (Payne, 2000), and in acute inpatient settings this is very much the norm.

Clinical supervision

Due to the intensity of work, and complexity of the issues associated with individuals with histories of offending in forensic settings, the demand for clinical supervision is great. Coupled with this, the prevalence of assaults is probably an accepted fact of life for most staff working with this group of patients, but it must never be taken for granted and efforts must be made to reduce the high levels of associated stress (Kettles *et al.*, 2000).

In most settings, clinical supervision is carried out in a uni-professional manner – if evident at all. Of all the disciplines in forensic settings, it would seem that nursing is the 'poor relation' when it comes to accessing clinical supervision. Other professionals regularly put aside time for reflection, and their management structures allow for this time to be built into practice routinely. Nurses, on the other hand, have been slower to accept the need for supervision, yet nearly all of those who have been subject to the experience have derived some benefit (Walker, 2001). The major problem appears to be finding time available for clinical supervision. Wards cannot run with a reduced number of staff – the full complement must be available at all times – thus, accessing time is a challenge. This is thought to be the main reason for the limited use of clinical supervision for nurses in forensic inpatient settings.

The use of clinical supervision in acute settings is extremely important, particularly due to the fact that they attract many junior members of nursing staff. Often, acute settings are the first placement of choice for nurses, due to the variety of experience offered. At this stage in their career, nurses require opportunities to reflect on their practice and consolidate the skills learned throughout their training. There are invariably many situations that pose dilemmas for the less experienced practitioner. The forensic patient can sometimes seem to be more of a concern, simply because of the past history of offending behaviour. This can create difficulties in communication, for example, through fear of saying something wrong, or feeling unable to challenge the person in a given situation. Clinical supervision is an excellent medium through which these issues can be explored.

The provision of supervision for multi-professional teams, as a unit, also remains a challenge, and this is certainly an area that is worthy of consideration. There are emerging examples of multi-professional supervision, such as the provision of joint clinical supervision for cognitive behavioural therapy for psychosis, from psychology and a clinical nurse specialist in a high secure setting in Scotland. In this same setting, there are plans for psychology to provide supervision for a dedicated team of female staff working with a patient with particularly disturbed behaviours. This collaborative approach is an indication of good working practice. There are also reports of multi-professional supervision in community mental health teams, so perhaps the tide is changing.

Approach to risk assessment and risk management

The assessment and management of risk for forensic mental health patients is of particular relevance, regardless of the setting in which they are placed. It stands to reason that many patients who come to the attention of the mental health services present an element of risk to themselves or others. Bowers' (2005) scoping review of the literature on admission to acute inpatient psychiatric wards offers a very useful summary. Within this, he highlights dangerousness as the most obvious criterion for admission and acknowledges the wider references related to this subject (Pablo *et al.*, 1986; Prunier and Buongiorno, 1989; Miller, 1992; Abas *et al.*, 2003).

Clinicians must be aware that forensic patients do tend to present a greater degree of risk that many others. The role of the multi-professional teams is to work together to deliver high-quality care and share the common goal of reducing risk for the patient and public. They also have a very clear security role and are essentially required to prevent the patients concerned from leaving the secure environment and to prevent them from harming any other person within that secure environment (Bowers, 2005). In addition, for those patients who are a danger to themselves, the task of acute inpatient care is to prevent such patients from harming themselves by acts of commission or omission. Jones and Plowman (2005, p. 133) argue that 'the assessment of risk, particularly of harmful behaviour towards others, is now a vital and mandatory element of effective multidisciplinary work in mental health services'. It has also become necessary to think more carefully about the tools used to measure elements of risk and ensure they are evidence-based. The use of multi-professional research to develop and try to test such tools is fast becoming routine practice. The problem still lies with the ability to translate the research findings into practice.

Risk assessment and risk prediction are fast becoming areas of expertise and we are witnessing the growth of risk management organisations across the UK. A Risk Management Authority has recently been introduced to Scotland. This is a public body which has been set up to ensure the effective assessment, management and minimisation of risk of serious violent and sexual offenders. It will be a national centre for expert advice on offender risk assessment and management.

Multi-professional training

Integrated care for patients and clients is thought to rely on the provision of educational training that gives staff a clear understanding of how their own roles fit with those of others in health and social care (Department of Health, 1997). Masterton (2002) notes that a plethora of professionals, assisted by a myriad of different types of support worker, are involved in the delivery of contemporary health services. High-quality health and social care depend on health and social care professionals working well together. Yet arguably, in many ways, the professions involved remain curiously apart. They train separately (in most authorities), still keep separate patient records, report to different hierarchies, read different journals and use different terminology. They have different interests, priorities, perspectives and even languages. Stark *et al.* (2002) ask 'What are the educational implications of multi-professional teamwork?' and argue that educational preparation (in particular), but also practice and policy arenas, need to shift to a more realistic recognition of the mental health context. It is suggested (Masterton, 2002) that service and role developments require a readiness to cross traditional boundaries, not only in practice but in education too. As the work of the health professionals continues to change, new configurations of staff emerge in the primary and secondary care sectors and flexible careers become the norm; this will require significant changes in the types of education and training that are provided.

There is an interesting and ongoing debate surrounding inter-professional education. The latter is said to occur when two or more professions learn with, from and about one another to facilitate collaboration in practice. It is a subset of multi-professional education during which professions learn side by side. Inter-professional and multi-professional education are being heralded as the means to achieve collaborative practice (Masterton 2002). Educators and policy makers think that inter-professional education breaks down some of the traditional and unhelpful demarcations between the health and social care professions, facilitates cultural change and promotes successful team-working. It is also thought to provide opportunities for health and social care professionals to learn with, from and about each other, and to develop the knowledge, skills and attitudes required for collaboration. The intention is not to create a generic worker but to use specialist skills and knowledge effectively (Annandale and Vanclay, 1997). The intended outcome is the facilitation of increased respect and mutual understanding, the acquisition of new competencies and the development of new solutions (Council of Europe, 1995). There still requires to be much thought in this area and evaluation will be essential, especially from a service user's perspective, since they are on the receiving end of the care.

Service users' perception of the multi-professional team

A search for service users' perceptions on multi-professional working proved to be quite difficult, since there was little written about the subject. However, the results of the study presented here highlight some key points that could easily be applicable to any psychiatric setting.

A fairly recent paper by Warne *et al.* (2000) explored a group of mental health service users' perceptions of their experiences and contact with the multi-professional team. The study was carried out in eight regions across England, revealing a poor correlation between service users' views of service professionals with regard to multi-professional team working. Whereas most service professionals reported that they understood their role and the role of others in the multi-professional team, many of the service users were not aware of their being a 'team' who provided their care.

In order to make some sense of the survey results, further questions were asked and it soon became apparent that the use of power affected certain aspects of the service users' experience; in particular, who had this power was a key factor in the service users' accounts of their experiences (Warne and Stark, 2004). At the Community Mental Health Team, the service users initially described the mental health professionals they came into contact with in a way that suggested that there was a clearly delineated hierarchy of organisational power. For example, the consultant psychiatrist was consistently seen as the most powerful member of the team. Whilst these perceptions were couched in terms of a form of ultimate power (over service users' current situation and immediate futures), the ward manager was also seen as a person who wielded power, albeit as a possible agent of the psychiatrist. The most 'helpful' member of the team, according to the majority of users, was the mental health nurse and, although not strictly a member of the core Community Mental Health Team (in terms of contact with health care professionals), the general practitioner (GP) was seen as being the least 'helpful'. The person they had most contact with was the social worker and least contact was with the psychiatrist. Therefore, the person who provided the most contact was not always seen as being the most helpful when service users reflected on the totality of their experiences. The community psychiatric nurses (CPNs) were seen as having an important integrating role, someone who could act as an intermediary between the user and other professionals.

Generally, most other staff involved in the service users' care were seen to be subordinate to the psychiatrist. However, there was some evidence to suggest that if service users had made a complaint, and a manager had dealt with this, then this manager was also accorded a top place within this power hierarchy. The perception of who had power was dependent upon the perceived organisational position of the individual and their apparent level of authority (whether this individual could effect change or not). This notion of a hierarchy of power, as expressed above, is congruent with the perceptions of service users noted elsewhere (Rodgers *et al.*, 1993; Edwards, 1995).

Conclusion

Many issues related to multi-professional working, described in this chapter, merit further discussion. The ever-changing climate of mental health provision dictates that we keep ourselves up to date with new trends and developments in work practice. We must, therefore, remain open-minded in our approach and embrace new concepts when they are presented. The current mindset advocates that effective treatment of mental illness relies upon a clearly formulated and defined package of multidisciplinary or multi-professional care, involving all the various available forms of appropriate assessment, intervention and treatment, including pharmacological and psychosocial approaches (Wix and Humphreys, 2005). The close collaboration of the team at each stage of the process is particularly important when dealing with forensic patients with multiple problems. It takes all the skills and resources of the team to deal with such patients and there is perhaps an element of blurring of roles. Good planning, good communication, a flexible approach and clear lines of accountability help in the smooth running of any multi-professional working environment, but all of the aforementioned are essential components for a successful team.

References

Abas, M., Vanderpyl, J., Le Prou, T., Kydd, R., Emery, B. and Foliaki, S. A. (2003). Psychiatric hospitalisation: reasons for admission and alternatives to admission in South Auckland, New Zealand. *Australian and New Zealand Journal of Psychiatry*, **37**, 620–5.

Annandale, S., Vanclay, L. (1997) *Developing Inter-professional Education in the South and West.* SW Regional Office of the Department of Health, Bristol.

Bowers, L. (2005) Reasons for admission and their implications for the nature of acute inpatient psychiatric nursing. *Journal of Psychiatric Mental Health Nursing*, **12**(2), 231–6.

Bradbury, N. (1996) *Joint Working: Why is it so Difficult?* North Birmingham Mental Health Trust, Birmingham.

Council of Europe (1995). *Multi-professional Education of Health Personnel.* Council of Europe Press, Strasbourg.

Department of Health (1997) *The New NHS: Modern, Dependable.* HMSO, London.

Department of Health (2001) *National Service Framework for Older People.* Department of Health, London.

Edwards, K. (1995) A preliminary study of users' and nursing students' views of the role of the mental health nurse. *Journal of Advanced Nursing*, **21**, 222–9.

Falk, K., Allebeck, P. (2002) Implementing assertive community care for patients with schizophrenia: a case study of co-operation and collaboration between mental health care and social services. *Scandinavian Journal of Caring Sciences*, **16**(3), 280–6.

Jones, J. and Plowman, C. (2005) Risk assessment: a multidisciplinary approach to estimating harmful behaviour in mentally disordered offenders. In: *Multidisciplinary Working in Forensic Mental Health Care* (eds. S. Wix and M. Humphreys) Elsevier, China.

Kettles, A. M. and Robinson, D. K. (2000) From a reactive past into the proactive new millennium. In: *Forensic Nursing and Multidisciplinary Care of the Mentally Disordered Offender* (eds. D. K. Robinson and A. M. Kettles). Jessica Kingsley, London.

King's Fund London Commission (1997) *Transforming Health in London.* King's Fund, London.

Leathard, A. (1994) *Going Inter-professional: Working Together for Health and Welfare.* Routledge, London.

Masterton, A. (2002) Cross-boundary working: a macro-political analysis of the impact on professional roles. *Journal of Clinical Nursing*, **11**(3), 331–9.

Miller, R. D. (1992) Need-for-treatment criteria for involuntary civil commitment: impact on practice. *American Journal of Psychiatry*, **149**, 1380–4.

Miller, C., Ross, N. and Freeman, M. (1999) *Shared Learning and Clinical Teamwork: New Directions in Education for Multi-professional Practice*. English National Board for Nurses, Midwives and Health Visitors, London.

National Board of Health and Welfare (1997) *Good Psychiatric Care on Equal Terms* (Summary in English). Socialstyrelsen, Stockholm.

National Board of Health and Welfare (1999) *Welfare and Freedom of Choice. Final Report from the Evaluation of the 1995 Psychiatric Care Reform* (Summary in English). Socialstyrelsen, Stockholm.

Norman, I. and Edward, P. (1999) Working together in adult community mental health services: an inter-professional dialogue. *Journal of Mental Health*, **8**(3), 217–30.

Norman, I., Peck, E. and Richards, H. (1998) *Interprofessional Working in Adult Community Mental Health Services: Setting a Positive Agenda*. King's Fund, London.

Ovretveit, J., Mathias, P. and Thomson, T. (1997) *Inter-professional Working for Health and Social Care*. Macmillan, Basingstoke.

Owens, P., Carrier, J. and Horder, J. (1995) *Interprofessional Issues in Community and Primary Health Care*. Macmillan, Basingstoke.

Pablo, R. Y., Kadlec, K. E. and Arboleda-Florez, J. (1986) The readmission of psychotic patients to a general hospital psychiatry unit. *General Hospital Psychiatry*, **8**, 190–7.

Payne, M. (2000) *Teamwork in Multiprofessional Care*. Macmillan, London.

Prunier, P. and Buongiorno, P. A. (1997) Guidelines for acute inpatient psychiatric treatment review. *General Hospital Psychiatry*, **11**, 278–81.

Quinn, S. M. (1988) *The Principles and Practice of Nurse Education*, 2nd edn. Chapman & Hall, London.

Reed, J. (1994) *Report of the Working Group on High Security and Related Psychiatric Provision (The Reed Review)*. Department of Health, London.

Rogers, A., Pilgrim, D. and Lacey, R. (1993) *Experiencing Psychiatry: Users' Views of Services*. Macmillan, London.

Stark, S., Stronach, I. and Warne, T. (2002) Teamwork in mental health: rhetoric and reality. *Journal of Psychiatric Mental Health Nursing*, **9**(4), 411–18.

Walker, H. (2003) An audit of clinical supervision in a forensic setting. *RCN Bulletin*, Spring.

Warne, T. and Stark, S. (2004) Service users, metaphors and teamworking in mental health. *Journal of Psychiatric and Mental Health Nursing*, **11**(6), 654–61.

Warne, T., Skidmore, D., Stark, S. and Stronach, I. (2000) Implications of current mental health policy for the practice and education of the mental health workforce. *Mental Health Care*, **4**, 48–52.

Wix, S. and Humphreys, M. (eds.) (2005) *Multidisciplinary Working in Forensic Mental Health Care*. Elsevier, Edinburgh.

CHAPTER 17

Psychosocial interventions

Helen Walker and Mike Doyle

Introduction

The vast majority of patients who require treatment in forensic settings, such as low, medium or high security units, suffer from schizophrenia (Thomson *et al.*, 1997), and the interventions used to treat this group have to be considered carefully. Schizophrenia can be a severe and chronic illness characterised by lack of insight and poor compliance with treatment (Pekkala, 2005). The severity of the illness can result in major upheaval in people's lives, causing considerable distress to the sufferer and carers alike. There are numerous approaches to the treatment and management of this condition, including the use of psychotropic medication. Despite advances in the pharmacological intervention for schizophrenia, pharmacological treatment alone is insufficient to help with the psychological and social impact of the illness on patients, their families and carers (Gillam, 2002). Psychosocial functioning limitations continue to be a major source of disability in schizophrenia (Meuser, 2000). This is perhaps one of the reasons why a range of Psychosocial Interventions (PSIs) have been recommended for use.

The National Institute for Health and Clinical Excellence (NICE) Guidelines for Schizophrenia (National Institute for Health and Clinical Excellence, 2002) recommended that psychological treatments should be an indispensable part of the treatment options for service users and their carers. The NICE Guidelines recommend that, in particular, two of the strands of psychosocial interventions should be routinely available for service users and their carers. These two strands are cognitive behavioural therapy and family interventions. Psychosocial interventions of this type have been shown to be effective in reducing distress, improving functioning and shortening hospital stays for service users who have a diagnosis of schizophrenia (Jones, 2004). The overall aim of PSIs is to ensure that service users and their families have routine access to a range of interventions that can decrease distress and improve quality of life.

Staff need to have appropriate training, supervision and support, and services should have the commitment and vision to embrace these interventions as part of routine care. It is essential that implementation of PSIs takes account of acute issues such as time constraints, engagement of challenging service users, developing therapeutic relationships and working with risk and individuals with personality disorder.

What are psychosocial interventions?

Psychosocial interventions (see Box 17.1) are a form of service provision that includes a wide range of interventions. In mainstream mental health services, typical components of PSIs are (Gamble and Brennan, 2006):

- Cognitive behavioural therapy
- Family interventions
- Relapse prevention
- Case management incorporating PSI principles (i.e. focusing upon social and psychological issues)

Psychosocial interventions are underpinned by a value base that involves:

- Collaboration between the user and the clinician/practitioner
- Collaboration with carers and families
- Recovery and self-determination
- Consideration of social context

Box 17.1 Psychosocial interventions

Coping strategy enhancement	Coping with distress resulting from hallucinations and delusions
Relapse prevention	Early warning sign detection and drawing up of action plans
Belief modification	Modifying delusions and beliefs about voices
Problem solving	Systematic approach to solving problems and dilemmas
Family interventions	Increasing patient activity and decreasing contact with family, stress management, problem solving
Medication management	Assessment and management of side-effects, self medication strategies
Anger management	Self-monitoring, relaxation, cognitive restructuring, stress inoculation
Motivational interviewing	Encouraging hope and motivation to participate in therapy
Case management	Assertive outreach, contingency planning, early intervention, relapse prevention, therapeutic alliance

- Social inclusion
- Focusing on the service user's strengths and solutions
- Increasing choice and control for the service user

(Gamble and Brennan, 2006).

Review of the research

The NHS Centre for Reviews and Disseminations (2000) carried out a literature search to explore the effectiveness of PSIs. A review of the research supported the claims that these approaches, when integrated to other systems of care, can reduce and/or shorten the duration of relapse, reduce distress associated with positive symptoms of schizophrenia, reduce hospital stays and improve functioning. Providing PSIs for service users and their families should, therefore, improve choice and assist in promoting hope and optimism for recovery.

A rigorous systematic review that considered 30 research papers on CBT for schizophrenia, found that CBT significantly increased discharge rate and improved mental state when compared to standard care alone (Jones, 2004). A similar review by Pharoah *et al.* (2003) found that family interventions for schizophrenia decreased relapse rates, encouraged compliance with medication and increased individuals' social functioning, while reducing problematic expressed emotion.

A small study by Ewers *et al.* (2002) showed that training forensic staff in these approaches could increase knowledge, change attitudes and decrease burnout rates. Training staff to utilise these approaches enables them to offer even more to service users and their families, and this can increase clinicians' own level of hope and job satisfaction. Reduced hospital stays also have potential financial benefits for services.

Integrating and implementing PSIs into services should benefit services users, their families and staff groups, while providing potential financial benefits for the wider organisation.

National policy context

The National Service Framework for Mental Health (Department of Health, 1999), and subsequent implementation guidance (Department of Health, 2002) and *The National Service Framework for Mental Health. Five Years On* (Department of Health, 2004) emphasise the need for developing new services, with a focus on people with serious mental illness and/or complex problems.

Since the National Service Framework for Mental Health was published, specialist services have started to develop, including assertive outreach services, crisis resolution and early intervention teams for people with psychosis. This emphasis, combined with a philosophy of recovery and organisational changes to support the integration of health and social care, rests on an assumption that effective biopsychosocial interventions will be available for people experiencing a serious mental illness.

The National Institute for Health and Clinical Excellence (2002) published clinical guidelines for treating and managing people with schizophrenia. The NICE guidelines include guidance for professionals and teams involved in providing treatment and promoting recovery within primary care and in specialist mental health services. Recommendations are made that treatment and care should be provided by crisis resolution, home treatment, early intervention and community mental health teams, as well as in acute day hospitals and within inpatient units. Pharmacological, psychological, social, occupational and educational interventions should be provided in collaboration with service users and their families.

It is also recommended that cognitive behavioural therapy (CBT) should be available as a treatment option. Such treatment should be given for more than six months and involve more than 10 planned treatment sessions. Family interventions should be available to the families of people with schizophrenia.

In summary, the NICE guidelines make it clear that psychological treatments should be an indispensable part of the treatment options available for service users and their families in an effort to promote recovery. The guidance states that interventions should be used in order to reduce the service user's and family's distress and promote greater quality of life, prevent relapse, reduce symptoms, increase insight and promote adherence to medication.

The NICE guidelines recommended that:

> Family interventions ... be offered to 100% of families of individuals with schizophrenia who have experienced a recent relapse, are considered to be at risk of relapsing, or who have persistent symptoms, and are living in close contact with their family.
>
> 100% of individuals who are experiencing psychotic symptoms should be offered CBT. (NICE, 2002, pp. 54–5)

Within the UK, a number of complementary psychosocial interventions with a growing evidence base are used. Cognitive behavioural therapy (CBT), psycho-education and family interventions are the three approaches considered to have the strongest evidence base in Scotland (SIGN, 1998). Whereas CBT, behavioural interventions, family interventions, individual family and group work are interventions promoted by (NICE, 2002) and recommended for use in England.

The advantages of these interventions in forensic psychiatry are still open to debate, but there is increasing research evidence to support their use. One of the greatest difficulties with any new intervention is the practical barriers associated with getting the activity into routine clinical practice. Psychosocial interventions in mental health practice are no exception. The use of PSIs in acute settings would be particularly advantageous to the forensic patient who is already familiar with this way of working. Clinicians must, however, be cautious and make sure they are adequately prepared to deliver the interventions and have the skills to deal with this group of individuals with complex needs.

Cognitive behavioural therapy

Over the past twenty years, cognitive behavioural theories and therapies have been developing rapidly. For most of that time, however, they have been applied to emotional disorders such as depression and anxiety. More recently, cognitive behavioural treatments have now been developed for most disorders encountered in psychiatric practice (Hawton, 1999). Gradually, through careful single-case designs, and more recently through randomised trials, evidence has accumulated to suggest that cognitive behavioural therapy (CBT) can be used with people diagnosed as having psychosis. Progress is such that it has become an integral part of the treatment for psychosis in some areas of the UK. CBT has been able to demonstrate the most consistent benefits for patients suffering from chronic psychotic illness. The majority of earlier research has been in the form of case studies or case series (Haddock *et al.*, 1996; Chadwick and Lowe, 1990; Kingdon and Turkington, 1991), which have demonstrated that psychological treatments can be effective with individuals with chronic psychosis.

Several controlled trials have suggested that cognitive behavioural interventions can result in a reduction of psychotic and associated symptoms that are resistant to medication in chronic schizophrenia (Tarrier *et al.*, 1993; Garety and Hemsley, 1994; Haddock and Slade, 1996; Kuipers *et al.*, 1997) and a single trial has shown reduction of symptoms in acute schizophrenia (Drury *et al.*, 1996). A 25% reduction in 'symptom severity', measured by standard psychiatric rating scales, has been reported as a result of CBT (Kuipers *et al.*, 1997), produced mainly by changes in unusual beliefs. It is worth noting that this is similar to the effects of the medication Clozapine (Kane *et al.*, 1998).

Although these trials were small and all suffered from methodological limitations, particularly a lack of blind assessment, they represent encouraging evidence that cognitive behavioural interventions can have considerable benefits in reducing persistent hallucinations and delusions (Tarrier *et al.*, 1998). Two studies found that people continue to improve even after therapy ends (Kuipers *et al.*, 1998; Sensky *et al.*, 2000) and, in terms of cost of treatment, it appears likely that CBT is cost-effective (Kuipers *et al.*, 1998) in the long run. There is also evidence that people who are hospital inpatients with acute and severe problems may benefit from a psychological intervention based on the same principles as used for patients in outpatient settings (Drury *et al.*, 1996; Haddock *et al.*, 1998).

More recent work by Tarrier and colleagues (Tarrier and Wykes, 2004) highlights that the last 15 years have seen a significant development in the use of CBT for psychosis, in the treatment of schizophrenia, with 20 randomised controlled trials having been published. A review of these studies indicates modest effect sizes, with the strongest evidence available for chronic patients. The cautious conclusion drawn by Tarrier and Wykes (2004) is that, overall, there is good evidence for the efficacy and effectiveness of CBT for psychosis in the treatment of schizophrenia.

Although the evidence presented here depicts a fairly positive picture, there are very few randomised controlled trials to substantiate the findings. Indeed, one of the most recent randomised controlled trials in Scotland points to a less favourable conclusion than those presented earlier in the text, in terms of improvement in outcome (Durham *et al.*, 2003). The conclusions that were drawn from the study indicated that CBT delivered by clinical nurse specialists is a helpful adjunct to routine care for some people with chronic psychosis. Their results noted only modest treatment effects, but CBT gave significantly greater improvement in overall symptom severity than supportive psychotherapy or treatment as usual, combined. Clinically significant improvements were achieved by 7/21 with CBT (33%), 3/19 with supportive psychotherapy (16%) and 2/17 with treatment as usual (12%).

The limited available evidence leads us to be somewhat cautious in our conviction of the efficacy of CBT for psychosis. At the same time, we ought to keep an open mind, because the intervention – CBT for psychosis – is still very much in its infancy and perhaps the picture might change over the coming years.

One of the key points made by some authors is the importance of using experienced clinicians to deliver CBT (Wykes *et al.*, 2005; Durham *et al.*, 2003) and the absolute necessity of supervision for clinicians. Staff need to be mindful of the need for experienced professionals, clinical supervision and the considerable length of time it can take to build a trusting therapeutic relationship with patients.

Individual family and group work with patients and carers

The idea of working with families of individuals with severe mentally illness in order to affect the course of the illness goes back at least as far as the early 1950s. In the earlier days, it was offered to single families, and was, unfortunately, rooted in the notion that families had in some way caused the illness of their relative and that the illness itself was more of a metaphor for trouble in the family than a biological reality (McFarlane *et al.*, 1995). Consequently, families understandably resented the notion they had caused the illness and were difficult to engage in family work. Over the years, investigators began to see the vital role that families played in outcome after a schizophrenic episode had occurred, which led to a review of the way families were involved. This saw a shift towards attempting to engage families collaboratively, sharing illness information and suggesting behaviours that promote recuperation, as well as coping strategies to reduce their sense of burden (Leff *et al.*, 1983). The group of interventions that emerged became known as 'family psycho-education'. The approach recognises schizophrenia as a brain disorder that is only partially remedied by medication, and that families can have a significant effect on their relative's recovery. Today, family work can be offered to single families on their own or to a group of families, depending upon their preference (National Institute for Health and Clinical Excellence, 2002).

The National Institute for Health and Clinical Excellence guidelines (2002) offer a concise and readable description of family interventions. They explain that schizophrenia affects both the individual and his or her family or partners; therefore, working with the family or partner can be very helpful to the patient and carers. Family work (including carers and partners working together) can also reduce the chance of further breakdowns. It is especially helpful for people who have had several breakdowns. It has been shown to be more effective if the treatment lasts for more than six months and includes more than 10 treatments. A systematic review by Mari and Streiner (1996) of family interventions for people with schizophrenia confirms that such interventions reduce relapse rates, rehospitalisation and costs of treatment, while increasing compliance with medication. In addition to this, there is evidence to suggest improved quality of life of the sufferer and their relative (Barrowclough *et al.*, 1992).

Although there is a need to provide specific family interventions, such as education about the illness and strategies which focus on high levels of negative expressed emotion, for example (Leff *et al.*, 1990), it is clear that what families need most is to be listened to, and for our mental health services to provide respite care to assist them in coping with what amounts to a considerable and often lifetime burden (Gournay, 1995).

Ten years ago, several reviewers noted the minimal spread of the family interventions beyond the research settings (Marshall, 1995; Anderson and Adams, 1996), and it was suggested that the challenge was to devise psychosocial interventions sustainable in routine practice (Burns, 1997). Barrowclough *et al.*, (1998) believed that part of this challenge was to develop the means of assessing the level of need for psychosocial interventions in carers supporting patients in the community. In spite of this strong evidence base, there is limited evidence that PSI approaches to the treatment of psychosis are being offered routinely in mental health services. A number of reasons why this is the case have been identified, including lack of time, diversity of interests, conflicting pressures, uncertainty regarding roles, weak infrastructure for workforce planning and therapist attrition following training (Brown, 2001; Fadden, 1997). It appears that staff trained in PSI interventions, no matter how motivated, cannot effectively implement those interventions without changes within the organisational systems in which they work. This, in turn, can lead to workplace frustration, stress and burnout.

Stigma associated with mental illness and offending remains and people admitted to forensic units still bear the burden of being seen by some members of the public as having an unsavoury reputation. This is one of the fundamental reasons for providing factual information about what is considered a severe and enduring psychotic illness. Nowadays, clinicians in all psychiatric units are being encouraged to inform and educate their patients and respective carers about psychosis. This requires acquisition of knowledge on the part of the practitioner and a level of expertise that enables them to undertake this task with a certain proficiency. Delivering information about psychosis can be an ominous task, whether the audience is a patient, carer or fellow professional. The subject can seem 'woolly' and definitions somewhat vague. The process of information giving has been a point of interest for decades, yet there would still seem to be unanswered questions over the timing and most effective method of delivery.

The term *psycho-education* in the context of treating patients with psychotic disorder refers to the clinical technique of educating the patient and his or her family about the nature and probable cause of psychotic illness, the treatment options available and the resources of the healthcare and community services. Smith *et al.* (1992) reported that up to 30 years ago it was 'common practice' for individuals suffering from a variety of disorders to receive information about their illness. The benefits of education, being well understood, are thought to include improving treatment compliance and reducing treatment costs (Roccella, 1976); facilitating early detection of relapse (Newman and Fuenning, 1977); and improving individuals' understanding of their illness (Gillum, 1974). Yet even with evidence of improvement, there has been little impact on psychiatry. Bisbee's (1979) theory was that long-held stereotypes of the 'psychiatric patient' may account for this resistance; for example, that the individual is unable to understand complex concepts, or that education may increase fear and stigma associated with the illness and encourage the acting out of a 'sick role'.

Over the past 20 years, a range of educational packages have been developed with the aim of improving outcome, social functioning and medication adherence through increasing understanding of the illness and the potential benefits of medication (Cunningham-Owens *et al.*, 2001). These interventions tend to be multi-sessional, and require some training to administer. One of the most striking aspects of the treatment of schizophrenia is the disjunction between the strength of what is known of the efficacy of family psychosocial and psycho-educational methods of treatment and the poor availability of these treatments in ordinary clinical settings (Penn and Meuser, 1996).

However, a recent review suggested that overall, the result of educational interventions in schizophrenia remains far from conclusive (Merinder, 2000). What is evident is that there is no clear guidance on the most appropriate format or structure for educational interventions in schizophrenia, their optimal duration or what selection criteria can be applied to allow targeting of those who will benefit most (Merinder, 2000). From this review, it is fairly obvious that clinicians need to focus their attention on improving their knowledge of delivering psycho-education: i.e. what works best? A finding from Vallina-Fernandez *et al.* (2001) indicated that psycho-education, as part of a package, for example, alongside psychotherapy, is a more effective way to provide information.

Psycho-education programmes should essentially have a purpose, and it is important to establish at the outset what clinicians hope to gain from delivering this intervention. The impact of providing education programmes can be considered from patients', carers' and professional viewpoints. As previously mentioned, there are indications that patients might comply better with medication, which has been of particular interest because of its relationship with relapse, but the effects of education beyond compliance have been neglected (Atkinson *et al.*, 1996). Psycho-education for families – and the impact on people with schizophrenia; for example, reduced hospitalisation – was reported by Cassidy *et al.* (2001). There are additional reports of training in psycho-education preventing burnout in nurses caring for people with schizophrenia (Ewers *et al.*, 2002). Findings from previous studies indicate that psycho-education could also have a positive impact on levels of insight (David, 1990; Walker *et al.*, 2005), patient attitudes towards taking medication (Kelly and Scott, 1990), and improved knowledge (Eckman *et al.*, 1992; Merinder, 2001).

Whilst there would appear to be many advantages of psycho-education, it is important to consider the potential disadvantages. Often patients enter into these programmes with very limited knowledge of the illness itself or the potential impact it may have on their lives. The work of Cunningham-Owens *et al.* (2001) indicated that there was an increase in suicidal ideation with increased insight. With this in mind, it is particularly important to give careful consideration to the delivery of the programme and to ensure that clinicians are sensitive to the feelings of patients. Whilst the focus of how to deliver psycho-education programmes is important, equal consideration must be given to the outcome measures used to evaluate the clinical effectiveness of the programmes (Feldmann *et al.*, 2002)

In acute settings, there are many opportunities to deliver psycho-education and this is perhaps one of the most crucial times for patients, enabling them to understand what is causing their problematic behaviour and confusing thoughts. Consideration should also be given to the various means through which information can be distributed: for example, through one-to-one discussion, information leaflets, engagement in psycho-education groups or the use of CD-ROMs. It is worth noting that people have individual learning styles and the choice of delivery method to optimise learning is quite specific to each person.

Monitoring the implementation and effectiveness of psychosocial interventions

In the authors' experience, a range of methods can be used to evaluate improvements in patient care, including:

- Participating in national audits
- Inviting service users to participate in assessing the clinical environment and services

- Exchanging visits with other mental health services to share ideas for good practice and achieving change
- Initiating local 'continuous quality improvement' projects
- Developing integrated care pathways
- Consulting mental health staff
- Setting objectives and monitoring training needs during staff appraisals
- Regularly reviewing local priorities in collaboration with mental health care staff, service users and/or informal carers
- Obtaining the views of service users e.g. through focus groups, interviews
- Establishing, maintaining and continuously reviewing a system for recording, monitoring and acting upon complaints
- Evaluating the usefulness and outcomes of staff training
- Devising good practice statements pertinent to PSI

These are simply suggestions, and can be used on their own or in conjunction with more robust research projects; thus they are worthy of consideration.

General barriers to implementation

Reference has been made to the limited implementation of PSI across the UK, despite the evidence to support its use. It is, therefore, necessary to try to understand why this might be happening and why there is such a gap between evidence and practice. Examples quoted in the literature are: a lack of partnership between researcher and clinician (Goldfried and Wolfe, 1996; Barlow, 1996); absence of appropriate knowledge and/or clinical skills within the relevant workforce (Lancashire *et al.*, 1996); characteristics of the organisation, institution or workplace in constraining such new developments (Corrigan and McCracken, 1995); and clinical techniques being more difficult to learn and implement than is generally realised. It is also understood that, in order to progress from innovation to practice, it is necessary that new treatments be seen as clinically relevant, be empirically validated, meet prioritised needs and be taught in a way that is accessible enough to staff to readily and faithfully acquire the knowledge and skills (Liberman and Eckman, 1989). Box 17.2 highlights the obstacles to effective PSIs in forensic services.

Summary

Considerable developments have taken place in our understanding of psychotic disorders over the last few decades. This has contributed to the development of treatments aimed at successfully ameliorating psychotic symptoms and their associated disabilities (Haddock *et al.*, 1996). There is growing evidence that psychosocial factors contribute significantly to the course and outcome of schizophrenia (Telles *et al.*, 1995) and are thus a viable approach.

Box 17.2 Obstacles to effective PSIs in forensic services

Clinical	Organisational
■ High risk status	■ Preoccupation with security
■ Impression management	■ Therapy vs. discipline/control duties
■ Positive role of anger and aggression	■ Lack of management commitment
■ Long histories of failure and rejection	■ High stress and expressed emotion among staff
■ Low motivation for change	■ Therapeutic pessimism – 'nothing works'
■ Treatment resistance/avoidance	■ Political override – 'what's the point?'
■ Underlying personality disorder	

There are considerable demands on mental health professionals to deliver evidence-based treatments for individuals with severe and enduring psychotic illnesses. The provision and implementation of PSI require a sound knowledge of the evidence base for treatments and available skills in implementing these interventions.

As well as providing an exciting opportunity for clinical research and training to staff, the PSI initiative fits in with the principles of clinical effectiveness, evidence-based practice and clinical governance. With regard to clinical effectiveness, it will facilitate effective clinical practice within any setting through:

- The development of knowledge and skills
- Improving processes and outcomes of care

With regard to evidence-based practice, it will encourage 'doing the right things right', as well as ensuring that knowledge and skill are targeted at individual needs. Lastly, with regard to clinical governance, organisations are responsible for providing an identifiable and accountable service that supports a wide range of clinical staff in delivering high-quality care based on evidence.

References

Anderson, J. and Adams, C. (1996) Family interventions in schizophrenia: an effective but underused treatment. *British Medical Journal*, **313**, 505–6.

Atkinson, J. M., Coia, D. A., Harper Gilmour, W. and Harper, J. (1996) The impact of education groups for people with schizophrenia on social functioning and quality of life. *British Journal of Psychiatry*, **168**, 199–204.

Barlow, D. (1996) Health care policy, psychotherapy research and the future of psychotherapy. *American Psychologist*, **51**(10), 1050–8.

Barrowclough, C. and Tarrier, N. (1992) *Families of Schizophrenic Patients: Cognitive Behavioural Intervention*. Chapman & Hall, London.

Barrowclough, C., Marshall, M., Lockwood, A., Quinn, J. and Sellwood, W. (1998) Assessing relatives' needs for psychosocial interventions in schizophrenia: a relatives' version of the Cardinal Needs Schedule (RCNS). *Psychological Medicine*, **28**, 531–42.

Bisbee, C. C. (1979) Patient education in psychiatric illness. *Journal of Orthomolecular Psychiatry*, **8**(4), 239–47.

Brown, M. (2001) Learning centres. A new approach for service improvement. *Psychiatric Bulletin*, **25**(5), 163–5.

Burns T. (1997) Psychosocial interventions. *Current Opinion in Psychiatry*, **10**, 36–9.

Chadwick, P. and Lowe, C. F. (1990) The measurement and modification of delusional beliefs. *Journal of Consulting and Clinical Psychology*, **58**, 225–32.

Cassidy, E., Hill, S. and O'Callaghan, E. (2001) Efficacy of a psychoeducational intervention in improving relatives' knowledge about schizophrenia and reducing hospitalization. *European Psychiatry*, **16**(8), 446–50.

Cunningham-Owens, D., Carroll, A., Fattah, S., Clyde, Z., Coffey, I. and Johnstone, E. C. (2001) A randomized, controlled trial of a brief interventional package for schizophrenic patients. *Acta Psychiatrica Scandinavica*, **103**(5), 362–9.

David, A. S. (1990) Insight and psychosis. *British Journal of Psychiatry*, **156**, 798–808.

Department of Health (1999) *National Service Framework for Mental Health: Modern Standards and Service Models*. Department of Health, London.

Department of Health (2001) *Implementation Guidance for Mental Health*. Department of Health, London.

Department of Health (2002) *Mental Health Policy Implementation Guide. National Minimum Standards for General Adult Services in Psychiatric Intensive Care Units (PICU) and Low Secure Environments*. The Stationery Office, London.

Department of Health (2004) *The National Service Framework for Mental Health. Five Years On*. Department of Health, London.

Corrigan, P. W. and McCracken, S. G. (1995) Refocusing the training of psychiatric rehabilitation staff. *Psychiatric Services*, **46**, 1172–7.

Drury, V., Birchwood, M., Cochrane, R. and McMillan, F. (1996) Cognitive therapy and recovery from acute psychosis: a controlled trail. II: Impact on recovery time. *British Journal of Psychiatry*, **169**, 602–7.

Durham, R. C., Guthrie, M., Morton, R. V., Reid, D. A., Treliving, L. R., Fowler, D. and MacDonald, R. R. (2003) Tayside–Fife clinical trial of cognitive behavioural therapy for medication-resistant psychotic symptoms: results to 3-month follow up. *British Journal of Psychiatry*, **182**, 303–11.

Eckman, T. A., Wirshing, W. C., Marder, S. R., Johnston-Cronk, K. Zimmerman, K. (1992) Techniques for training schizophrenic patients in illness self-management: a controlled trial. *American Journal of Psychiatry*, **149**, 1549–55.

Ewers, P., Bradshaw, T., McGovern, J. and Ewers, B. (2002) Does training in psychosocial interventions reduce burnout rates in forensic nurses? *Journal of Advanced Nursing*, **37**(5), 470–6.

Fadden, G. (1997) Implementation of family interventions in routine clinical practice following staff training programmes: a major cause for concern. *Journal of Mental Health*, **6**(6), 599–612.

Feldmann, R., Hornung, W. P., Prein, B., Buchkremer, G. and Arolt, V. (2002) Timing of psychoeducational psychotherapeutic interventions in schizophrenic patients. *European Archives of Psychiatry & Clinical Neuroscience*, **252**(3), 115–19.

Gamble, C. and Brennan, G. (eds.) (2006) *Working With Serious Mental Illness. A Manual for Clinical Practice*, 2nd edn. Baillière Tindall, Elsevier, Edinburgh.

Garety, P. A. and Hemsley, D. R. (1994) *Delusions: Investigations into the Psychology of Delusional Reasoning*. Oxford University Press, Oxford.

Gillam, T. (2002) Schizophrenia: care for the 21st century. *Nursing Times*, **98**(40), 36–7.

Gillum, R. (1974) Patient education. *Journal of the National Medical Association*, **66**, 156–9.

Goldfried, M. R. and Wolfe, B. C. (1996) Psychotherapy practice and research: repairing a strained alliance. *American Psychology*, **51**(10), 1007–16.

Gournay, K. (1995) Changing patterns in mental health care. *Psychiatric Care*, **12**(3), 93–5.

Gournay, K. (2000) Role of the community psychiatric nurse in the management of schizophrenia. *Advances in Psychiatric Treatment*, **6**, 243–51.

Haddock, G. and Slade, P. (1996) *Cognitive-Behavioural Interventions with Psychotic Disorders*. Routledge, London.

Haddock, G., Tarrier, N., Spaulding, W., Yusupoff, L., Kinney, C. and McCarthy, E. (1998) Individual cognitive-behaviour therapy in the treatment of hallucinations and delusions: a review. *Clinical Psychology Review*, **18**, 821–38.

Hawton , K., Salkovskis, P. M., Kirk, J. and Clark, D. M. (1999) *Cognitive Behaviour Therapy for Psychiatric Problems: a Practical Guide*. Oxford University Press, New York.

Jones, A. (2004) Perceptions on the standardisation of psychiatric work; development of a care pathway. *Journal of Psychiatric and Mental Health Nursing*, **11**(6), 705–13.

Jones, C., Cormac, I., Silveira da Mota Neto, J. I. and Campbell, C. (2004) Cognitive behaviour therapy for schizophrenia. *Cochrane Database Systematic Review*. 18 October (4), CD000524.

Kane, J. M., Honingfeld, G., Singer, J. and Meltzer, H. (1998) Clozapine for the treatment-resistant schizophrenic: a double blind comparison with chlorpromazine. *Archives of General Psychiatry*, **45**, 789–96.

Kelly, G. R. and Scott, J. E. (1990) Medication compliance and health education among outpatients with chronic mental disorders. *Medical Care*, **28**, 1181–97.

Kingdon, D. G. and Turkington, D. (1991) Preliminary report. The use of cognitive behavioural therapy and a normalising rationale in schizophrenia. *Journal of Nervous and Mental Disease*, **179**, 207–11.

Kuipers, E., Garety, P. A., Fowler, D., Dunn, G., Bebbington, P., Freeman, D. and Hadley, C. (1997) London–East Anglia randomised controlled trail of cognitive-behavioural therapy for psychosis. I: Effects of treatment phase. *British Journal of Psychiatry*, **171**, 319–27.

Kuipers, E., Fowler, D., Garety, P. A., Chisholm, D., Freeman, D., Dunn, G., Bebbington, P. and Hadley, C. (1998) London–East Anglia randomised controlled trail of cognitive-behavioural therapy for psychosis. III: Follow-up and economic evaluation at 18 months. *British Journal of Psychiatry*, **173**, 61–8.

Lancashire, S., Haddock, G., Butterworth, T., Tarrier, N. and Baguley, I. (1996) Training mental health professionals to use psychosocial interventions with people who have severe mental health problems. *Clinician*, **14**, 32–40.

Leff, J., Kuipers, L., Berkowitz, R., Vaughn, C. and Sturgeon, D. (1983) Life events, relatives' expressed emotion and maintenance neuroleptics in schizophrenic relapse. *Psychological Medicine*, **13**(4), 799–806.

Leff, J., Berkowitz, R., Shavitm N., Strachan, A., Glass, I. and Vaughn, C. (1990) A trial of family therapy versus a relatives' group for schizophrenia: two year follow-up. *British Journal of Psychiatry*, **157**, 571–7.

Liberman, R. P. and Eckman, T. (1989) Dissemination of skills training modules to psychiatric facilities. Overcoming obstacles to the utilisation of a rehabilitation innovation. *British Journal of Psychiatry*, **155**(suppl. 5), 117–22.

Mari, J. J. and Streiner, D. (update 23 February 1996) The effects of family intervention on those with schizophrenia. In: *Schizophrenia module: Cochrane Database of Systematic Review* (eds. C. Adams, J. Anderson and J. J. Mari). (Available in the Cochrane Library, London; *British Medical Journal*, 1996).

Marshall, M. (1995) Case management: a dubious practice. Underevaluated and ineffective, but now government policy. *British Medical Journal*, **312**, 523–4.

McFarlane, W. R., Lukens, E., Link, B., Dushay, R., Deakins, S. A., Newark, M., Dunne, E., Horen, B. and Toran, J. (1995) Multiple-family groups and psychoeducation in the treatment of schizophrenia. *Archives of General Psychiatry*, **52**, 679–87.

Merinder, L. B. (2001) Patient education in schizophrenia: a review. *Acta Psychiatrica Scandinavica*, **102**(2), 98–106.

Meuser, K. T. (2000) Cognitive functioning, social adjustment and long-term outcome in schizophrenia. In: *Cognition in Schizophrenia* (eds. T. Sharma and P. Harvey). Oxford University Press, New York.

National Institute for Health and Clinical Excellence (2002) *Schizophrenia: Core Interventions in the Treatment and Management of Schizophrenia in Primary and Secondary Care*. NICE, London.

Newman, I. and Fuenning, S. (1977) Health education: potential for patient care. *Nebraska Medical Journal*, 226–30.

NHS Centre for Reviews and Disseminations (2000) Psychosocial interventions for schizophrenia. *Effective Health Care*, **6**(3).

Pekkala, E. and Merinder, L. (2005) *Psychoeducation for Schizophrenia*. Cochrane Database of Systematic Reviews 2.

Penn, D. and Meuser, K. (1996) Research update on the psychosocial treatment of schizophrenia. *American Journal of Psychiatry*, **153**, 607–17.

Pharoah, F. M., Rathbone, J., Mari, J. J. and Streiner, D. (2003) *Family Intervention for Schizophrenia*. Cochrane Database of Systematic Reviews 4.

Roccella, E. (1976) Potential for reducing health care costs by public and patient education. *Public Health Reports*, **91**, 223.

Sensky, T., Turkington, D., Kingdon, D., Scott, J. L., Scott, J., Siddle, R., O'Carroll, M. and Barnes, T. R. (2000) A randomised controlled trail of cognitive-behaviour therapy for persistent symptoms in schizophrenia resistant to medication. *Archives of General Psychiatry*, **57**(2), 165–72.

SIGN (1998) *Psychosocial Interventions in the Management of Schizophrenia: a National Clinical Guideline*. Scottish Intercollegiate Guidelines Network Secretariat, Edinburgh.

Smith, J., Birchwood, M. and Haddrell, A. (1992) Informing people with schizophrenia about their illness: the effect of residual symptoms. *Journal of Mental Health*, **1**, 61–70.

Tarrier, N. and Wykes, T. (2004) Is there any evidence that cognitive behavioural therapy is an effective treatment for schizophrenia? A cautious or cautionary tale? *Behaviour Research and Therapy*, **42**(12), 1377–401.

Tarrier, N., Beckett, R., Harwood, S., Baker, A., Yuspoff, L. and Ugartebrau, I. (1993) A trial of two cognitive behavioural methods of treating drug-resistant symptoms in schizophrenic outpatients: I. Outcome. *British Journal of Psychiatry*, **162**, 524–32.

Tarrier, N., Yuspoff, L., Kinney, C. and Wittoski, A. (1998) Some reasons why patients suffering from chronic schizophrenia fail to continue in psychological treatment. *Behavioural and Cognitive Psychotherapy*, **26**, 177–81.

Telles, C., Karno, M., Mintz, J., Paz, G., Arias, M., Tucker, D. and Lopez, S. (1995) Immigrant families coping with schizophrenia. Behavioural family intervention versus case management in a Spanish-speaking population. *British Journal of Psychiatry*, **167**, 473–9.

Thomson, L. G. D., Bogue, J., Humphreys, M., Owens, D. and Johnstone, E. C. (1997) The State Hospital Survey: a description of psychiatric patients in conditions of special security in Scotland. *Journal of Forensic Psychiatry*, **8**(2), 263–84.

Vallina-Fernandez, O., Lemos-Giraldez, S., Rodger, V. *et al.* (2001) An integrated psychological treatment program for schizophrenia. *Psychiatric Services*, **52**(9), 1165–7.

Walker, H., Connaughton, J. and Wilson, I. (2005) *Thesis: Psycho-education for psychosis in forensic psychiatry: an evaluation of the 'Coping With Mental Illness' course*. The State Hospital Carstairs, Scotland.

Wykes, T., Hayward, P., Thomas, N., Green, N., Surguladze, S., Fannon, D. and Landau, S. (2005) What are the effects of group cognitive behaviour therapy for voices? A randomised control trial. *Schizophrenia Research*, **77**, 201–10.

CHAPTER 18

Conclusions: fifteen themes, action and research for the future

Richard Byrt, Alyson McGregor Kettles and Phil Woods

Introduction

Throughtout this book, the authors have tried to offer up-to-date and, where possible, research-based accounts of aspects of nursing and multidisciplinary assessment and care for forensic patients in acute mental health settings.

We hope, within this short chapter, to highlight some of the main themes which have emerged. Some key areas of care have been presented and discussed in this book. We have tried to address some of the contributions made by forensic and other mental health nurses to the professional care, interventions and treatment of patients with a forensic history who are nursed in acute mental health environments. Insights from practice and related writing in this area can provide a basis for the development of ideas, thinking and future research related to ways in which nurses' roles and interventions can enable the best possible care to be given to the person in this situation (Kettles *et al.*, 2006).

Evidence from a number of central government and local inquiries suggests that there is a continuing tendency to apply only generic mental health concepts directly to the care of people in forensic and other mental health environments, but to ignore issues concerning risk assessment and management related to offending behaviours. It is detrimental to the individual forensic patient, as well as to others who may be at risk, if problems related to offending are ignored, or seen as a relatively unimportant issue requiring secondary interventions (Jones and Plowman, 2005; Peay, 1996; Ritchie *et al.*, 1994).

Emerging themes

The range of topics covered in this book indicates the many areas of nursing and multidisciplinary assessments and interventions relevant to the care of forensic, and, in many instances, other patients receiving care in acute mental health settings. Relevant issues that have been considered in this book include the following.

- **Theme 1: All nursing and multidisciplinary assessments and interventions for forensic patients are concerned with the overlapping aims of:**
  - Ensuring safety and prevention and reduction of risk of harm to self and others
  - Relieving distress
  - Respecting the individual's unique needs, and his/her shared humanity and diversity (see Chapter 1)

- **Theme 2: Mental health models to inform nursing care**. There is a need for nursing and multidisciplinary interventions for forensic patients in acute mental health settings to be informed by models and therapeutic frameworks of care which achieve the three aims highlighted in Theme 1, above. Examples include Barker's Tidal Model (Barker, 2002) and others outlined in this book, such as low conflict high therapy nursing in Chapter 8; therapeutic community principles (Chapter 4); and psychosocial interventions informed by stress vulnerability models (Chapters 4 and 17).

- **Theme 3: System change**. In the future, staff need to begin working towards changes given in the timetables from the National Reviews of Mental Health Nursing (Department of Health, 2006a; Scottish Executive Health Department, 2006) The following could benefit forensic patients in acute settings and enhance nurses' professional development:
  - Staff rotation between different services, in order to learn skills and perspectives.
  - The opportunity to follow the patient through their journey from the onset of an acute mental health problem to recovery in the community.
  - Improved educational opportunities.
  - The use of models of care that are specific to mental health.

  It has been suggested that all these factors can contribute to changes in the system of care that will be beneficial to the patient (Department of Health, 2006a; Scottish Executive Health Department, 2006).

- **Theme 4: Attitude change**. Several studies of service users' views have highlighted the importance to patients of staff attitudes in both acute (Duxbury and Whittington, 2005; Secker and Harding, 2002; Secker *et al.*, 2004) and forensic mental health settings (Bowers, 2002; Meehan *et al.*, 2006; Mercer *et al.*, 1999).

- **Theme 5: Engagement and communication with patients**. The literature suggests the value of increased therapeutic working with patients, with dedicated time set aside for this (Dodds and Bowles, 2002; Kent, 2005). As staff are educated to fulfil need, this is likely to become the norm. Carol Watson and Alyson McGregor Kettles, in Chapter 2, have outlined the potential for staff working in acute mental health services to improve the quality of the care they provide. In addition, much of the literature highlights the importance of therapeutic communication to forensic and other mental health patients (Bowers, 2002; Duxbury and Whittington, 2005; Faulkner, 2004; Meehan *et al.*, 2006; Secker *et al.*, 2004; see Chapters 3 and 4). The need for nurses' engagement and communication during observation of patients has been emphasised (Jones and Jackson, 2004; Kettles and Woodally, 2006).

- **Theme 6: The importance of valid and reliable risk assessment and management in increasing the safety of the individual and others** is emphasised in much of the literature (Doyle and Duffy, 2006; Morgan and Wetherall, 2004) and by Mike Doyle and Michael Coffey (Chapter 6) and other authors in this book. Holistic assessments, related to the individual's needs, are also relevant to minimising risk, as well as relieving the individual's distress and respecting him/her as an individual (Doyle and Duffy, 2006). This includes measuring the individual's health and social functioning, considered by Phil Woods and Alyson McGregor Kettles in Chapter 7.

- **Theme 7: Several authors have indicated the need for increased understanding of diversity issues; and implementation of culturally sensitive and culturally competent care**, based on respect for the individual and his/her unique needs. The latter include those related to ethnicity, culture, spirituality, gender, sexual orientation, gender identity, age, varying physical, sensory and intellectual abilities and specific problems (Addo, 2006; Anderson and Bruce, 2003). Cultural and diversity issues are considered in Chapters 13 and 14.

- **Theme 8: Also increasingly emphasised in the literature is the provision of ward social and physical environments that are safe**, relieve individuals' stress and distress; and are beneficial in other ways, e.g. through the application of psychosocial interventions and therapeutic community principles (Bowers *et al.*, 2002; Byrt, 2006; see Chapters 3 and 4) and 'low conflict, high therapy nursing' (Bowers *et al.*, 2006; see Chapter 8).

- **Theme 9: Partnership working with the patient, his/her carers and community-based and other professionals and agencies** is expected to increase, in line with Government policy (Department of Health, 2005, 2006b). Chapter 11 by Linda Hart and Wendy Ifill's contribution in Chapter 8 remind us of the crucial need to consider service users' views and to enable their participation. Helen Walker considers the importance of multi-professional working in Chapter 17.

  The available evidence suggests that the carers are the ones who are currently not sufficiently consulted (Byrt and Dooher, 2003), but Alyson McGregor Kettles and Paula Hall in Chapter 9, and Michael Coffey and his co-authors in Chapter 10, have shown the need for appropriate information to be made available to community colleagues. Several recent central government policy documents stress the need to provide acute services in partnership with service users and carers and with local community and voluntary organisations, e.g. in relation to services that are sensitive to the needs of individuals from minority ethnic groups (Department of Health, 2005) and women (Department of Health, 2006b).

- **Theme 10**: This imperative to involve local community groups in services is partly aimed at **increasing social inclusion** (Repper and Perkins, 2004) of individuals faced with the dual stigma of mental health problems and histories of offending (Bartlett, 2004). In relation to recovery models of care, it can be argued that the aim of interventions, in acute and other mental health settings, is not only to reduce symptoms associated with distress and reoffending. In addition, it is about enabling individuals to lead their lives in accordance with their goals, beyond the role of 'client', and with freedom from discrimination and access to life opportunities available to most of the population (Repper, 2004; Roe *et al.*, 2004; Sayce, 2000). In addition, we suggest that nurses who work in acute mental health settings with forensic patients could be seen as having a primary prevention role in combatting stigma and raising public (and perhaps political) awareness of issues concerning these individuals' problems, strengths, care and recovery (Kettles *et al.*, 2006).

- **Theme 11: Improvements in crisis care** include alternatives to enable the individual to live at home (Chapter 9) and the establishment of crisis houses and other alternatives in the community (Mental Health Foundation and Sainsbury Centre for Mental Health, 2002; Care Services Improvement Partnership, 2006) (see Chapter 4).

- **Theme 12: There is a need for the development of specialist nursing and multidisciplinary assessments and interventions**, including those concerned with:
  - Individuals with needs related to specific mental health problems, including:
    - People with personality disorders (whose needs have often not been met in generic mental health services: NIMHE and Department of Health, 2003; see Chapter 12)
    - Individuals with problematic substance use (Kettles and Woodally, 2006)
    - Individuals with schizophrenia (Chapters 4 and 16)
  - The application of specialist approaches, including cognitive – behavioural therapy, psychosocial interventions and therapeutic community principles (Chapters 4 and 17)
  - Preventing and reducing violence and aggression (Chapter 5)
  - Preventing and reducing suicide and self-harm (Chapters 6 and 12)

- **Theme 13**: Carol Watson and Alyson McGregor Kettles (Chapter 2) and several other authors in the book have emphasised the need for **high quality education, support and clinical supervision** to enable nurses to work with forensic patients in acute settings.

- **Theme 14: Research**. There is continuing need for evaluative studies in forensic services, but in some respects the need for nursing research is even greater in acute mental health settings (Bowers, 2005; Woods and Richards, 2003). There is also an argument for some research that crosses boundaries to enable understanding of the meaning of care for both staff and patients in the different settings (Coffey, 2006) and how transition through different settings affects people (Skelly, 2001).

- **Theme 15**: Finally, in line with recommendations of the Mental Health Nursing Reviews for Scotland, England and Wales (Department of Health, 2006a; Scottish Executive Health Department, 2006), **developments in nursing policy** are needed to further practice development and care of people who are forensic patients in acute mental health settings.

Mental health nursing is continuing to develop, with, in some services, the growth of evidence-based approaches to provide the best possible care for people suffering from a variety of mental health problems. Recent changes include the use of recovery models of care (Kelly and Gamble, 2005; Repper, 2004; Roe *et al.*, 2004), integrated continuous whole systems care, and service users and carers being supported fully as active partners in care (Edwards, 2005). These developments and related policies are coming to fruition, as services move towards integrated care and as mental health nurses recognise the way forward in care provision (Barker, 2003; Department of Health, 2006a; Norman and Ryrie, 2004; Scottish Executive Health Department, 2006).

Conclusion

We hope that the outcome of this text will be the following:

- That what is known about care can be appropriately used in practice to the benefit of those people with a forensic history who find themselves in an acute mental health setting.
- That this text helps in the education of both acute and forensic mental health staff who work with patients in a variety of settings, and contributes to improved communication between staff in these diverse services, with positive consequences for patient care.
- That the literature presented here helps to inform the way forward and contributes to the development of appropriate policy, services and interventions.

We hope that you have enjoyed reading this book as much as we have enjoyed writing and editing parts of it. We will close with two thought-provoking comments by individuals with experience as service users:

> ... It is absolutely vital that we remember what it feels like to be at the receiving end of acute mental health care. Many accounts have been written about the experience of being admitted to an acute psychiatric ward.... They make difficult reading, not least because the loss of status and identity, the distress and discrimination associated with mental ill-health, is often compounded by the attitudes and experiences encountered in hospital... (Faulkner, 2004, p. 79, citing Faulkner, 1998; Rose, 2000; and Lloyd-Jones, 2001).

> I think the best professionals involved in my care have walked alongside me, opening themselves to the mystery that is schizophrenia. They have gained my trust, sharing and supporting my inner search for meaning and understanding of self in relation to illness. We have certainly learned about medication, but we have also learned to predict stressors and avert relapse, seeing my well-being as a result of many influences on my life. They have helped me try to integrate the strange upwellings of psychotic material and to deal with the fear and unease caused by relapse. They have not always been certain, but rather, experimenters like myself, carefully watching what was happening at a specific time with my own particular form of schizophrenia, before choosing an intervention (Champ, 1999, pp. 123ff).

References

Addo, M. (2006) Culture, spirituality and ethical issues in caring for clients with personality disorder. In: *Forensic Mental Health Nursing: Interventions with People with 'Personality Disorder'* (ed. National Forensic Nurses' Research and Development Group), Chapter 5. Quay, Salisbury.

Barker, P. (2002) The tidal model: the healing potential of metaphor within the patient's narrative. *Journal of Psychosocial Nursing and Mental Health Services*, **40**(7), 42–50.

Barker, P. (ed.) (2003) *Psychiatric and Mental Health Nursing: The Craft of Caring*, Chapter 32. Arnold, London.

Bartlett, A. (2004) Fashions in psychiatric care: implications for sense of self. In: *Every Family in the Land: Understanding Prejudice and Discrimination Against People with Mental Illness* (ed. A. H. Crisp), Chapter 49. Royal Society of Medicine Press, London.

Bowers, L. (2002) *Dangerous and Severe Personality Disorder: Response and Role of the Psychiatric Team.* Routledge, London.

Bowers, L. (2005) Reasons for admission and their implications for the nature of acute inpatient psychiatric nursing. *Journal of Psychiatric and Mental Health Nursing*, **12**(2), 231–6.

Bowers, L., Crowhurst, N., Alexander, J., Callaghan, P., Eales, S., Guy, S., McCann, E. and Ryan, C. (2002) Safety and security policies on psychiatry acute admission wards: results from a London-wide survey. *Journal of Psychiatric and Mental Health Nursing*, **9**, 427–33.

Bowers, L., Brennan, G., Flood, C., Lipang, M. and Oladapo, P. (2006) Preliminary outcomes of a trial to reduce conflict and containment on acute psychiatric wards: City Nurses. *Journal of Psychiatric and Mental Health Nursing*, **13**, 165–72

Byrt, R. (2006) Nursing interventions in therapeutic communities. In: *Forensic Mental Health Nursing: Interventions with People with 'Personality Disorder'* (ed. National Forensic Nurses' Research and Development Group), Chapter 14. Quay, Salisbury.

Byrt, R., Dooher, J. (2003) 'Service users' and 'Carers' and their desire for empowerment. In: *Empowerment and the Health Service User* (eds. J. Dooher and R. Byrt), Chapter 1. Quay, Salisbury.

Care Services Improvement Partnership (2006) *10 High Impact Changes for Mental Health Services.* Department of Health, London.

Champ, S. (2000) A most precious thread. In: *From the Ashes of Experience. Reflections on Madness, Survival and Growth* (eds. P. Barker, P. Campbell and B. Davidson), Chapter 7. Whurr, London.

Coffey, M. (2006) Researching service user views in forensic mental health: a critical review. *Journal of Forensic Psychiatry and Psychology*, **17**(1), 73–107.

Department of Health (2005) *Delivering Race Equality in Mental Health Care. An Action Plan for Reform. Inside and Outside Services and The Government's Response to the Independent Inquiry Into the Death of David Bennett.* Department of Health, London.

Department of Health (2006a) *From Values to Action: The Chief Nursing Officer's Review of Mental Health Nursing.* Department of Health, London.

Department of Health (2006b) *Supporting Women into the Mainstream. Commissioning Women Only Community Day Services.* Department of Health, London.

Dodds, P. and Bowles, N. (2001) Dismantling formal observation and refocusing nursing activity in acute psychiatry: a case study. *Journal of Psychiatric and Mental Health Nursing*, **8**(2), 183–8.

Doyle, M. and Duffy, S. (2006) Assessing and managing risk to self and others. In: *Forensic Mental Health Nursing: Interventions with People with 'Personality Disorder'* (ed. National Forensic Nurses' Research and Development Group), Chapter 10. Quay, Salisbury.

Duxbury, J. and Whittington, R. (2005) Causes and management of patient aggression and violence: staff and patient perspectives. *Journal of Advanced Nursing*, **50**(5), 469–78.

Edwards, K. (2005) *Partnership Working in Mental Health Care. The Nursing Dimension*. Elsevier Churchill Livingstone, Edinburgh.

Faulkner, A. (2004) Strategies for surviving acute care. In: *Acute Mental Health Nursing: From Acute Concerns to the Capable Practitioner* (eds. M. Harrison, D. Howard and D. Mitchell), Chapter 4. Sage, London.

Jones, J. and Jackson, A. (2004) Observation. In: *Acute Mental Health Nursing: From Acute Concerns to the Capable Practitioner* (eds. M. Harrison, D. Howard and D. Mitchell), Chapter 8. Sage, London.

Jones, J. and Plowman, C. (2005) Risk assessment: a multidisciplinary approach to estimating harmful behaviour in mentally disordered offenders. In: *Multidisciplinary Working in Forensic Mental Health Care* (eds. S. Wix and M. Humphreys). Elsevier Churchill Livingstone, Edinburgh.

Kelly, M. and Gamble, C. (2005) Exploring the concept of recovery in schizophrenia. *Journal of Psychiatric and Mental Health Nursing*, **12**, 245–51.

Kent, M. (2005) My mental health. *Mental Health Practice*, **8**(8), 22.

Kettles, A. M. and Woodally, J. (2006) Observation and engagement with people with personality disorder. In: *Forensic Mental Health Nursing: Interventions with People with 'Personality Disorder'* (ed. National Forensic Nurses' Research and Development Group), Chapter 12. Quay, Salisbury.

Kettles, A. M., Woods, P. and Byrt, R. (2006) Conclusions: themes, action and research for the future. In: *Forensic Mental Health Nursing: Interventions with People with 'Personality Disorder'* (ed. National Forensic Nurses' Research and Development Group), Chapter 16. Quay, Salisbury.

Meehan, T., McIntosh, W. and Bergen, H. (2006) Aggressive behavior in high-secure settings: the perceptions of patients. *Journal of Psychiatric and Mental Health Nursing*, **13**(1), 19–25.

Mental Health Foundation and Sainsbury Centre for Mental Health (2002) *Being There in a Crisis: A Report of the Learning from Eight Mental Health Crisis Services*. Mental Health Foundation and Sainsbury Centre for Mental Health, London.

Mercer, D., Mason, T. and Richman, J. (1999) Good and evil in the crusade of care. *Journal of Psychosocial Nursing and Mental Health Services*, **37**(9), 13–17.

Morgan, S. and Wetherell, A. (2004) Assessing and managing risk. In: *The Art and Science of Mental Health Nursing: a Textbook of Principles and Practice* (eds. I. Norman and I. Ryrie), Chapter 8. Open University Press, Maidenhead.

National Institute for Mental Health in England and Department of Health (2003) *Personality Disorder. No Longer a Diagnosis of Exclusion*. Department of Health, London.

Norman, I. and Ryrie, I. (eds.) (2004) *The Art and Science of Mental Health Nursing: a Textbook of Principles and Practice*. Open University Press, Maidenhead.

Peay, J. (1996) *Inquiries After Homicide*. Duckworth, London.

Repper, J. and Perkins, R. (2004) Social inclusion and acute care. In: *Acute Mental Health Nursing: From Acute Concerns to the Capable Practitioner* (eds. M. Harrison, D. Howard and D. Mitchell). Sage, London.

Ritchie, J., Dick, D. and Lingham, R. (1994) *The Report of the Inquiry into the Care and Treatment of Christopher Clunis*. HMSO, London.

Roe, D., Chopra, M., Wagner, B., Katz, G. and Rudnick, A. (2004) The emerging self in conceptualising and treating mental illness. *Journal of Psychosocial Nursing and Mental Health Services*, **42**(2), 33–40.

Sainsbury Centre for Mental Health (2006) *The Search for Acute Solutions. Improving the Quality of Care in Acute Psychiatric Wards*. Sainsbury Centre for Mental Health, London.

Sayce, L. (2000) *From Psychiatric Patient to Citizen: Overcoming Discrimination and Social Exclusion*. Macmillan Press, Basingstoke.

Scottish Executive Health Department (2006) *Rights, Relationships and Recovery: The Report of the National Review of Mental Health Nursing in Scotland*. Scottish Executive, Edinburgh.

Secker, J. and Harding, C. (2002) African and African Caribbean users' perceptions of inpatient services. *Journal of Psychiatric and Mental Health Nursing*, **9**, 161–7.

Index